DEDICATION

To all parents trying their best to make smart choices for their children

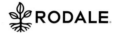

We inspire and enable people to improve their lives and the world around them

For more of our products visit rodalestore.com or call 800-848-4735

Book design by George Karabotsos

Photographs by Orly Catz (pages 40–41, 72–73, 76–77, 78–79, 88–89); Jeff Harris, photographer; Roscoe Betsill, stylist (cover photos, 13–18, 286–287); Michael LoBiondo, photographer; John Hartley, stylist (pages 44–45, 56–57, 64–65, 82–83, 96–97, 104–105); all other photos © Mitch Mandel and Tom MacDonald/Rodale Images; Melissa Reiss, stylist

Library of Congress Cataloging-in-Publication Number: 2008032482
ISBN: 978–1–60961–898–8 paperback

2   4   6   8   10   9   7   5   3   1

This special edition was printed for Kohl's Department Stores, Inc. (for distribution on behalf of Kohl's Cares, LLC, its wholly owned subsidiary) by Rodale Inc.

978–1–60961–898–8 • Kohl's • 1–60961–898–X • 123386 • 4/12–5/12

CONTENTS

ACKNOWLEDGMENTS

This book is the product of thousands of meals, hundreds of conversations with experts and concerned parents, and the collective smarts, dedication, and raw talent of dozens of individuals. Our undying thanks to all of you who have inspired this project in any way. In particular:

Steve Murphy, who captains the ship called Rodale Inc. with grace, courage, and remarkable vision. Thanks for continuing to make this the best publishing company on the planet.

The Rodale family, whose dedication to improving the lives and well-being of their readers is apparent in every book and magazine they put their name on.

George Karabotsos, whose vision has turned a jumble of words and numbers into something that's impossible to put down.

Stephen Perrine, with whom we've conferred over many a fast-food lunch and who never met an exclamation mark he didn't like.

Clint Carter, whose heroic efforts helped make sense out of a daunting database of numbers and ingredients.

The entire *Men's Health* editorial staff: a smarter, more inspiring group of writers, editors, researchers, designers, and photo directors does not exist, in the magazine world or beyond.

To the Rodale book team: Karen Rinaldi, Chris Krogermeier, Sara Cox, Tara Long, Marc Sirinsky, Mitch Mandel, Susan Eugster, Jennifer Giandomenico, Steve Schirra, and Nancy Bailey. Your extraordinary sacrifices of time and sanity brought another project to reality in record time.

The doctors, researchers, and nutritionists whose expertise helped inform this book: David Katz, MD; Beth Wallace, RD; and Mary Story, PhD, RD, among others.

Special thanks to: Adam Campbell, Mark Michaelson, Willy Gutierrez, John Dixon, Laura White, and Jaclyn Colletti.

And to the people who matter most to us in this world: families, friends, and our lovely partners, Melissa and Lauren.

Sorry for all the talk about calorie counts.

—Dave and Matt

The Choice Is Yours

You have already made a million smart choices for your children.

From the moment you discovered you were an expectant parent, you began to change your life. You thought hard about your finances, setting aside some frivolous expenses in order to save for a new future. You looked at your home, your neighborhood, your life and thought—is this a good place for a child to grow up? And you made some hard choices there, as well.

That's what being a parent is all about—making choices, not on your own behalf, but on behalf of another. It's a difficult job, and you should be proud of what you've already achieved.

But not every choice is clear-cut. Feeding your kids well, and keeping them healthy, is a particular challenge—especially in today's fast-food culture.

Fortunately, being a parent, and making smart choices, has just gotten easier. Because you have in your hands a revolutionary new guide that is going to arm you, and your son or daughter, in the battle against an emerging threat to your children's health and happiness—the threat of obesity. **EAT THIS, NOT THAT! FOR KIDS!** is your essential guide to making smart nutritional choices no matter where or when you're faced with them.

The New Challenge for Parents

Being a parent has always been hard, but it seems that here in the early stages of the 21st century, it's gotten harder than ever—and not just because we've traded drive-ins for drive-bys, *Father Knows Best* for *Flavor of Love*, and role models like Joni Mitchell and Joe Montana for Britney Spears and Barry Bonds.

It's gotten harder because America's restaurants and food marketers are putting our children in danger.

Consider this: Since the 1970s, the obesity rate in this country has doubled, with two-thirds of our population now overweight. The health condition most directly tied to obesity—diabetes—eats up one in every five dollars Americans spend on health care, and a recent study at Harvard found that obesity may soon surpass tobacco as the number-one cause of cancer deaths.

And no matter how frightening that may sound, the statistics are even worse for our children. The percentage of overweight youths age 12 to 19 in the United States has nearly quadrupled between 1976 and 2004. Indeed, 17 percent of this country's youth are now overweight or obese.

To put it another way: Do you remember what you and your friends looked like when you were growing up? Think back, and then look around: Do the children you see in your neighborhood look like that?

No. The children are different. Your children may be different. Think about it: No matter what your weight may have been growing up, your child faces four times the risk of obesity as you did.

HOW CAN THIS BE?

You're probably ready to finger the same bad guy that most parents point to: the pop culture boogeyman. When we were kids, we cared more about fishing nets than the Internet, played our tennis games on actual courts instead of virtual ones, and even walked to our friends' homes on the other side of the neighborhood (remember when they used to have sidewalks in neighborhoods?). Sure, the jocks dominated the sports teams, but you didn't have to be a jock to ride a bike or zip around on a skateboard. Even the slackers and the rockers at least got some exercise toting electric guitars and amps around town, instead of doing all their rocking out on Guitar Hero.

Have our kids cut down on their physical exercise? Sure. The Centers for Disease Control found that daily participation in school physical education among adolescents dropped from 42 percent in 1991 to 33 percent in 2005. It also found that a mere 36 percent of kids are currently meeting their recommended levels of activity each week.

But before you blame the rise in childhood obesity on our budding couch potatoes sending roots down into the upholstery, consider this: Only 15 percent of our daily calorie burn comes from exercise. The majority of the calories we burn off each day are eaten up by the simple acts of growing and breathing and maintaining our bodies, and from the digestion of food. That's why you see even kids dedicated to sports having to struggle with their weight.

So what's causing this crisis? And what, exactly, is happening to our children?

Here's the truth: It's not the TV, and it's not the Internet, and it's not the video games or the cell phones or the iPods. It's not the culture that's endangering our children's health.

It's the food.

The Hidden Health Danger

When a child's weight begins to grow out of proportion, so does his risk of disease—both in childhood and in his or her later life. Consider:

- The most common form of diabetes is called Type 2 or "adult-onset" diabetes and is caused primarily by years of poor eating habits. But "adult onset" no longer fits because for the first time in history, we realize that children can come down with it, too. Indeed, doctors have reported seeing children as young as 4 with the disease, and the American Diabetes Association says it is approaching catastrophic proportions in teens. The Centers for Disease Control recently predicted that one in three children born in the year 2000 will develop diabetes at some point in his or her lifetime. The laundry list of diabetes' complications? Blindness. Heart attack. Stroke. Amputation.

- Researchers at the National Institute of Child Health and Human Development found that overweight kids were more likely to suffer bone fractures and 30 percent more likely to suffer from joint or muscle pain than children of normal weight.

- The Centers for Disease Control found that almost 60 percent of overweight children have at least one cardiovascular disease risk, including high cholesterol, high blood pressure, and abnormal glucose tolerance. Twenty-five percent of overweight kids displayed at least two of these risk factors.

- A link between body weight and asthma in children has emerged in recent years. A 2008 study in the *Journal of Asthma* found that a disproportionate percentage of children with asthma were overweight, and that overweight sufferers of asthma had more severe cases than those of normal weight. And according to *Pediatric Respiratory Reviews*, obesity in children is also associated with obstructive sleep apnea syndrome, which can contribute to high blood pressure and cardio-vascular disease.

- Indeed, even an old complaint of middle-age curmudgeons, kidney stones, has begun to surface with regularity in children, according to researchers at Johns Hopkins Medical Institutions. The reason: too much salt in their diets and water being replaced with sugary sodas and juice boxes.

Those are some strange and scary statistics, but the reality of our children's obesity epidemic is unavoidable. It's right there in front of us—at the school, in the playground, and too often, in our own homes.

But how is this happening? How are our children being supersized? And why do we seem powerless to stop it?

Attack of the Frankenfoods

Here's an eye-opener: The Centers for Disease Control found that American kids eat more than 150 additional calories *every day* than they did in 1989.

Let's run the math on that one. It takes 3,500 calories to create an extra pound of body weight. That means every 20 days, the average American child eats enough extra calories to weigh a pound more than his 1989 contemporary. Over the course of a year, that's enough to add 18 pounds of extra heft to your child's frame.

How can this be? Are children today simply that much more gluttonous? Are parents that much more lax? Did somebody farm out all our new home construction to Hansel and Gretel Architects, Inc.?

Well, consider this: It's not just our kids who are eating vastly more calories. In 1971, the average American male consumed 2,450 calories a day; the average woman, 1,542. But by the year 2000, American men were averaging about 2,618 daily calories (up 7 percent), while women were eating 1,877 calories (a whopping 18 percent increase, or 335 more calories every day!). The real truth of the matter is this: The food that we consume today is simply different from the food that Americans ate 20 or 30 years ago. And the reasons are as simple as they are sneaky:

✖ **WE'VE ADDED EXTRA CALORIES TO TRADITIONAL FOODS.** In the early 1970s, food manufacturers, looking for a cheaper ingredient to replace sugar, came up with a substance called high-fructose corn syrup (HFCS). Today, HFCS is in an unbelievable array of foods—everything from breakfast cereals to bread, from ketchup to pasta sauce, from juice boxes to iced tea. According to the FDA, the average American consumes 82 grams of added sugars every day, which contribute an empty 317 calories to our diets. HFCS no doubt shares some of the blame; as a cheap by-product with a long shelf life, the food industry is finding all sorts of new foods in which to hide sugar. So Grandma's pasta sauce now comes in a jar, and it's loaded with stuff just perfect for adding meat to your bones—and flab on your belly.

✖ **WE'VE BEEN TRAINED TO SUPERSIZE IT.** It seems like Economics 101: If you can get a lot more food for just a few cents more, then it makes all the sense in the world to upgrade to the "value meal." And because food is so inexpensive for manufacturers to produce on a large scale, your average fast-food emporium makes a hefty profit whenever you supersize your meal—even though you're getting an average of 73 percent more calories for only a 17 percent increase in cost. The problem is the way we look at food—we should be looking at cutting down on our calories, not adding to them. In fact, if we were really smart, fast food shops would be charging us more for the smaller portions!

✖ **WE'VE LACED OUR FOOD WITH TIME BOMBS.** A generation ago it was hard for food manufacturers to create baked goods that would last on store shelves. Most baked goods require oils, and oil leaks at room temperature. But since the 1960s, manufacturers have been baking with—and restaurateurs have been frying with—something called trans fats. Trans fats are cheap and effective: They make potato chips crispier and Oreo cookies tastier, and they let fry cooks make pound after pound of fries without smoking up their kitchens. The downside: Trans fats increase your bad cholesterol, lower your good cholesterol, and greatly increase your risk of heart disease.

✖ **WE'RE DRINKING MORE CALORIES THAN EVER.** A study from the University of North Carolina found that we consume 450 calories a day from beverages, nearly twice as many as 30 years ago. This increase amounts to an extra 23 pounds a year that we're forced to work off—or carry around with us. Many of the calories come from HFCS in our drinks—especially, when it comes to kids, in our "fruit" drinks that are often nothing more than water, food coloring, and sweetener. In fact, anything you have for your kids to drink in your fridge right now—unless it's water, milk, or a diet soda—probably has HFCS in it. Go ahead—read the label.

✖ **WE DON'T KNOW WHAT'S IN OUR FOOD.** More and more, marketers are adding new types of preservatives, fats, sugars, and other "new" food substances to our daily meals. But often, they go unexplained (what is "xanthan gum" anyway?) or, in the case of restaurant food, unmentioned. Unless we're eating it right off the tree, it's hard to know what, exactly, is in that fruity dish.

All of these disturbing trends in our food supply are a lot to chew on—but chew on them we do. Indeed, some of the food that restaurants and packaged-goods manufacturers are marketing to our children are so unbelievably bad for our kids, you have to take a step back and ask, "Do these people have any idea what they're doing?" Consider that the recommended daily calorie intake for a 12-year-old is 2,000, and that his recommended intake of sodium is no more than 2,200 milligrams of sodium. Then, consider this:

AT RUBY TUESDAY'S, the Kid's Turkey Minis & Fries pack 893 calories and 47 grams of fat. Talk about deceptive! Who would have guessed that two tiny turkey burgers could pack as many calories as a Double Whopper? Want dessert with that? The Strawberries and Ice Cream come with 914 calories and 50 grams of fat.

AT COSÍ'S, the Kids Pepperoni Pizza will feed your child 911 calories, 43 grams of fat, and a seemingly heart-stopping 2,731 milligrams of sodium—that's as much salt as you'd find in 15 small bags of potato chips!

AT ON THE BORDER, the Kids Bean & Cheese Nachos comes with a 980-calorie price tag. On top of that, this plate of chips and cheese has a full day's worth of sodium and as much saturated fat as 29 strips of bacon!

Unfortunately, there's no way to tell which Bart Simpson—size meals come with Homer-size loads of calories, sodium, and fat. Unlike packaged-goods manufacturers, who are required to post detailed nutritional information on their boxes, bags, and cans, restaurant chains don't labor under any nutritional disclosure regulations. A handful do list such information on their Web sites—major chains who deserve kudos for helping parents make informed choices include Chili's, Panera Bread, and Uno Chicago Grill. But nutritional information at most sit-down and fast-food restaurants is murkier than a Florida election.

And if you're shocked at how bad much of today's "kids menus" are, you're not alone. Most of us don't labor under the illusion that ice cream snacks and fast-food burgers are healthy—the occasional sinful indulgence is part of living, even for (or especially for) kids. But most parents could never guess how bad many of today's kids' meals really are. In a 2006 study published in the *American Journal of Public Health,* consumers presented with obviously high-calorie restaurant foods still underestimated the nutritional heft of the items by an average of 600 calories.

That's why **EAT THIS, NOT THAT! FOR KIDS!** is your secret weapon. We've analyzed kids offerings from all of the major chains, taken a hard look at packaged foods and snacks, and uncovered the real truth about what America is really feeding its children. And the great news: You can have a major impact on your children's health and future simply by making a handful of smart choices.

And as a parent, that's what you're already good at: making choices for your children. All you need is the right information at the right time.

And now you have it.

For more great food swaps, nutritional secrets, weight-loss strategies, and the latest breaking news on how to keep you and your family feeling great, go to **eatthis.com**

Our Children's Future

A child who's overweight is 15 times more likely to be overweight as an adult. What does that really mean in terms of your child's health? Take a look at the numbers:

Overweight people are:

- **50 percent more likely to develop heart disease** (obese: up to 100 percent)
- **Up to 360 percent more likely to develop diabetes** (obese: up to 1,020 percent)
- **16 percent more likely to die of a first heart attack** (obese: 49 percent)
- **Roughly 50 percent more likely to have total cholesterol above 250** (obese: up to 122 percent)
- **14 percent less attractive to the opposite sex** (obese: 43 percent)
- **Likely to spend 37 percent more a year at the pharmacy** (obese: 105 percent)
- **Likely to stay 19 percent longer in the hospital** (obese: 49 percent)
- **20 percent more likely to have asthma** (obese: 50 percent)
- **Up to 31 percent more likely to die of any cause** (obese: 62 percent)
- **19 percent more likely to die in a car crash** (obese: 37 percent)
- **120 percent more likely to develop stomach cancer** (obese: 330 percent)
- **Up to 90 percent more likely to develop gallstones** (obese: up to 150 percent)
- **590 percent more likely to develop esophageal cancer** (obese: 1,520 percent)
- **35 percent more likely to develop kidney cancer** (obese: 70 percent)
- **14 percent more likely to have osteoarthritis** (obese: 34 percent)
- **70 percent more likely to develop high blood pressure** (obese: up to 170 percent)

We Can Change the Future

Children who struggle with weight issues today can grow up to lead healthy, active lives. How do I know? Because I used to be one of the "fat kids" myself.

As a boy growing up in a small town in Pennsylvania, I, too, struggled with weight issues. I made bad choices—choosing fast food over smart food, then trying to starve myself to get my body in the shape I wanted it in. Sure enough, I'd get hungry again—or sad, or lonely, or just bored—and there I'd be, barking orders into a clown's mouth once again. My brother, Eric, used to invite his friends over to watch my dietary indiscretions: "Don't disturb the big animal," he'd tell his buddies. "It's feeding."

Several things happened that changed my life for the better. I joined the high school wrestling team, which made me cognizant of my weight and my fitness. I paid my way through college by joining the Navy Reserve, where I learned the importance of discipline and the life-or-death impact of staying in shape. And I came to work at *Men's Health* magazine, where I've spent the last 15 years studying nutrition and fitness and learning more than I ever thought possible about the role that our diets play in our overall health.

And then, in 1998, my life changed forever. My father, Bohdan, died of a stroke at the age of 52.

My father struggled with his weight all his life—starting in his teen years. I remember him, even in his 30s, laboring to catch his breath as he climbed a simple flight of stairs.

His death drove it all home for me: If we allow the bad stuff into our diets, if we trust the chain restaurants and mass-food marketers with our health—and if we don't raise questions such as "what's really in this?" and "how is this food affecting my body," we risk so much. We risk being able to do the things we like. To be proud of the way we look and feel. To live to see our children and our grandchildren grow.

EAT THIS, NOT THAT! FOR KIDS! is designed to help you and your children avoid that fate. With the simple photo-driven information and intensively researched nutritional data in these pages, you'll finally have control of your diet, your body, your life. And more important, you'll pass that gift on to your children.

The tough choices won't end here. As a parent, you'll be called upon to give your kids advice, solace, and guidance for the next, oh, 60 years or so. But one aspect of parenthood—making smart nutritional choices for your children—is going to be a whole heck of a lot easier.

So turn the page, and let's get started on building a better future for ourselves and our children.

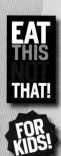

FEEDING THE FUTURE

Feeding the Future

Imagine you and I, and all our friends and relatives, and our children, are on a big boat in the middle of the ocean. And the boat is taking on water. On one side of the boat, you and I and our friends and families and a whole bunch of other folks are bailing as fast as we can. We're working hard, thinking smart, trying to save all of our lives and keep the ship afloat. On the other side of the boat is a smaller group working just as hard, punching holes in the hull. And no matter how much progress the big group makes, it just can't compensate for the damage the smaller group is doing.

Frustrating, right? Well, that's sort of the way I feel when I think about the battle against obesity and what America's food marketers are doing to us, to our children, and to our country.

Like most parents, you probably try hard to get your kids to eat healthy. You play "green bean airplane" with your toddler's spoon. ("Here comes the plane, open the hangar!") You read the labels in the grocery store, always on the lookout for bad stuff. You keep an eye on their snack consumption and do all you can to urge them to try new things. And you worry, too, about your own fitness levels: Every year, Americans spend an estimated $42 billion on diet books; $18.5 billion on health club memberships; and $5.2 billion on diet foods and weight loss programs. We're all trying to exercise, to eat healthy, and to keep ourselves slim, and in doing so, we're trying to set a good example for our children.

But no matter how hard those of us on this side of the boat try, there's a group of folks on the other side of the boat punching holes in our efforts. And those are the food marketers who make money by getting our children to eat junk.

According to media industry estimates, advertisers spend $900 million every year on television shows aimed at children under 12. And more than two-thirds of that advertising is for food products: fast-food meals with action figures and dolls; sugary cereals with cartoon spokespeople; "juice" drinks that have about as much to do with actual fruit as Swedish Fish have to do with mackerel. The average child between 8 and 18 spends 3 hours a day in front of the television, and according to the Federal Trade Commission, kids ages 2 to 11 will see 26,000 TV ads this year—22 percent of them marketing food.

Now think about the messages that your child is receiving about food. Think about the fun and happy lands portrayed on TV advertisements, where cartoon characters come to life and magic carpet rides become a reality as soon as he or she opens a box of Sugary Sweet Mouthrot Cereal, or whatever today's big craze might be. The more advertisers promise this golden land of happiness, and associate it in our children's minds with junk food, the more our children will want to follow those promises—again and again—in hopes of finding themselves there, in Sugary Sweet Mouthrot Paradise Land. The message—that junk food equals instant happiness—is one that sticks with a child for all his life. Our "eat this, feel better" culture just promotes more unhealthy nutritional habits for years to come.

And the worst part of it all may be this: The foods that advertisers are selling to kids, the stuff that supposedly is going to make them happier, has in fact the opposite result. No kid feels happy when he's nodding off in class at the end of a sugar high, getting picked last in gym class because he's too heavy to make basic athletic moves, or skipping social events because he's ashamed of the way his body looks.

In other words, it's a setup: Our society is promising our children one thing and delivering something completely different. As a result, the nonpartisan consumer group Trust for America's Health has warned, "Today's children are likely to be the first generation to live shorter, less-healthy lives than their parents."

It doesn't have to be this way. We can bail all we want, but we can't keep our kids' ship from sinking if fast-food marketers are going to keep punching holes in our hull.

But there is something we can do.

We can teach our children how to swim.

Doggie Paddling Through the Nutritional Ocean

One of the biggest mistakes we make when we think about "watching our weight" is to assume that our first goal is to eat less. In fact, what we really need to concentrate on is eating more—not more food or calories, but more nutrients. Because while our consumption of calories is way up, our consumption of essential nutrients, including vitamins, minerals, and fiber, is actually down. That's right. We're eating more food, but we're eating fewer nutrients! Refined grains, added fats and sugars, hard-to-pronounce chemical ingredients—all conspire to bloat our waistlines, but add nothing to our nutritional bottom lines. It's like we're filling our piggy banks with pennies and overlooking the $100 bills lying around us.

A parent's first instinct, when she sees her child gaining weight, is to deny him or her those extra snacks and nibbles. But that's a losing strategy, just like any fad diet. One of the reasons diets fail is because nobody likes to feel as though they are denying themselves—in a land of plenty, we don't want to feel left out. And children are no different. Why should some other kid get a snack and our child miss out? Besides, skipping a snack is a guaranteed way to feel hungry, and a child's hunger is a VIP first-class ticket to Candy Aisle Meltdown.

Instead of even thinking about cutting down on your child's food intake, think of expanding his or her palette. Here are some simple rules that will teach your child to swim—no matter how rough the nutritional seas may get.

RULE #1:
NEVER SKIP BREAKFAST. EVER.

Yes, mornings are crazy. But they're also our best hope at regaining our nutritional sanity. A 2005 study synthesized the results of 47 studies that examined the impact of starting the day with a healthy breakfast. Here's what they found.

Children skipped breakfast more than any other meal. Skipping is more prevalent in girls, older children, and adolescents.

People who skip breakfast are more likely to take up smoking or drink-

ing, less likely to exercise, and more likely to follow fad diets or express concerns about body weight. Common reasons cited for skipping were lack of time, lack of hunger, or dieting.

- On the day of the surveys, 8 percent of 1- to 7-year-olds skipped, 12 percent of 8- to 10-year-olds skipped, 20 percent of 11- to 14-year-olds skipped, and 30 percent of 15- to 18-year-olds skipped.

Bad news. And sure, it would seem to make sense that skipping breakfast means eating fewer calories, which means weighing less. But it doesn't work that way. Consider:

- Breakfast eaters tend to have higher total calorie intakes throughout the day, but compared to skippers, they also received significantly more fiber, calcium, and other micronutrients. Breakfast eaters also tended to consume less soda and French fries and more fruits, vegetables, and milk.
- Breakfast eaters were approximately 30 percent less likely to be overweight or obese. (And think about that—kids who eat breakfast eat more food, but weigh less!)

RULE #2:
SNACK WITH PURPOSE

There's a big difference between mindless munching and strategic snacking. Snacking with a purpose means reinforcing good habits, keeping the metabolic rate high, and filling the gaps between meals with the nutrients a child's body craves.

- In the 20 years leading up to the 21st century (1977 to 1996), salty snack portions increased by 93 calories, and soft drink portions increased by 49 calories. This data comes from the Nationwide Food Consumption Survey and the Continuing Surveys of Food Intake, which together create a sample of 63,380 people ages 2 and older. So when you give your kid an individual bag of chips and a soda—the same snack you might have enjoyed when you were 10—he's ingesting 142 more calories than you did. Feeding him that just twice a week means he'll weigh about a pound more than you did within a year.

Need snack ideas? Try popcorn. The 2005 Dietary Guidelines for Americans lists it as a viable means by which to increase whole-grain consumption. (This doesn't work if the popcorn's saturated with butter and salt.) A study of popcorn consumers published in the *Journal of the American Dietetic Association* found that popcorn eaters had a 22 percent higher intake of fiber and 250 percent higher intake of whole grains than noneaters. Other great choices include not just the low-cal stuff (vegetables and fruit) but more filling fare like unsalted nuts and even dark chocolate, which is packed with antioxidants and even some fiber. The point is not to deny food, but to teach our children to crave foods that are healthy for them. One parent I know has a great rule for her kids: They must always ask permission to have a snack, but they never need permission to reach for a piece of fruit. She says it has helped train her kids to go the easy route—and that just happens to be the healthy route.

RULE #3:
BEWARE OF PORTION DISTORTION

Snacks aren't the only thing that's increased wildly in portion size. Since 1977, hamburgers have increased by 97 calories, French fries by 68 calories, and Mexican foods by 133 calories, according to a study by the University of North Carolina at Chapel Hill.

Eat This Pyramid, Not That One

The USDA has its pyramid, of course, but the iconic image young students learn so well in our school system leaves a lot to be desired in terms of specifics. According to the vagaries of the image, a serving of white rice and quinoa both count the same toward the daily recommended six servings, despite the fact that one is packed with fiber, healthy fat, and essential amino acids (quinoa) and the other is a nutritional black hole (rice).

It's time for parental discretion. One-quarter of all vegetables consumed by kids are French fries, and according to a government study of 4,000 kids between the ages of 2 and 19, the overwhelming bulk of their nutrients comes from fruit juice and sugary cereals. While those might have a place in the USDA's pyramid, they have no place in ours. It's still important for your kids to go about constructing their pyramids each day—you just need to be sure they have the right building blocks.

FATS AND OILS

Eat This
Healthy fats: olive oil, canola oil, monounsaturated fats from nuts, avocado, salmon

Not That!
Unhealthy fats: Stick margarine, lard, palm oil, anything with partially hydrogenated oil

DAIRY (2 TO 3 1-CUP SERVINGS)

Eat This
2 percent milk, string cheese, cottage cheese, plain yogurt sweetened with fresh fruit

Not That!
Chocolate milk, ice cream, hot cheese dip, yogurt with fruit on the bottom

MEAT, POULTRY, FISH, EGGS, AND BEANS (2 TO 3 2-OUNCE SERVINGS)

Eat This
Grilled chicken breast, roast pork tenderloin, sirloin steak, scrambled, boiled, or poached eggs, stewed black beans, almonds, unsweetened peanut butter

Not That!
Chicken fingers, crispy chicken sandwiches, cheeseburgers, strip or rib-eye steak, peanut butter with added sugars

VEGETABLES (5 ½-CUP SERVINGS)

Eat This
Sautéed spinach, steamed broccoli, romaine or mixed green salads, roasted mushrooms, grilled pepper and onion skewers, baby carrots, tomato sauce, salsa, homemade guacamole

Not That!
French fries, potato chips, onion rings, eggplant parmesan

FRUIT (3 ½-CUP SERVINGS)

Eat This
Sliced apples or pears, berries, grapes, stone fruit like peaches, plums, and apricots, 100 percent fruit smoothies

Not That!
More than one 8-ounce glass of juice a day; more than a few tablespoons of dried fruit a day; smoothies made with sherbet, frozen yogurt, or added sugar

GRAINS (6 1-OUNCE SERVINGS)

Eat This
Brown rice, whole grain bread, quinoa, whole grain pasta, oatmeal

Not That!
White rice, white bread, pasta, muffins, tortillas, pancakes, waffles, heavily sweetened cereal

- A study published in the *American Journal of Preventive Medicine* looked at 63,380 individuals' drinking habits over a span of 19 years. The results show that for children ages 2 to 18, portions of sweetened beverages increased from 13.1 ounces in 1977 to 18.9 ounces in 1996.

One easy way to short-circuit this growing trend? **Buy smaller bowls and cups.** A recent study at the Children's Nutrition Research Center in Houston, Texas, shows that 5- and 6-year-old children will consume a third more calories when presented with a larger portion. The findings are based on a sample of 53 children who were served either 1- or 2-cup portions of macaroni and cheese.

RULE #4:
DRINK RESPONSIBLY

Too many of us keep in mind the adage "watch what you eat," and we forget another serious threat to our children's health: We don't watch what we drink. One study found that that sweetened beverages constituted more than half (51 percent) of all beverages consumed by fourth through sixth grade students. The students who consumed the most sweetened beverages took on approximately 330 extra calories per day, and on average they ate less than half the amount of real fruit than did their nondrinking or light-drinking peers.

One important strategy is to keep cold, filtered water in a pitcher in the fridge. You might even want to keep some cut-up limes, oranges, or lemons nearby for kids to flavor their own water. A UK study showed that in classrooms with limited access to water, only 29 percent of students met their daily needs; free access to water led to higher intake.

- The *American Journal of Preventive Medicine* looked at four studies that showed 73,345 individuals' drinking habits over a span of 24 years. They found that for children ages 2 to 18, the amount of calories from soft drinks as a percentage of total calories more than doubled from 3 to 6.9 percent. The same is true for fruit drinks, which increased from 1.8 to 3.4 percent. And total calories from sweetened beverages increased from 4.8 to 10.3 percent. The percentage of calories from milk, on the other hand, decreased from 13.2 to 8.3 percent.

- A study using the national survey Continuing Survey of Food Intakes by Individuals found that consumption of real fruit juice is higher than other beverages only for very young children. By the age of 5, the consumption of fruit drinks, -ades, and sodas surpassed that of real fruit juice. As children get older, the gap between soda consumption and real fruit drinks continues to grow until, for the 14- to 18-year-old demographic, children are drinking only one-fifth as much fruit juice as soda (3.7 ounces juice, 18 ounces soda).

As it is with all things, a parent's example is a critical determinant as to whether a child will drown him- or herself in soda. A Minnesota study showed that children were 3 times more likely to drink soda five or more times per week when their parents regularly drank soda.

- A USDA report shows that soft drink availability doubled between 1970 and 1995.

The importance of drinking milk is overrated, right? Nope. In fact, growing boys and girls create at least 40 percent of their adult bone mass during adolescence, and 73 percent of the calcium in the US food supply comes from dairy foods. Children who do not receive adequate amounts of this critical mineral are at an increased risk of bone disease later in life.

RULE #5:
EAT MORE WHOLE FOODS AND FEWER SCIENCE EXPERIMENTS

Here's a rule of healthy eating that will serve you well when picking out foods for your family: The shorter the ingredient list, the healthier the food. (One of the worst foods we've ever found, the Baskin Robbins Heath Shake, has 73 ingredients—and, by the way, a whopping 2,310 calories and more than three days' worth of saturated fat! Whatever happened to the idea that a milkshake was, um, milk and ice cream?) And don't think that you're the only one who's confused: The FDA maintains a list of more than 3,000 ingredients that are considered safe to eat, and any one of them could wind up in your next box of mac 'n' cheese.

- According to USDA reports, most of the sodium in the American's diet comes from packaged and processed foods. Naturally occurring salt accounts for only 12 percent of total intake, while 77 percent is added by food manufacturers.

RULE #6:
SET THE TABLE

Children in families with a more structured mealtime exhibit healthier eating habits. Among middle-school and high-school girls, those whose families ate together only one or two times per week were more than twice as likely to exhibit weight control issues compared with those who ate together three or four times per week.

Of course, the notion of 6 PM dinnertime and then everyone into their pjs is a quaint one, but it hardly fits within a society where both Mom and Dad work, where the office may call at any time day or night, and where our kids have such highly scheduled social lives that the delineation between "parent" and "chauffeur" is sometimes difficult to parse. While we can't always bring the family together like Ozzie Nelson's (or, heck, even like Ozzy Osbourne's), we can make some positive steps in that direction. One busy family I know keeps Sunday night dinner sacred—no social plans, no school projects, no extra work brought home from the office. And although it's not ideal, keeping the family ritual just once a week gives parents the opportunity to point out what is and isn't healthy at the dinner table.

Another smart move: **Get your kids involved in cooking.** Make a game of trying to pack the most healthful ingredients into your meals. A Texas study showed that children can be encouraged to eat more fruits and vegetables by giving them goals and allowing them to help in preparation. In a classroom curriculum program called *Squire's Quest!*, 671 fourth-grade students were asked to select a fruit, fruit-juice, or vegetable recipe to prepare at home. Among those who completed the study, the average increase was one serving per day of fruit or vegetables. Those who completed more of the recipes showed the biggest improvements.

RULE# 7:
KICK THE SUGAR HABIT

Take a look at the label on your loaf of sliced bread. Then take a look at the label on your ketchup. Now, for the coup de grâce, take a look at the label on a package of Twizzlers, or Jolly Ranchers, or Nerds. As different as they may seem, chances are these foods all contain the same ingredient: high-fructose corn syrup, or HFCS. According to the USDA, high-fructose corn syrup constitutes more than 40 percent of the caloric sweeteners

What Our Kids Need Each Day

	1-3 YEARS	4-8 YEARS	9-13 YEARS	14-18 YEARS
CALORIES	1000–1400	1400–1600	1800–2200 (B)	2200–2400 (B)
			1600–2200 (G)	2000 (G)
FAT	33–54 grams	39–62	62–85	61–95 (B) 55–78 (G)
SATURATED FAT	<12–16 grams	<16–18	<20–24 (B) <18–22 (G)	<24–27 (B) <22 (G)
SODIUM	1000–1500 mg	1200–1900	1500–2200	1500–2300
CARBS	130 grams	130	130	130
FIBER	19 grams	25	31 (B) 26 (G)	38 (B) 26 (G)
PROTEIN	13 grams	19	31 (B) 26 (G)	52 (B) 46 (G)

used in US foods and beverages. Now consider this: In 1970, high-fructose corn syrup accounted for less than 1 percent of all caloric sweeteners.

Why is this so bad? It's not because HFCS is more dangerous for you than sucrose; in fact, most recent data suggests that the body metabolizes HFCS in the same way it does ordinary sugar. No, the major concern is that HFCS—a derivative of corn that's cheaper to produce than sugar and has a longer shelf life—is being added to foods that you'd never imagine would need sugar. But as Americans have been trained to develop a more intense sweet tooth, marketers have begun adding cheap sugar substitutes into

everything from tomato sauce to wheat bread. And that pads everything we eat with extra calories. Today, the average American consumes 132 calories' worth of HFCS every day.

To completely avoid HFCS, you'd have to give up eating packaged foods, and that's just not practical for most families. Instead, become a savvy label reader (learn how on page 154) and eliminate foods not just with HFCS, but with any form of sugar at the top of the ingredient list.

RULE# 8:
EAT THE RAINBOW
Kids need a colorful diet. Turn the page to find out why.

Eat the Rainbow

Better nutrition starts not with cutting out the bad, but with adding in the good. Fill your children's meals with healthful, high-quality food and you'll eventually squeeze out the bad stuff.

I'm not going to pretend that getting a child to eat what's good for him isn't sometimes a struggle. "A lot of parents tell me, 'My kids don't like healthy foods,'" says David Katz, MD, an associate clinical professor of epidemiology and public health at Yale Medical School. "'Finicky' is not an excuse. You never hear a parent say, 'My child doesn't like to look both ways before he crosses the street.' They tell him to do it. More kids today will die of complications from bad foods they eat than they will from tobacco, drugs, and alcohol."

So how do you teach the basics of nutrition to a 7-year-old? Even we grownups have trouble understanding which vitamins and minerals we need more of and which complicated chemical ingredients we need to avoid.

Well, here's a simple trick: Just teach your kids to eat as many different colors as they can. And no, I'm not talking about mixing the red, green, and purple Skittles. I'm talking about adding as much of a mix of fruits and vegetables as possible. That's because the colors represented in foods are indicators of nutritional value—and different colors mean different vitamins and minerals.

Not everything on this list is going to appeal to your child's appetite. But there's enough variation here that he or she can squeeze one food from each category into a day's worth of eating. For a fun project, make a multicolor checklist, and have your kid check off each color as he or she eats it throughout the day.

Or do what our parents did and sell them on the kid-friendly benefits trapped inside of spinach, carrots, and the like. Each group of produce offers seriously cool "superpowers" that appeal to kids' deepest desires to dominate math quizzes and monkey bars alike. Feel free to sell these as hard as you want. Hey, even if it didn't end up making you as strong as Popeye, you still ate your spinach, right?

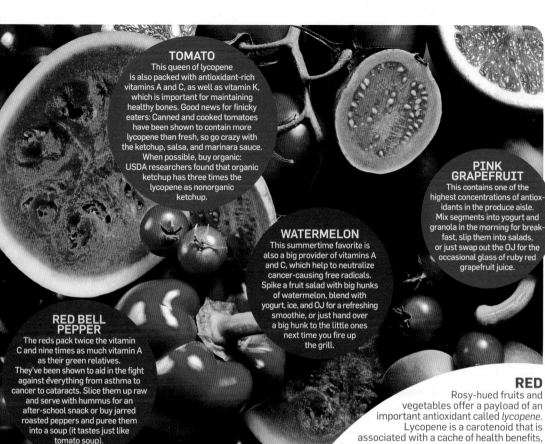

TOMATO

This queen of lycopene is also packed with antioxidant-rich vitamins A and C, as well as vitamin K, which is important for maintaining healthy bones. Good news for finicky eaters: Canned and cooked tomatoes have been shown to contain more lycopene than fresh, so go crazy with the ketchup, salsa, and marinara sauce. When possible, buy organic: USDA researchers found that organic ketchup has three times the lycopene as nonorganic ketchup.

PINK GRAPEFRUIT

This contains one of the highest concentrations of antioxidants in the produce aisle. Mix segments into yogurt and granola in the morning for breakfast, slip them into salads, or just swap out the OJ for the occasional glass of ruby red grapefruit juice.

WATERMELON

This summertime favorite is also a big provider of vitamins A and C, which help to neutralize cancer-causing free radicals. Spike a fruit salad with big hunks of watermelon, blend with yogurt, ice, and OJ for a refreshing smoothie, or just hand over a big hunk to the little ones next time you fire up the grill.

RED BELL PEPPER

The reds pack twice the vitamin C and nine times as much vitamin A as their green relatives. They've been shown to aid in the fight against everything from asthma to cancer to cataracts. Slice them up raw and serve with hummus for an after-school snack or buy jarred roasted peppers and puree them into a soup (it tastes just like tomato soup).

GUAVA

Like most lycopene vessels, guava is packed with vitamins A and C. It also contains heart-healthy omega-3 fatty acids and belly-filling fiber. Get your hands on these in the produce aisle of larger supermarkets or Latin grocers, or simply stock a bottle of guava nectar in the fridge.

RED

Rosy-hued fruits and vegetables offer a payload of an important antioxidant called *lycopene*. Lycopene is a carotenoid that is associated with a cache of health benefits, including protecting the skin from sun damage and decreasing the risk of heart disease and certain forms of cancer. Lycopene is most strongly concentrated in the most red of all red fruits: the tomato. What is surprising, though, is that cooked and processed tomatoes have higher lycopene concentrations, so don't shy away from the salsa or marinara sauce. **SUPERPOWER:** Red food makes you dash like the Flash! There's a reason he wore red: Lycopene-rich foods have been shown to decrease symptoms of wheezing, asthma, and shortness of breath in people when they exercise.

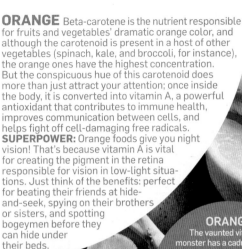

ORANGE Beta-carotene is the nutrient responsible for fruits and vegetables' dramatic orange color, and although the carotenoid is present in a host of other vegetables (spinach, kale, and broccoli, for instance), the orange ones have the highest concentration. But the conspicuous hue of this carotenoid does more than just attract your attention; once inside the body, it is converted into vitamin A, a powerful antioxidant that contributes to immune health, improves communication between cells, and helps fight off cell-damaging free radicals.

SUPERPOWER: Orange foods give you night vision! That's because vitamin A is vital for creating the pigment in the retina responsible for vision in low-light situations. Just think of the benefits: perfect for beating their friends at hide-and-seek, spying on their brothers or sisters, and spotting bogeymen before they can hide under their beds.

WINTER SQUASH

A true party bag of nutrients, winter squash is a great source of a dozen different vitamins, including a host of B vitamins, folate, manganese, and fiber. What does that all mean? It means feed it to your kid! And lots of it! The best way is to cut the squash into 1-inch wedges and bake at 375°F for 40 minutes, until soft and caramelized.

ORANGE

The vaunted vitamin C monster has a cadre of critical phytonutrients known to lower blood pressure and contain strong anti-inflammatory properties. Juice is fine, but the real fruit is even better. The secret, though, is that the orange's most powerful healing properties are found in the peel; use a zester to grate the peel over bowls of yogurt, salads, or directly into smoothies.

CANTALOUPE

The surge of vitamin A is important not just for the eyes, but also for healthy lungs, and the megadose of vitamin C helps white blood cells ward off infection. Sliced cantaloupe and yogurt make a killer breakfast, or combine the two in a food processor with a touch of honey and lemon and puree into a soup, which makes a great low-cal dessert.

SWEET POTATO

The best part about sweet potatoes, outside of the beta-carotene, is that they're loaded with fiber. That means they have a gentler effect on your kid's blood sugar levels than regular potatoes. Substitute baked sweet potatoes for baked potatoes, mash them up like you would an Idaho, or make fries out of them by tossing spears with olive oil and roasting in a 400°F oven for 30 minutes.

CARROT

The snack of choice for Bugs Bunny happens to be the richest carotene source of all. Baby carrots are perfect plain for dipping or snacking on, of course, but also try shredding carrots into a salad or marinara for a hit of natural sweetness, or roasting them slowly in the oven with olive oil and salt.

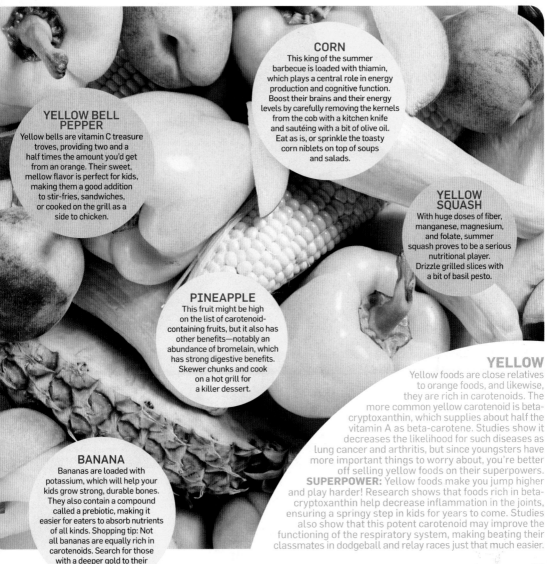

CORN

This king of the summer barbecue is loaded with thiamin, which plays a central role in energy production and cognitive function. Boost their brains and their energy levels by carefully removing the kernels from the cob with a kitchen knife and sautéing with a bit of olive oil. Eat as is, or sprinkle the toasty corn niblets on top of soups and salads.

YELLOW BELL PEPPER

Yellow bells are vitamin C treasure troves, providing two and a half times the amount you'd get from an orange. Their sweet, mellow flavor is perfect for kids, making them a good addition to stir-fries, sandwiches, or cooked on the grill as a side to chicken.

YELLOW SQUASH

With huge doses of fiber, manganese, magnesium, and folate, summer squash proves to be a serious nutritional player. Drizzle grilled slices with a bit of basil pesto.

PINEAPPLE

This fruit might be high on the list of carotenoid-containing fruits, but it also has other benefits—notably an abundance of bromelain, which has strong digestive benefits. Skewer chunks and cook on a hot grill for a killer dessert.

BANANA

Bananas are loaded with potassium, which will help your kids grow strong, durable bones. They also contain a compound called a prebiotic, making it easier for eaters to absorb nutrients of all kinds. Shopping tip: Not all bananas are equally rich in carotenoids. Search for those with a deeper gold to their edible flesh.

YELLOW

Yellow foods are close relatives to orange foods, and likewise, they are rich in carotenoids. The more common yellow carotenoid is beta-cryptoxanthin, which supplies about half the vitamin A as beta-carotene. Studies show it decreases the likelihood for such diseases as lung cancer and arthritis, but since youngsters have more important things to worry about, you're better off selling yellow foods on their superpowers.

SUPERPOWER: Yellow foods make you jump higher and play harder! Research shows that foods rich in beta-cryptoxanthin help decrease inflammation in the joints, ensuring a springy step in kids for years to come. Studies also show that this potent carotenoid may improve the functioning of the respiratory system, making beating their classmates in dodgeball and relay races just that much easier.

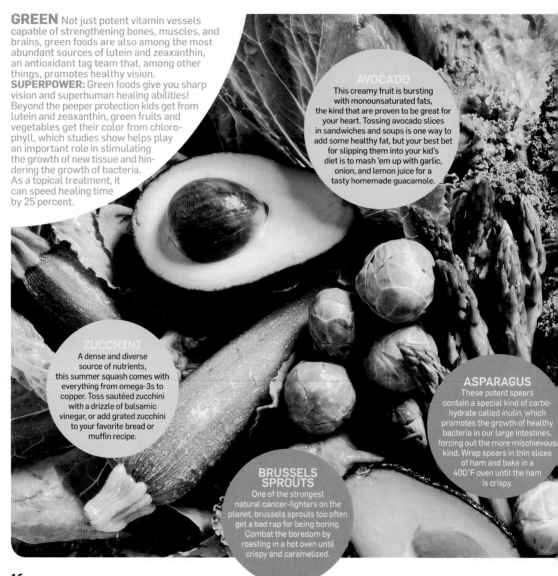

GREEN Not just potent vitamin vessels capable of strengthening bones, muscles, and brains, green foods are also among the most abundant sources of lutein and zeaxanthin, an antioxidant tag team that, among other things, promotes healthy vision.

SUPERPOWER: Green foods give you sharp vision and superhuman healing abilities! Beyond the peeper protection kids get from lutein and zeaxanthin, green fruits and vegetables get their color from chlorophyll, which studies show helps play an important role in stimulating the growth of new tissue and hindering the growth of bacteria. As a topical treatment, it can speed healing time by 25 percent.

AVOCADO
This creamy fruit is bursting with monounsaturated fats, the kind that are proven to be great for your heart. Tossing avocado slices in sandwiches and soups is one way to add some healthy fat, but your best bet for slipping them into your kid's diet is to mash 'em up with garlic, onion, and lemon juice for a tasty homemade guacamole.

ZUCCHINI
A dense and diverse source of nutrients, this summer squash comes with everything from omega-3s to copper. Toss sautéed zucchini with a drizzle of balsamic vinegar, or add grated zucchini to your favorite bread or muffin recipe.

ASPARAGUS
These potent spears contain a special kind of carbohydrate called *inulin*, which promotes the growth of healthy bacteria in our large intestines, forcing out the more mischievous kind. Wrap spears in thin slices of ham and bake in a 400°F oven until the ham is crispy.

BRUSSELS SPROUTS
One of the strongest natural cancer-fighters on the planet, brussels sprouts too often get a bad rap for being boring. Combat the boredom by roasting in a hot oven until crispy and caramelized.

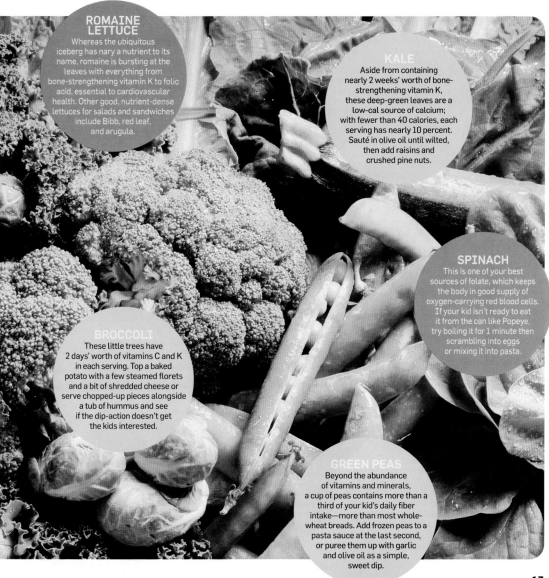

ROMAINE LETTUCE

Whereas the ubiquitous iceberg has nary a nutrient to its name, romaine is bursting at the leaves with everything from bone-strengthening vitamin K to folic acid, essential to cardiovascular health. Other good, nutrient-dense lettuces for salads and sandwiches include Bibb, red leaf, and arugula.

KALE

Aside from containing nearly 2 weeks' worth of bone-strengthening vitamin K, these deep-green leaves are a low-cal source of calcium; with fewer than 40 calories, each serving has nearly 10 percent. Sauté in olive oil until wilted, then add raisins and crushed pine nuts.

SPINACH

This is one of your best sources of folate, which keeps the body in good supply of oxygen-carrying red blood cells. If your kid isn't ready to eat it from the can like Popeye, try boiling it for 1 minute then scrambling into eggs or mixing it into pasta.

BROCCOLI

These little trees have 2 days' worth of vitamins C and K in each serving. Top a baked potato with a few steamed florets and a bit of shredded cheese or serve chopped-up pieces alongside a tub of hummus and see if the dip-action doesn't get the kids interested.

GREEN PEAS

Beyond the abundance of vitamins and minerals, a cup of peas contains more than a third of your kid's daily fiber intake—more than most whole-wheat breads. Add frozen peas to a pasta sauce at the last second, or puree them up with garlic and olive oil as a simple, sweet dip.

EGGPLANT

A pigment called *nasunin* is concentrated in the peel of the eggplant, and studies have shown it has powerful disease-fighting properties. Simplify eggplant parmesan by baking 1/2-inch-thick slices and layering them with marinara and cheese.

BLACKBERRY

One cup of berries contains 5 percent of your child's daily folate and half the day's vitamin C. Try pureeing blackberries, then combining with olive oil and balsamic vinegar for a super healthy salad dressing.

BEET

This candy-sweet vegetable derives most of its color from a cancer-fighting pigment called *betacyanin*. The edible root is replete with fiber, potassium, and manganese. Toss roasted beet chunks with toasted walnuts and orange segments, or grate them raw into salads.

RADISH

Nutritional benefits vary among the many varieties of radishes, but they share an abundance of vitamin C and a tendency to facilitate the digestive process. Try serving thinly sliced radishes on a bagel with low-fat cream cheese and black pepper.

BLUEBERRY

The most abundant source of anthocyanins has more antioxidant punch than red wine, and it helps the body's vitamin C do its job better. Sprinkle blueberries into oatmeal, cereal, or yogurt, or mix with almonds and a few chocolate chips for a quick trail mix.

BLUE/PURPLE

Blue and purple foods get their colors from the presence of a unique set of flavonoids called *anthocyanins*. Flavonoids in general are known to improve cardiovascular health and prevent short-term memory loss, but the deeply pigmented anthocyanins go even further. Researchers at Tufts University have found that blueberries may make brain cells respond better to incoming messages and might even spur the growth of new nerve cells, providing a new meaning to smart eating. **SUPERPOWER:** Blue foods make you the smartest kid in the class!

PURPLE GRAPE

Some researchers believe that, despite their high-fat diets, the French are protected from heart disease by their mass consumption of grapes and wine. Look for a deeper shade of purple—that's an indication of a high flavonoid concentration. Try freezing grapes in the dead of summer for a cool, healthy treat.

PLUM

Another rich source of antioxidants, plums have also been shown to help the body better absorb iron. Roast chunks in the oven and serve warm over a small scoop of vanilla ice cream.

18

What Our Kids Aren't Eating

In the grips of an obesity crisis, it might be counterintuitive to talk about encouraging our children to eat more. But according to the *Journal of the American College of Nutrition,* only 25 percent of kids met the daily recommendations for fruit and vegetable intake, which in turn creates an array of nutrient deficiencies that can have lasting health implications. Combat the problem by turning the missing nutrients into a treasure hunt with your kids.

WHAT'S MISSING	WHO'S MISSING IT	WHERE TO FIND IT
CALCIUM Vital for building strong, dense bones. Also important in many cell and muscle functions	Calcium's a concern for children of all ages, but especially among young children and girls between 9 and 13	Green leafy vegetables, broccoli, oranges, milk and other dairy products
IRON Helps our bodies produce energy, as well as maintain a healthy immune system	Infants and adolescent girls	Lean red meat, legumes, tofu, green vegetables, mushrooms, and tomatoes
VITAMIN D Builds strong bones and teeth, fights inflammation, and protects against diabetes, heart disease, and cancer	More than half of all children have inadequate levels of vitamin D in their blood.	Milk, eggs, salmon, and shrimp. For infants, the American Academy of Pediatrics recommends providing vitamin D supplements.
VITAMIN E Promotes healthy cell communication, fights off free radicals, and guards our skin against ultraviolet light	For children ages 1 to 8, only 48 percent meet their daily requirements.	Sunflower seeds, almonds, olives, papaya, spinach, and blueberries
FIBER Normalizes blood sugar levels to fight against diabetes, maintains cholesterol levels, and aids satiety	According to a USDA report, only 3 percent of children eat an adequate amount of fiber.	Whole fruits (not juice), whole grains, beans, lentils, peas, berries, cauliflower, spinach, and carrots

AT THEIR FAVORITE RESTAURANTS

EAT THIS NOT THAT!

FOR KIDS!

Eat Out, Eat Right

Being a parent is hard. Being a parent who's trying to feed her kids healthy fare is even harder.

But being a parent who wants to feed her kids healthy fare at today's restaurants? Nearly impossible.

First, there's the simple logistical challenge of keeping kids—especially little ones—fed and happy on the road. They don't adhere to scheduled mealtimes. They don't adhere to accepted standards of polite behavior. Traveling with little children is like being the road manager for a gaggle of crazed rock stars—they won't listen to reason, their demands are impossible, and when they've worked up an appetite, they want it satisfied now.

And let's face it—a kid's palate is not what you'd call sophisticated. Most young kids have two major food groups: stuff that's beige (fries, chicken fingers, crackers, and bananas), and stuff that has cartoon characters on the box.

Kids don't make mealtimes easy for their parents.

But neither do today's restaurants. Oh sure, most offer "kids' menus," which almost always include the same five choices—pasta, grilled cheese, burgers, mac and cheese. Nothing that's going to set the nutritional world on fire there, but it's not much different than what we ate as kids, right? How bad could such fare be?

The answer is: really, really bad. In fact, even though we try to feed our kids the same type of stuff we remember eating when we were growing up, in reality, today's food is just plain different. According to the New York City Department of Health and Mental Hygiene, fast food and other chain restaurants have allowed their portion sizes and calorie counts to grow faster than Lindsay Lohan's arrest record.

Consider the average fast-food dinner of burger, fries, and a soda—just what Fonzie and Richie ate at Arnold's Drive-In in the '50s and '60s, just what you and I ate when we were kids in the '70s and '80s. But since the 1970s, that simple meal has morphed into something grotesque: The typical serving size for soft drinks has increased by 49 calories; for French fries by 68 calories; and for hamburgers by 97 calories. Eating this standard fast-food meal once a week will give you 11,128 more calories a year—or 3 pounds of extra body weight—than the same meal did when we were kids.

The reasons for this caloric bonanza are complex, but they come down to sheer numbers: Restaurants in general, and chain restaurants in particular, want to create the largest foods they can for the lowest cost. Then they pass those giant portions and low prices on to their customers, and the meals seem like a bargain. And chain restaurants are a bargain—if you're shopping for flab. That's because the cheapest cost comes from the cheapest ingredients: starch, sugar (especially high-fructose corn syrup), salt, and grease (especially trans fats). Because big farms grow high-yield crops (read: soy, corn, and wheat; cows, pigs, and chickens) and don't bother with crops that are hard to grow (read: vegetables and fruit), the cheapest ingredients are also the most calorie-dense and nutrition-

thin. That's why—against what would seem to be all logic—you can buy a Big Mac for half the cost of a fresh cantaloupe.

It's also why, even though only one in four meals is prepared in restaurants, a whopping 35 percent of our weekly caloric intake is consumed there—up from 23 percent in the 1970s. Sure, we eat out more, and take out more, than we did when you and I were kids—it's a by-product of our crazy, two-income, 24/7 lifestyle, which happens to be the same lifestyle that's made cooking at home much more of a rarity than it once was. But the number of calories being pumped into us by restaurants is out of proportion with the actual number of meals we eat there. To put it another way: Restaurants make up only one-quarter of our meals, but account for more than one-third of our calories. (And, incredibly, eating out now sucks up 47 percent of Americans' food dollars.)

And the drive-through calories are piling up even faster for those of us not yet old enough to drive. According to researchers from Harvard Medical School, consumption of fast food by children 4 to 19 years old increased by a remarkable fivefold in

2 decades, from 2 percent of their total calorie intake in the late 1970s to 10 percent by the mid 1990s. (If you are what you eat, the typical American adolescent is 10 percent McNugget.) According to a study in the *Journal of Pediatrics*, children who eat fast food not only consume more calories, fat, carbohydrates, and added sugar, they also drink more soda, consume less milk, and eat fewer fruits and vegetables than kids who lay off the Unhappy Meal. Sadly, not many of our kids are ignoring the clown: In a study of 1,474 middle school students by the Harvard School of Public Health, 66 percent had eaten fast food in just the past 7 days!

Now, we all know that fast food is often bad for us. And, interestingly enough, American dining trends aren't pointing to the big burger pusher with the crown. More and more, we're turning to the big chain sit-down restaurants: Olive Garden, Don Pablo's, T.G.I. Friday's, and the like. Indeed, some economists forecast that between 2000 and 2020, spending at sit-down, or full-service, restaurants will grow three times as fast as spending at fast-food restaurants.

You'd think that would be a good thing. Waiters, tablecloths, and salad forks ought to indicate that we're eating healthier than if we're scarfing down dinner with one hand on the steering wheel, no?

Well, no. See, we've all come to the conclusion that fast food is bad for us. But few of us realize that sit-down restaurants are just as culpable in the supersizing of American children.

Part of the problem is that sit-down meals just feel healthier—and they aren't. In fact, we conducted a survey of over 40 chain restaurants and found that the average entrée at a sit-down restaurant has 345 more calories than a fast-food entrée. And worse, there's no way for the typical American to tell just how unhealthy these choices are. Unlike packaged-goods manufacturers, whose supermarket wares are required by law to contain detailed nutritional information on their labels, restaurant chains don't labor under any nutritional disclosure regulations. Some of them do list nutritional information on their Web sites—major chains who trust their customers to make informed choices include Burger King, Quizno's, and Romano's Macaroni Grill. But if you can decipher the nutritional makeup of a typical chicken nugget, then please, feel free to also explain to me how, exactly, the electoral college works.

In fact, many restaurants' foods are so bad for us that, even when we know they're unhealthy, we still don't understand just how belly-bloating, artery-choking, and energy-sucking they really are. As mentioned before—and it certainly bears repeating—consumers presented with obviously high-calorie restaurant foods still underestimated the nutritional heft of the items by an average of 600 calories. (Eating 600 unexpected calories just once a week would add an extra 30,000 calories annually to one's diet—enough to add 9 pounds to your weight every year!)

Don't believe me? Let's test the theory. Come with me to a restaurant that's probably somewhere in your neighborhood: Chili's Grill & Bar. You know it? It's a national, family-friendly chain that caters to fajita and burger lovers. Now settle in and take a look at the menu. No, not the grown-ups' menu—the kids' menu. Let's try, hmmm . . . how about the Pepper Pals Country-Fried Chicken Crispers?

Chicken fingers are a staple of the harried parent's food artillery, right up there with Goldfish crackers and Cheerios. It's hardly a health food,

but how bad can it be? For example, an entire bag of breaded Chicken Breast Tenders from Tyson has 880 calories, 48 grams of fat, and 1,400 milligrams of sodium. Not great, but that's 20 tenders.

So how many calories, and how much sodium and fat, does a single serving of chicken fingers at Chili's have? The same? Double? More?

Turns out just three Crispers have a mind-boggling 610 calories and 41 grams of fat. Factor in the fries and ranch dipping sauce that's offered with this meal and suddenly your kid is taking in 1,100 calories, 1,980 milligrams of sodium, and more fat (82 grams) than you'd find in seven Krispy Kreme glazed doughnuts. I'm not making this stuff up.

In the following pages, you're going to find dozens more shocking revelations about what restaurateurs are shilling to America's children. But you're also going to find hundreds of smart swaps you can make to keep your own kids safe from these dietary time bombs.

More and more, the local family restaurant is where your child's future health will be determined. Stay vigilant, stay savvy, stay smart.

You can make a difference.

600 CALORIES

Romano's Macaroni Grill's Mac 'n' Cheese has as much saturated fat as 20 strips of bacon.

The 20 Worst Kids' Foods in America

The restaurant industry has declared war on our kids' waistlines. It's time for parents to fight back.

WORST BREAKFAST CEREAL

20 Cap'n Crunch® (1 cup)

146 calories
2 g fat (1 g saturated)
16 g sugars
1 g fiber

The Cap'n's cereal didn't make the list because it's loaded with fat or calories; it made the list by being among the most dominant sources of empty calories in a child's diet. Aside from the small amount of added vitamins, which are mandated by the government, this cereal is an amalgam of worthless food particles and chemicals. Buyer beware: Most cereals marketed to kids suffer similar problems.

Eat This Instead!

Cascadian Farm® Clifford Crunch (1 cup)

100 calories
1 g fat (0 g saturated)
6 g sugars
5 g fiber

WORST SIDE

19 Bob Evans® Smiley Face Potatoes

524 calories
31 g fat (6 g saturated)
646 mg sodium
57 g carbohydrates

Not even an extended bath in hot oil could wipe the grins from the faces of these creepy-looking potatoes. When eating out, side dishes make or break a meal, and with more fat and calories than Bob's Sirloin Steak, this side falls woefully into the latter category. Let this be a lesson to all the kids out there: Just because they're smiling doesn't mean they're nice.

Eat This Instead!

Home Fries

186 calories
7 g fat (1 g saturated)
547 mg sodium
27 g carbohydrates

WORST PB&J

18 Cosi's® Kids Peanut Butter and Jelly

560 calories
26 g fat* (5 g saturated)
65 g carbohydrates*

Normally a nutritional safe haven, the American classic enters the danger zone at Cosí. Somehow, the sandwich chain manages to create a PB&J with 60 percent more calories than their own Gooey Grilled Cheese. Add in the chips that come with this meal and you're at 700 calories—before the drink.

*Numbers based on estimates. Cosí will not provide fat and carbohydrate counts for this sandwich.

Eat This Instead!

Kids Turkey Sandwich

289 calories
7 g fat (1 g saturated)
48 g carbohydrates

WORST PASTA MEAL

17 Romano's Macaroni Grill® Kids Macaroni 'n' Cheese

600 calories
31 g fat (20 g saturated)
1,720 mg sodium

This dish used to be double the size and caloric impact, but after we attacked it in the first *Eat This, Not That!*, they finally cut the massive portion size down. Thanks, Macaroni Grill. (P.S. It's still a disaster.)

Eat This Instead!
Spaghetti & Meatballs with Tomato Sauce

500 calories
20 g fat (8 g saturated)
1,520 mg sodium

WORST HOME-STYLE MEAL

16 Boston Market's™ Kids' Meatloaf with Sweet Potato Casserole and Cornbread

650 calories
30 g fat (11 g saturated)
910 mg sodium

This slab-o-meat begins as beef and ends as a science project, with 55 ingredients that include the understandable (cheese cultures), the detestable (partially hydrogenated cottonseed oil), and the unpronounceable (azodicarbonamide). Don't let your kid be the lab rat.

Eat This Instead!
Kids' Roasted Turkey with Green Bean Casserole and Cornbread

300 calories
7.5 g fat (2.5 g saturated)
948 mg sodium

WORST SANDWICH

15 Au Bon Pain® Kids' Grilled Cheese

670 calories
41 g fat (25 g saturated)
1,060 mg sodium

Au Bon Pain turns a simple sandwich into a complicated mess, with as much saturated fat as 25 strips of bacon. As a rule of thumb, avoid all of Au Bon Pain's kids' sandwiches, as every one of them contains more than 500 calories.

Eat This Instead!
Kids' Macaroni and Cheese

220 calories
14 g fat (9 g saturated)
650 mg sodium

WORST PREPARED LUNCH

14 Oscar Mayer® Maxed Out Turkey & Cheddar Cracker Combo Lunchables

680 calories
22 g fat (9 g saturated)
1,440 mg sodium

The Maxed Out line is the worst of the lackluster Lunchables, with a back label that looks like a chemistry textbook index. Oscar even crams in 61 grams of sugar—more than you'll find in two packs of Reese's Peanut Butter Cups!

Eat This Instead!
Hillshire Farm® Deli Wrap Smokehouse Ham & Swiss Wrap Kit

260 calories
11 g fat (4 g saturated)
960 mg sodium

WORST FAST-FOOD MEAL

13 Burger King's® Kids Double Cheeseburger and Kids Fries

740 calories
42 g fat (17 g saturated, 4.5 g trans)
1,410 mg sodium

BK's dubious double burger earns the distinction of being the fattiest meal for an on-the-go kid, with nearly a day's worth of saturated fat for the average 8-year-old.

Eat This Instead!
4-piece Chicken Tenders® with Strawberry-Flavored Applesauce

280 calories
11 g fat (3 g saturated)
440 mg sodium

WORST BREAKFAST

12 Denny's® Big Dipper French Toastix™ with whipped margarine and syrup

770 calories
71 g fat (13 g saturated)
107 g carbohydrates

It's hard to deny that breakfast is the most important meal of the day, but that doesn't mean you should make your kids eat it twice in one sitting. At this size, four French Toastix is three too many.

Eat This Instead!
Smiley-Alien Hotcakes with sugar-free syrup and Anti-Gravity Grapes

313 calories
3 g fat (0.5 g saturated)
71 g carbohydrates

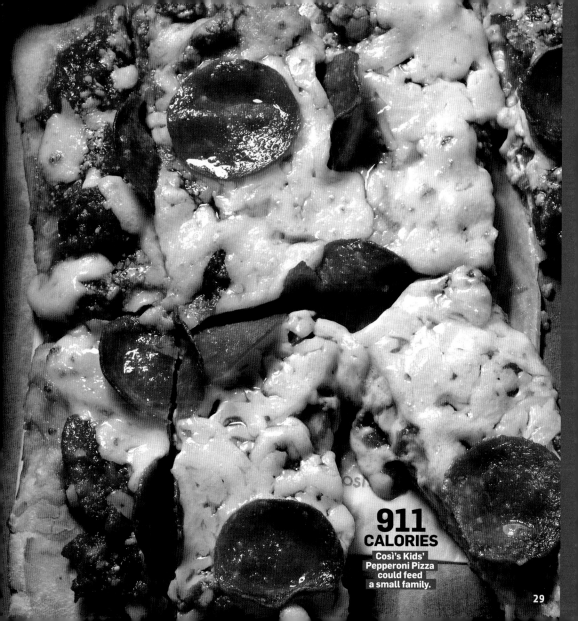

911 CALORIES

Cosi's Kids' Pepperoni Pizza could feed a small family.

29

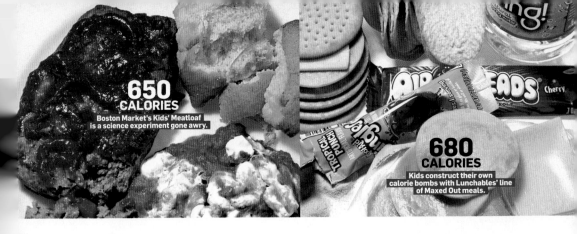

650 CALORIES
Boston Market's Kids' Meatloaf is a science experiment gone awry.

680 CALORIES
Kids construct their own calorie bombs with Lunchables' line of Maxed Out meals.

WORST FROZEN SUPERMARKET MEAL

11 DiGiorno® For One Garlic Bread Crust Pepperoni Pizza

840 calories
44 g fat (16 g saturated, 3.5 g trans)
1,450 mg sodium

This is why parents need to spend the time reading nutrition labels. The name says it's made to satisfy a single appetite, yet it contains a child's full day of saturated fat and a giant glob of trans fat baked into the crust. Whether fresh or frozen, keep your pizza thin crust and pepperoni-free.

Eat This Instead!
Red Baron® Thin & Crispy Four Cheese Pizza

300 calories
14 g fat (8 g saturated)
600 mg sodium

WORST DESSERT

10 Uno Chicago Grill's® Kid's Sundae

840 calories
36 g fat (18 g saturated)
98 g sugars

You wouldn't let your kid finish dinner at home with three Baby Ruth® candy bars, would you? Then don't let him tackle this caloric equivalent after dinner at Uno. Weighing in at a hulking three-quarters of a pound, this abominable sundae is twice as big as the Kid's Pasta, and twice as caloric as his entire meal should be.

Eat This Instead!
Kid's Slush

140 calories
0 g fat
32 g sugars

WORST MEXICAN MEAL

9 On the Border's® Kids' Beef Soft Taco Mexican Dinner with Rice and Refried Beans

840 calories
35 g fat (14 g saturated)
2,760 mg sodium
91 g carbohydrates

The taco (yes, this scale-tipping meal has just one taco) alone has 19 grams of fat, and there are 11 grams more stowed in the beans. Taken together, the taco, beans, and rice provide enough calories for two kids' meals and enough sodium to preserve a small city.

Eat This Instead!
Kids' Grilled Chicken with Black Beans

310 calories
9 g fat (3 g saturated)
1,230 mg sodium
20 g carbohydrates

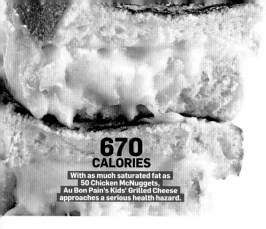

670 CALORIES
With as much saturated fat as 50 Chicken McNuggets, Au Bon Pain's Kids' Grilled Cheese approaches a serious health hazard.

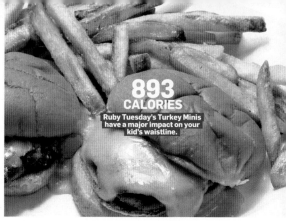

893 CALORIES
Ruby Tuesday's Turkey Minis have a major impact on your kid's waistline.

WORST FINGER FOOD

8 Denny's® Little Dippers with Marinara and Fries

860 calories
43 g fat (17 g saturated)
1,679 mg sodium
80 g carbohydrates

Dippable foods are usually dangerous, and this one meal combines three of the worst of them: nuggets, mozzarella sticks, and fries. The treacherous trio packs a punishing wallop of calories, fat, carbs, and sodium. For a meal that doesn't require a fork to eat, this option, containing half of a kid's daily calories, is toxic.

Eat This Instead!
Moons & Stars Chicken Nuggets with Moon Crater Mashed™ Potatoes and Gravy

335 calories
19 g fat (6 g saturated)
897 mg sodium
29 g carbohydrates

WORST BURGER

7 Ruby Tuesday's® Kids Turkey Minis & Fries

893 calories
47 g fat
88 g carbohydrates

In a perfect world, ground turkey is leaner than ground beef and a turkey burger is a decent thing to feed your kid. But Ruby Tuesday finds a way to confound all expectations by cramming half a day's worth of calories into these tiny burgers. We chose the turkey version because it presents itself as a healthier alternative to the beef burgers, but in reality it has just 14 fewer calories.

Eat This Instead!
Petite Sirloin (7 oz) with Mashed Potatoes

460 calories
20 g fat
31 g carbohydrates

WORST PIZZA

6 Così's® Kids' Pepperoni Pizza

911 calories
43 g fat
2,731 mg sodium
112 g carbohydrates

Before your child eats this doughy, oversized pizza, consider strapping two boxes of mozzarella Bagel Bites® to her stomach to see if she likes the added bulk, because that's how many calories she stands to absorb. You're better off ordering in—even two slices of a 12-inch pepperoni pizza from Papa John's® is only 440 calories.

Eat This Instead!
Gooey Grilled Cheese

357 calories
21 g fat
759 mg sodium
26 g carbohydrates

WORST NACHOS

5 On the Border's® Kids Bean & Cheese Nachos

980 calories
57 g fat (29 g saturated)
1,850 mg sodium

The kids' portion is a scaled-down version of the massive, 1,900-calorie appetizer, but it still contains enough saturated fat to make a cardiologist shudder. By the time your kid makes it through the complimentary sundae, he'll have taken in 1,300 calories and 70 grams of fat.

Eat This Instead!
Crispy Chicken Tacos (2)

480 calories
24 g fat (10 g saturated)
1,240 mg sodium

WORST DRINK

4 Baskin-Robbins® Heath® Shake (small)

990 calories
46 g fat (28 g saturated)
113 g sugars

It's a marvel of modern food science that Baskin-Robbins can fit this much fat and sugar into a 16-ounce cup. It took 73 ingredients and a reckless sense of abandon to do so. All told, it has almost as many calories as five actual Heath bars.

Drink This Instead!
Strawberry Citrus Fruit Blast (small)

350 calories
1 g fat (0 g saturated)
85 g sugars

WORST CHINESE ENTRÉE

3 P.F. Chang's® Chicken Lo Mein

1,198 calories
67 g fat (11 g saturated)

P.F. Chang's doesn't offer a kids' menu, but for many parents, this traditional Chinese dish meets the criteria: thin noodles stir-fried and served with chicken. Problem is, Chang's take on this seemingly innocent Chinese staple packs more fat than five chocolate Krispy Kreme® doughnuts.

Eat This Instead!
Buddha's Feast Lunch Bowl with brown rice

541 calories
8 g fat (1 g saturated)

WORST APPETIZER

2 T.G.I. Friday's® Potato Skins (½ order)

1,430 calories*

What happened to the appetizer that simply roused the appetite? This monstrosity contains 80 percent of a 9-year-old child's daily caloric intake. Splitting a full order of skins among a family of four would still saddle each member with over 550 calories.

Eat This Instead!
Zen Chicken Pot Stickers

370 calories*

*T.G.I. Friday's will not provide nutritional information on anything other than calories.

THE WORST KIDS' MEAL IN AMERICA

1 Chili's® Pepper Pals® Country-Fried Chicken Crispers with Ranch Dressing and Homestyle Fries

1,110 calories
82 g fat (15 g saturated)
1,980 mg sodium
56 g carbohydrates

Most kids, if given the choice, would live on chicken fingers for the duration of their adolescent lives. If those chicken fingers happened to come from Chili's, it might be a pretty short life. A moderately active 8-year-old boy should eat around 1,600 calories a day. This single meal plows through 75 percent of that allotment. So unless he plans to eat carrots and celery sticks for the rest of the day (and we know he doesn't), find a healthier chicken alternative. Chili's Pepper Pals menu has one of the most extensive collection of kids' entrées and side dishes in America, all of which prove considerably healthier than this country-fried disaster.

Eat This Instead!
Pepper Pals® Grilled Chicken Platter with Cinnamon Apples

350 calories
11 g fat (3 g saturated)
870 mg sodium
38 g carbohydrates

524 CALORIES

As America's worst side dish for kids, Bob Evans Smiley Face Potatoes are no laughing matter.

Applebee's

REPORT CARD

F

Applebee's is one of a handful of restaurant-industry titans that refuses to give up the goods on their nutritional information. Until they tell diners what they're putting in their bodies, we'll be forced to fail them.

SURVIVAL STRATEGY
The 10-item menu in partnership with Weight Watchers® provides a smattering of nutritional analysis for each dish. It's a small step, but until Applebee's coughs up all the info, stick with these 10 dishes, or find another restaurant.

GREAT GROWN-UP GRUB

Italian Chicken & Portobello Sandwich

360 calories,
6 g fat
11 g fiber

This wheat-bun sandwich is spread with chunky marinara instead of fattening mayonnaise. Between the mushroom stack, rich in B vitamins, and the side of fresh fruit, you'll knock out a couple of servings of fruits and vegetables for the kids without breaking a sweat.

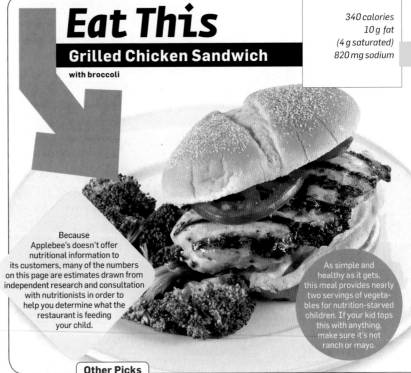

Eat This

Grilled Chicken Sandwich

with broccoli

340 calories
10 g fat
(4 g saturated)
820 mg sodium

Because Applebee's doesn't offer nutritional information to its customers, many of the numbers on this page are estimates drawn from independent research and consultation with nutritionists in order to help you determine what the restaurant is feeding your child.

As simple and healthy as it gets, this meal provides nearly two servings of vegetables for nutrition-starved children. If your kid tops this with anything, make sure it's not ranch or mayo.

Other Picks

Grilled Cajun Tilapia
with black bean and corn salsa

310 calories
6 g fat (0 g saturated)
1,025 mg sodium

Tortilla Chicken Melt

480 calories
13 g fat (4 g saturated)
935 mg sodium

Hot Fudge Sundae Dessert Shooter

310 calories
10 g fat (4 g saturated)
22 g sugars

690 calories
32 g fat
(9 g saturated)
950 mg sodium

Not That!

Chicken Fingers

with celery with ranch dressing

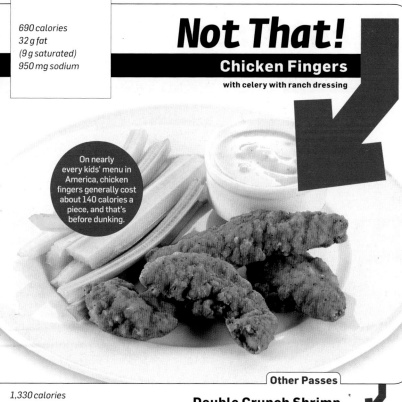

On nearly every kids' menu in America, chicken fingers generally cost about 140 calories a piece, and that's before dunking.

Other Passes

Double Crunch Shrimp
with fries, cole slaw, and cocktail sauce

1,330 calories
62 g fat (23 g saturated)
1,890 mg sodium

Honey Barbecue Chicken Sandwich

1,280 calories
58 g fat (21 g saturated)
1,970 mg sodium

Blue Ribon Brownie

1,290 calories
58 g fat (23 g saturated)
95 g sugars

11

The number of hours a kid would have to spend raking leaves in order to burn off the 2,027 calories in Applebee's Riblet meal with beans, coleslaw, and fries.

Arby's

Although the choices for kids are few, no entrée contains more than 275 calories, and the fruit-cup side earns the sandwich shop extra points. Too bad the rest of the menu is so lousy—most sandwiches suffer from spread overload or big-bread syndrome. And breakfast should be avoided altogether.

SURVIVAL STRATEGY
Lean roast beef is what they're known for, and it's never a bad way to go.

FOOD MYTH #1
Wheat bread is always healthier than white bread.

Not all wheat bread is 100 percent whole grain, which means your kid may not be getting the fiber benefits of true wheat breads. On top of that, manufacturers tend to add extra sugar to wheat bread to make it more appealing to eaters. The honey wheat bread on Arby's Market Fresh™ sandwiches contains vegetable shortening, high-fructose corn syrup, and 361 calories.

Eat This

Arby's Melt

303 calories
12 g fat
(5 g saturated)
921 mg sodium

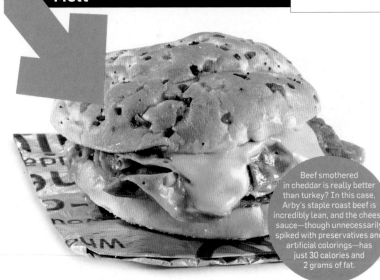

Beef smothered in cheddar is really better than turkey? In this case, Arby's staple roast beef is incredibly lean, and the cheese sauce—though unnecessarily spiked with preservatives and artificial colorings—has just 30 calories and 2 grams of fat.

Other Picks

Ham and Swiss Melt Sandwich

268 calories
5 g fat (2 g saturated)
1,042 mg sodium

Market Fresh™ Mini Turkey and Cheese Sandwich

244 calories
5 g fat (1 g saturated)
854 mg sodium

T.J. Cinnamons® Chocolate Twist

250 calories
12 g fat (4 g saturated)
12 g sugars

708 calories
30 g fat
(8 g saturated)
1,677 mg sodium

Not That!

Roasted Turkey and Swiss Sandwich

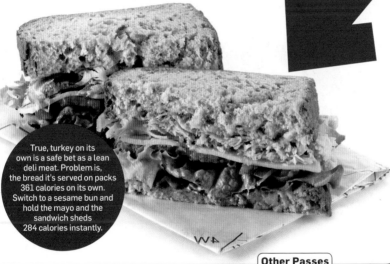

True, turkey on its own is a safe bet as a lean deli meat. Problem is, the bread it's served on packs 361 calories on its own. Switch to a sesame bun and hold the mayo and the sandwich sheds 284 calories instantly.

Other Passes

395 calories
17 g fat (3 g saturated)
1,002 mg sodium

Grilled Chicken Fillet Sandwich

272 calories
12 g fat (2 g saturated)
698 mg sodium

Kids Popcorn Chicken

377 calories
16 g fat (5 g saturated)
41 g sugars

Apple Turnover

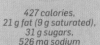

HIDDEN DANGER
Chicken Club Salad with Buttermilk Ranch

Just in case you were tempted to encourage your child to eat a "healthy" salad. Yes, there's popcorn chicken, bacon, and cheese polluting the innocent lettuce leaves, but the real damage comes from the ranch, which packs a whopping 34 grams of fat.

750 calories,
56 g fat
(12 g saturated)
1,551 mg sodium

UNHAPPY MEALS
Regular Jalapeño Bites®
with Bronco Berry Dipping Sauce®

427 calories,
21 g fat (9 g saturated),
31 g sugars,
526 mg sodium

There's not one berry in the Bronco Berry sauce—but lots of added sugar. The fat comes from the jalapeños' fried breading and cream-cheese filling. If your kid has a taste for spicy foods, go for Arby's Spicy Three Pepper Sauce®.

37

Au Bon Pain

The virtues of Au Bon Pain's nutritional transparency, which include on-location kiosks that provide the calorie counts, are unfortunately outweighed by the pitfalls of calorie-laden baked goods and a kids' sandwich lineup that doesn't include a single selection that comes in under 500 calories. Au Bon Pain Portions are, however, a beacon of health for kids and parents alike.

SURVIVAL STRATEGY
Skip over sandwiches and nudge your kids toward a hearty soup, or help them mix and match 200-calorie Portion plates.

SMART SIDES

Hummus and Cucumber

*130 calories,
8 g fat
(0 g saturated)
460 mg sodium*

The base of hummus is made from chickpeas, which has fiber that helps prevent your child's blood sugar level from rising too quickly after a meal. And don't fear the fat—it's the good kind.

Eat This

Honey Mustard Chicken

and cheddar, fruit, and crackers portions

*360 calories
13 g fat
(5 g saturated)
530 mg sodium*

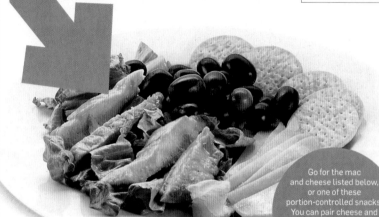

Go for the mac and cheese listed below, or one of these portion-controlled snacks. You can pair cheese and crackers with a variety of chicken options and still keep the calorie count under 400.

Other Picks

Kids Macaroni and Cheese

*220 calories
14 g fat (9 g saturated)
650 mg sodium*

Au Bon Pain Portions BBQ Chicken

*170 calories
2 g fat (0 g saturated)
340 mg sodium*

Bacon and Bagel

*340 calories
6 g fat (2 g saturated)
630 mg sodium*

670 calories
41 g fat
(25 g saturated)
1,060 mg sodium

Not That!
Kids Grilled Cheese Sandwich

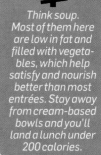

If the kids are going to order grilled cheese, you're better off staying in: The average homemade grilled cheese runs a reasonable 300 calories, with about 6 grams of saturated fat.

STEALTH HEALTH FOOD

Turkish Apricots
120 calories, 0 g fat, 4 g fiber

This exotic dried-fruit snack benefits from a ton of fiber and a rich reserve of beta-carotene. Plus, they're sweet enough to win any picky eater over.

Other Passes

310 calories
21 g fat (10 g saturated)
1,000 mg sodium

Broccoli and Cheddar Soup

550 calories
27 g fat (5 g saturated)
1,330 mg sodium

Kids Smoked Turkey Sandwich

510 calories
19 g fat (2 g saturated)
550 mg sodium

Blueberry Muffin

SUGAR SPIKES

Low-Fat Blueberry Yogurt with Fruit (small)

The Impact: 37 g sugars
The bulk of the sugar isn't from blueberries, but a mix of cane sugar and corn syrup sweeteners.

Baja Fresh

Baja's bad grade stems from an inability to serve a single kids' entrée with fewer than 500 calories and 900 milligrams of sodium. Add to that an array of appealing, cheesy entrées and sides likely to catch a kid's attention, and you see how hard it is to feed your kids well at this Cali-Mex chain.

SURVIVAL STRATEGY
Unless you can convince the tots to tackle a bowl of fiber-rich beans and salsa, then the only viable option (for them and you) is tacos.

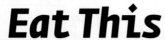

Eat This
Original Baja Chicken Tacos
(2)

420 calories
10 g fat
(2 g saturated)
460 mg sodium

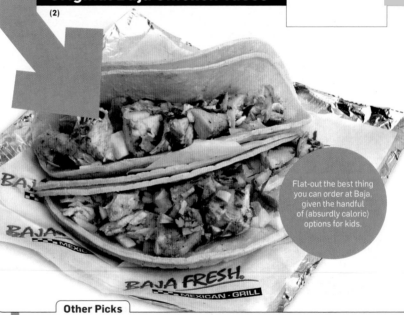

Flat-out the best thing you can order at Baja, given the handful of (absurdly caloric) options for kids.

SMART SIDES

Guacamole
110 calories,
9 g fat
(2 g saturated),
280 mg sodium

Scoop some guac into a taco or mix it with rice and beans. Aside from being one of the world's best condiments, the mashed avocados are packed with fiber, vitamin C, and healthy monounsaturated fats, which help the body regulate weight and metabolism.

Other Picks

Kids Mini Bean and Cheese Burrito with Chicken

590 calories
15 g fat (7 g saturated)
1,200 mg sodium

Steak Original Baja Tacos
(2)

460 calories
16 g fat (4 g saturated)
520 mg sodium

Rice and Beans Plate
with tortilla chips

630 calories
14 g fat (2.5 g saturated)
1,375 mg sodium

630 calories
33 g fat
(7 g saturated)
990 mg sodium

Not That!

Kids Chicken Taquitos

(served with ranch dressing)

Why Baja abandons their healthy homemade salsas for ranch dressing here is beyond us. If your kids must have taquitos, save them a few hundred calories and a boatload of fat by switching back over to the salsa.

Other Passes

1,200 calories
78 g fat (37 g saturated)
2,140 mg sodium

Cheese Quesadilla

520 calories
26 g fat (12 g saturated)
1,280 mg sodium

Steak Americano Soft Tacos
(2)

1,890 calories
108 g fat (40 g saturated)
2,530 mg sodium

Cheese Nachos

Genius
PARENT TRICK

Get your kids hooked on beans. Rice may have 40 fewer calories than beans at Baja, but calories from rice are driven by quick-burning carbohydrates, whereas a side order of pinto beans has an astounding 21 grams of fiber—enough to keep the young ones full and content until dinnertime.

HIDDEN DANGER
Steak Nachos

How bad can a plate of chips and cheese really be? Bad enough to be the caloric equivalent of four Big Macs®, with 2 full days' worth of saturated fat tangled in the heap. Even split among a family of four, this dish would still have a punishing impact.

2,120 calories,
118 g fat
(44 g saturated, 4.5 g trans),
2,990 mg sodium

41

Baskin-Robbins

It's hard to serve just ice cream and still make the grade, but Baskin-Robbins does nothing to help its case by serving up some of the fattiest scoops in the industry, plus 900-calorie soft serve concoctions, smoothies with more sugar than fruit, and, as of publication, the worst drink on the planet, a Heath® Premium Shake with 2,310 calories in a large serving!

SURVIVAL STRATEGY
Seek solace in Baskin's lighter side, where sherbets, sorbets, and low-sugar treats offer ample opportunity to feel indulgent without really being so.

CONE DECODER

● **WAFFLE:** 160 calories, 4 g fat (1 g saturated), 13 g sugars

● **SUGAR:** 45 calories, 0.5 g fat (0 g saturated fat), 3 g sugars

● **CAKE:** 25 calories, 0 g fat, 0 g sugars

Eat This

No Sugar Added Chocolate Chocolate Chip Ice Cream
in a waffle cone (1 scoop)

310 calories
9 g fat
(4.5 g saturated)
20 g sugars

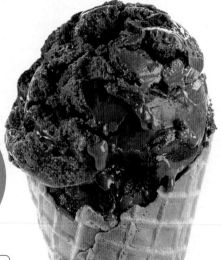

Even without added sugar, this mammoth chocolate cone will be more than enough to satisfy even the sweetest tooth out there. Cut the calories significantly by downsizing to a sugar cone.

Other Picks

Chocolate Ice Cream in a sugar cone (1 scoop)

305 calories
14.5 g fat (9 g saturated)
34 g sugars

Strawberry Sorbet in a cup (1 scoop)

130 calories
0 g fat
34 g sugars

Wild Mango Fruit Blast (small)

340 calories
1 g fat (0 g saturated)
82 g sugars

480 calories
24 g fat
(10 g saturated)
41 g sugars

Not That!

Peanut Butter 'n Chocolate Ice Cream

in a waffle cone (1 scoop)

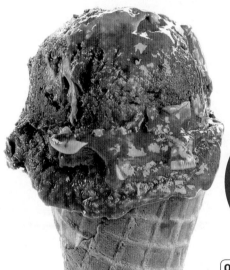

The worst ice cream you can order at Baskin-Robbins. Two scoops on this calamitous cone will saddle you with an entire day's worth of saturated fat.

Other Passes

620 calories
30 g fat (18 g saturated)
77 g sugars

Chocolate Shake
(small)

240 calories
12 g fat (7 g saturated)
26 g sugars

Cherries Jubilee Ice Cream in a cup (1 scoop)

440 calories
1.5 g fat (0 g saturated)
101 g sugars

Mango Fruit Blast Smoothie
(small)

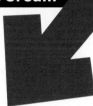

Genius
PARENT TRICK

Ordering an ice cream cake for the next birthday bash? Make it one of Baskin-Robbins's roll cakes, which provide slices that are neither as dense nor as giant as those cut from the more popular round and sheet cakes. The proof is in the numbers: A slice of chocolate chip from a round cake weighs in at 410 calories, while a slice of the same flavor from a roll cake has only 290 calories.

SUGAR SPIKES

Strawberry Banana Fruit Blast Smoothie (small)

*The Impact:
110 g sugars*

This smoothie contains the combined sugars of one scoop each of Rocky Road, French Vanilla, Chocolate Chip, and Very Berry Strawberry Ice Cream. We say skip the smoothie, pick one scoop, and count your savings.

Ben & Jerry's

The hippy-hued company's commitment to hormone-free Vermont milk and Fair Trade vanilla, cocoa, and coffee—ingredients that quell the sweet tooth while calming the conscience—is good news for your family. So is the fact that many single scoops fall below 250 calories. But at the end of the day, it's still just an ice cream shop.

SURVIVAL STRATEGY
Sorbet and frozen yogurt always trump the cream-and-candy scoops that Ben and Jerry's is known for. Rule of thumb: The more complicated an ice cream sounds, the worse it is for you.

GUILTY PLEASURES

Cherry Garcia® Low-Fat Frozen Yogurt (½ c)

*170 calories,
3 g fat (2 g saturated),
20 g sugars*

There's a reason this is on Ben & Jerry's top-selling flavors list. Bring home some of Jerry's cherry flavor, and it will keep you satiated without busting your belt.

Eat This

Strawberry Original Ice Cream

in a sugar cone (½ c)

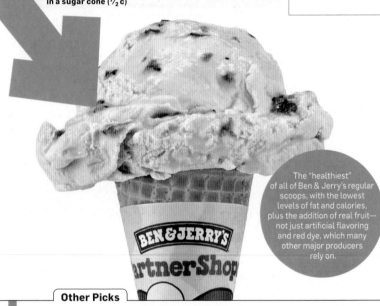

*215 calories
9.5 g fat
(6 g saturated)
22 g sugars*

The "healthiest" of all of Ben & Jerry's regular scoops, with the lowest levels of fat and calories, plus the addition of real fruit—not just artificial flavoring and red dye, which many other major producers rely on.

Other Picks

Chocolate Chip Cookie Dough Original Ice Cream (½ c)

*270 calories
14 g fat (9 g saturated)
24 g sugars*

Chocolate Fudge Brownie Frozen Yogurt (½ c)

*170 calories
2.5 g fat (0.5 g saturated)
23 g sugars*

Berry Berry Extraordinary Sorbet (½ c)

*100 calories
0 g fat
23 g sugars*

295 calories
15.5 g fat
(11 g saturated)
25 g sugars

Not That!
Chocolate Original Ice Cream

in a sugar cone (¹⁄₂ c)

In the classic showdown of chocolate versus strawberry, chocolate loses out with more of everything that hurts—calories, fat, sugar—and less of the one ingredient that helps: real fruit.

BEN & JERRY'S
artnerShop

Other Passes

340 calories
24 g fat (12 g saturated)
24 g sugars

Peanut Butter Cup
Original Ice Cream (¹⁄₂ c)

250 calories
12 g fat (8 g saturated)
25 g sugars

Chocolate Fudge Brownie
Original Ice Cream (¹⁄₂ c)

140 calories
1.5 g fat (1 g saturated)
20 g sugars

Black Raspberry Frozen Yogurt
(¹⁄₂ c)

SUGAR SP KES

Jamaican
Me Crazy Sorbet
(¹⁄₂ c)

The Impact:
29 g sugars

The sorbet is fat-free, but the sugar is sky-high. Try to keep your intake of added sugars to fewer than 65 grams a day. A 2004 study linked irregular blood-sugar levels with brain decay. Over a 4-year span, women who had diabetes were twice as likely as women with normal blood sugar to develop the signs of dementia.

Genius
PARENT TRICK

Ben & Jerry's uses real fruit in their smoothies, and if you ask, they'll let you create your own recipe. Ask them to start with sorbet and then have your child pick the fruit. The result will be relatively healthy and totally delicious, and the experience will teach your child to make good nutritional decisions.

Bob Evans

Bob Evans provides kids' meals with modest portions and a bounty of wholesome sides. You can run up a dangerously high calorie count, though, by matching the wrong entrées—chicken strips, mini cheeseburgers—with the wrong sides, namely the creepy Smiley Face Potatoes.

SURVIVAL STRATEGY: Opt for fruit, yogurt, and eggs over pancakes and French toast in the morning. At night, pair a few vegetable sides with lean turkey, chicken breast, or even pasta.

Genius
PARENT TRICK

Get your kids hooked on turkey sausage early. The Bob Evans turkey links are one-third bigger and have two-thirds less fat and calories than the pork sausage.

Eat This

Turkey Lurkey

with glazed carrots, mashed potatoes, and gravy

429 calories
16 g fat
(8 g saturated)
1,355 mg sodium

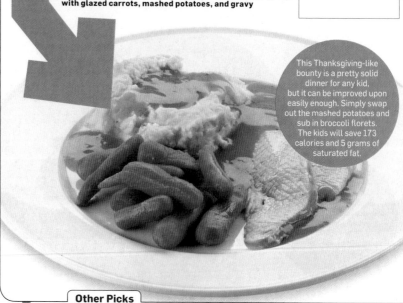

This Thanksgiving-like bounty is a pretty solid dinner for any kid, but it can be improved upon easily enough. Simply swap out the mashed potatoes and sub in broccoli florets. The kids will save 173 calories and 5 grams of saturated fat.

Other Picks

Kids Marinara Pasta

206 calories
5 g fat (1 g saturated)
858 mg sodium

Fit from the Farm Breakfast
with parfait

359 calories
12 g fat (3 g saturated)
707 mg sodium
33 g sugars

Fried Chicken Breast
with home fries and broccoli florets

503 calories
20 g fat (4 g saturated)
1,334 mg sodium

495 calories
38 g fat
(8 g saturated)
1,165 mg sodium

Not That!

Grilled Chicken Strips

with side salad with ranch

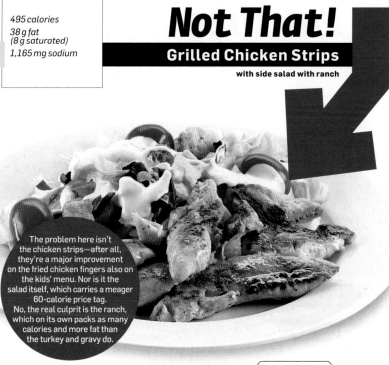

The problem here isn't the chicken strips—after all, they're a major improvement on the fried chicken fingers also on the kids' menu. Nor is it the salad itself, which carries a meager 60-calorie price tag. No, the real culprit is the ranch, which on its own packs as many calories and more fat than the turkey and gravy do.

Other Passes

Kids Macaroni and Cheese

320 calories
11 g fat (3 g saturated)
778 mg sodium

Kids Plenty-o-Pancakes
with syrup

750 calories
21 g fat (2 g saturated)
1,226 mg sodium
70 g sugars

Kids Mini Cheeseburgers
with Smiley Face Potatoes

830 calories
50 g fat (13 g saturated)
1,171 mg sodium

UNHAPPY MEALS
Slow-Roasted Chicken Pot Pie

908 calories,
60 g fat (16 g saturated),
2,847 mg sodium

Pot pies are scary stuff. The lean chicken and smattering of vegetables are overwhelmed by the buttery crust and viscous, creamy sauce.

GREAT GROWN-UP GRUB

Slow-Roasted Chicken-N-Noodles

296 calories,
16 g fat (3 g saturated),
846 mg sodium,
13 g protein

We've never met a kid who didn't appreciate a good bowl of chicken-noodle soup. This one's especially tasty, with a healthy mix of carrots, celery, and onions.

SMART **SIDES**
Cottage Cheese

115 calories,
5 g fat (3 g saturated),
14 g protein

Turn your kids into cottage converts. The protein contains all of the essential amino acids, so your child's body will be less likely to metabolize it into fat.

Boston Market

With more than a dozen healthy vegetable sides and lean meats like turkey and roast sirloin on the menu, the low-cal, high-nutrient possibilities at Boston Market are endless. But with nearly a dozen calorie-packed sides and fatty meats like dark meat chicken and meat loaf, it's almost as easy to construct a lousy meal.

SURVIVAL STRATEGY
There are three simple steps to nutritional salvation: 1) Start with turkey, sirloin, or rotisserie chicken. 2) Add two non-creamy, nonstarchy vegetable sides. 3) Ignore all special items, such as potpie and nearly all of the sandwiches.

SUGAR SPIKES

Sweet-Potato Casserole
The Impact:
39 g sugars

Sweet potatoes are one of nature's most nutritional treats, so why ruin them with boatloads of sugar, oil, and butter? This side dish has almost twice as much sugar as Boston Market's Apple Pie.

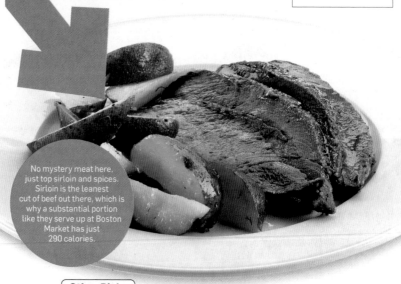

Eat This

Roasted Sirloin
with garlic dill new potatoes

430 calories
18 g fat
(7 g saturated)
560 mg sodium

No mystery meat here, just top sirloin and spices. Sirloin is the leanest cut of beef out there, which is why a substantial portion like they serve up at Boston Market has just 290 calories.

Other Picks

Rotisserie Chicken Open Face Sandwich

330 calories
9 g fat (2 g saturated)
1,540 mg sodium

Individual Roasted Turkey Meal

180 calories
3 g fat (1 g saturated)
635 mg sodium

Chicken Noodle Soup

170 calories
5 g fat (1.5 g saturated)
930 mg sodium

765 calories
49 g fat
(20.5 g saturated)
2,350 mg sodium

Not That!

Meatloaf

with mashed potatoes and gravy

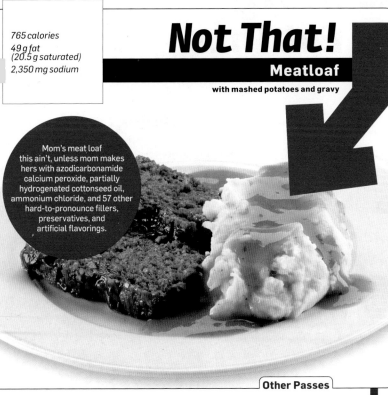

Mom's meat loaf this ain't, unless mom makes hers with azodicarbonamide calcium peroxide, partially hydrogenated cottonseed oil, ammonium chloride, and 57 other hard-to-pronounce fillers, preservatives, and artificial flavorings.

Other Passes

1,190 calories
77 g fat (18 g saturated)
2,110 mg sodium

Tuscan Herb Chicken Salad Sandwich

470 calories
28 g fat (15 g saturated)
690 mg sodium

Baked Whitefish

400 calories
40 g fat (8 g saturated)
980 mg sodium

Caesar Side Salad

UNHAPPY MEALS
Boston Sirloin Dip Carver

1,000 calories,
51 g fat
(15 g saturated),
1,690 mg sodium,
70 g carbohydrates

Boston Market's Carvers are a precarious lot. If you must, go for a half Carver, and then stick to chicken or turkey—not sirloin.

Genius
PARENT TRICK

Excluding the sandwiches, all Boston Market meals get a complimentary hunk of cornbread. Ask them to leave it off when you order; you'll save your child 180 calories and 12 grams of sugar, and she'll never even know it's missing.

Burger King

Burger King has only three legitimate kids' entrées on the menu, and none of them—French Toast Sticks, hamburger, chicken tenders—are particularly healthy. And while the recent addition of Apple Fries provides a much-needed healthy side alternative for kids, the menu is still sullied with trans fats. BK pledged to remove trans fats from the menu by the end of 2008, but so far, we've seen little action.

SURVIVAL STRATEGY
The best kids' meal? A 4-piece Chicken Tenders®, applesauce or Apple Fries, and water or milk. Beyond that, there is little hope of escaping unscathed.

7

The number of hours a child would have to sit in detention in order to burn off a large order of French fries.

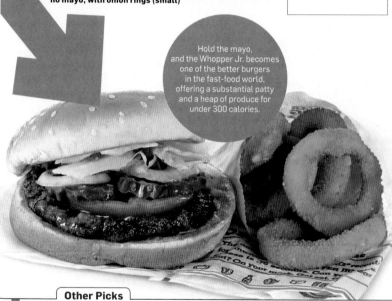

Eat This

Whopper Jr.®
no mayo, with onion rings (small)

430 calories
19 g fat
(6 g saturated,
1.5 g trans)
700 mg sodium
4 g fiber

Hold the mayo, and the Whopper Jr. becomes one of the better burgers in the fast-food world, offering a substantial patty and a heap of produce for under 300 calories.

Other Picks

Chicken Tenders®
(5 pieces)

210 calories
12 g fat (3 g saturated, 2 g trans)
600 mg sodium

Ham Omelet Sandwich

290 calories
13 g fat (4.5 g saturated)
870 mg sodium

Vanilla Milk Shake
(Value Size: 12 fl oz)

310 calories
11 g fat (7 g saturated)
43 g sugars

560 calories
29 g fat
(10 g saturated,
3.5 g trans)
1,160 mg sodium
3 g fiber

Not That!

Cheeseburger
with French fries (small)

Burger King bucks all established fast food rules by serving onion rings that actually have fewer calories than fries. In this case, a small order of rings will save you 90 calories and 2 grams of trans fats over the small fry.

DIPPING SAUCE DECODER (1 OZ EACH)

● **ZESTY ONION:**
150 calories, 15 g fat
(2.5 g saturated)

● **RANCH:**
140 calories, 15 g fat
(2.5 g saturated)

● **HONEY MUSTARD:**
90 calories,
6 g fat (1 g saturated)

● **BUFFALO:**
80 calories,
8 g fat (1.5 g saturated)

● **SWEET & SOUR:**
45 calories, 0 g fat

● **BARBECUE:**
40 calories, 0 g fat

Other Passes

510 calories
19 g fat (3.5 g saturated, 0.5 g trans)
1,180 mg sodium

Tendergrill® Chicken Sandwich

680 calories
24 g fat (6 g saturated, 3 g trans)
590 mg sodium

French Toast Sticks Kids Meal with syrup

610 calories
24 g fat (16 g saturated)
78 g sugars

Vanilla Oreo® Sundae Shake
(small: 16 fl oz)

Chick-fil-A

No kids' menu? No problem. With every single sandwich below 500 calories, a variety of healthy sides like fresh fruit that can be substituted into any meal, and nutritional brochures readily available for perusing at each location, Chick-fil-A earns the award for America's Healthiest Chain Restaurant for Kids.

SURVIVAL STRATEGY

Even the smartest kid in the class can still fail a test, so be on your toes at all times. Skip salads with ranch or Caesar dressings, any sandwich with bacon, and all milkshakes.

SUGAR SPIKES

Chocolate Hand-Spun Milkshake (20 oz)

The Impact:
107 g sugars

One of these hand-spun choco-bombs is the equivalent of 75 Milk Duds®. The chocolate syrup consists primarily of high-fructose corn syrup, corn syrup, and sugar.

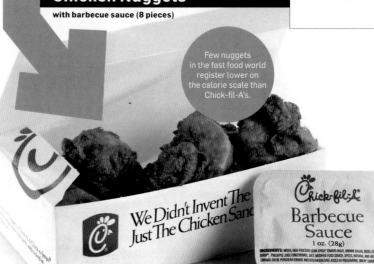

Eat This

Chicken Nuggets

with barbecue sauce (8 pieces)

305 calories
13 g fat
(2.5 g saturated)
1,020 mg sodium

Few nuggets in the fast food world register lower on the calorie scale than Chick-fil-A's.

Other Picks

Chargrilled Chicken Club Sandwich

380 calories
11 g fat (5 g saturated)
1,240 mg sodium

Chick-n-Minis™

280 calories
11 g fat (3.5 g saturated)
580 mg sodium

Icedream®

240 calories
6 g fat (3.5 g saturated)
42 g sugars

480 calories
16 g fat
(6 g saturated)
1,640 mg sodium

Not That!

Chicken Caesar Cool Wrap®

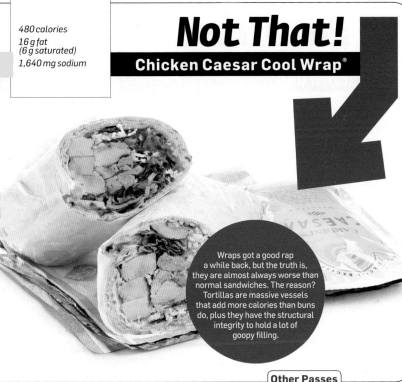

Wraps got a good rap a while back, but the truth is, they are almost always worse than normal sandwiches. The reason? Tortillas are massive vessels that add more calories than buns do, plus they have the structural integrity to hold a lot of goopy filling.

Other Passes

410 calories
16 g fat (3.5 g saturated)
1,300 mg sodium

Chicken Sandwich

490 calories
32 g fat (10 g saturated)
1,060 mg sodium

Sausage Biscuit

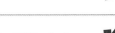

660 calories
27 g fat (16 g saturated)
89 g sugars

Vanilla Milkshake

SMART SIDES

Fruit Cup (medium)

70 calories,
0 g fat, 0 mg sodium,
17 g carbohydrates

Out of every five Americans, only one consumes the recommended daily amount of fruit. With progressive side options like this, you can help your child be a part of that healthy minority. These cups are prepared fresh on location, and they include apple slices, grapes, strawberries, and mandarin oranges—a bounty of natural energy for your child's body.

GREAT GROWN-UP GRUB

Chargrilled Chicken Sandwich

270 calories,
3 g fat (1 g saturated),
28 g protein,
37 g carbohydrates

Good luck finding a better chicken sandwich. This one has less than one-fifth of the fat in the McDonald's® Premium Grilled Chicken Club.

STEALTH HEALTH FOOD

Carrot & Raisin Salad

260 calories,
12 g fat (1.5 g saturated),
160 mg sodium

This salad will smack your kid's cellular and immune systems with a nutritious wallop of vitamin A.

Chili's

REPORT CARD

C-

Chili's gets the award for the longest, most diverse kids' menu we've seen, and many of the items on it represent reasonable nutritional options. Unfortunately, sodium is a major problem. And the adult menu, where older kids might be tempted to wander, is an abomination.

SURVIVAL STRATEGY
Choose wisely, as the difference between good (corn dog) and bad (chicken strips) can be 700 calories. On the adult menu, the Chicken Fajita Pita is a solid choice.

Genius PARENT TRICK

Think marinara. Not just for pasta, but also as a dip or a sandwich spread. Marinara is nearly fat-free and packed full of lycopene, an antioxidant that helps skin fight the sun's UV rays.

Eat This

Pepper Pals® Corn Dog

with mashed potatoes

440 calories
28 g fat (6 g saturated)
620 mg sodium

Surprisingly enough, Chili's corn dog is one of the healthiest options on the entire Pepper Pals menu, beating out the mac and cheese by 210 calories.

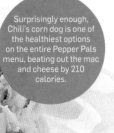

Other Picks

Pepper Pals® Little Mouth Burger

280 calories
15 g fat (5 g saturated)
300 mg sodium

6 Spicy Garlic & Lime Grilled Shrimp with black beans

295 calories
10 g fat (1.5 g saturated)
1,250 mg sodium

Dutch Apple Caramel Cheesecake Sweet Shot

230 calories
6 g fat (3 g saturated)
41 g carbohydrates

54

1,110 calories
82 g fat
(15 g saturated)
1,980 mg sodium

Not That!

Pepper Pals® Country-Fried Chicken Crispers

with ranch and Homestyle Fries

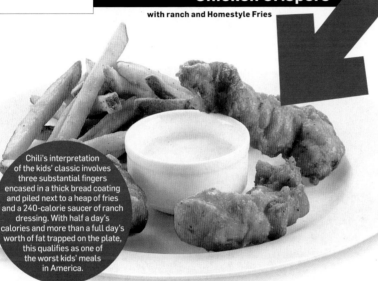

Chili's interpretation of the kids' classic involves three substantial fingers encased in a thick bread coating and piled next to a heap of fries and a 240-calorie saucer of ranch dressing. With half a day's calories and more than a full day's worth of fat trapped on the plate, this qualifies as one of the worst kids' meals in America.

Other Passes

420 calories
27 g fat (16 g saturated)
1,200 mg sodium

Pepper Pals® Grilled Cheese Sandwich

620 calories
26 g fat (13 g saturated)
1,720 mg sodium

Pepper Pals® Cheese Quesadilla
with rice

640 calories
27 g fat (16 g saturated)
92 g carbohydrates

Frosty Choc-A-Lot Shake
with chocolate sprinkles

UNHAPPY MEALS

Honey BBQ Ribs
with Honey BBQ Sauce

*1,060 calories,
65 g fat (24 g saturated),
4,460 mg sodium*

Kids might be attracted to these sickly sweet, fatty ribs, but if you let them indulge, they'll be eating the fat equivalent of 22 strips of bacon and the sodium equivalent of 13 large orders of McDonald's® French fries.

SMART SIDES

Black Beans with Pico de Gallo

*120 calories,
0 g fat, 660 mg sodium*

Black beans are rich in protein and fiber, and they have a high concentration of omega-3 fats. They're even better with a scoop of salsa.

STEALTH HEALTH FOOD

Guiltless Salmon

*480 calories,
14 g fat (3 g saturated)*

Salmon is one of the best sources of omega-3 fats, which are vital brain builders. One study found that children who took omega-3s for just 3 months showed big improvements in reading, spelling, and behavior.

Chipotle

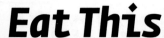

We noticed a sudden drop in calories on Chipotle's nutritional accounting right around the time New York City law forced chain restaurants to display calorie counts on their menu boards. Did they just suddenly downsize their mammoth portions? Not likely. It doesn't much matter, though, because the lack of options for kids means young eaters are forced to tussle with one of Chipotle's massive burritos or taco platters, which can easily top 1,000 calories.

SURVIVAL STRATEGY
Stick to the crispy tacos or burrito bowls, or saw a burrito in half.

570

The number of calories you'll save if you skip the chips. You'll also cut 27 grams of fat.

Eat This

Crispy Steak Tacos

with tomato salsa and romaine lettuce (3)

395 calories
14 g fat
(3.5 g saturated)
940 mg sodium

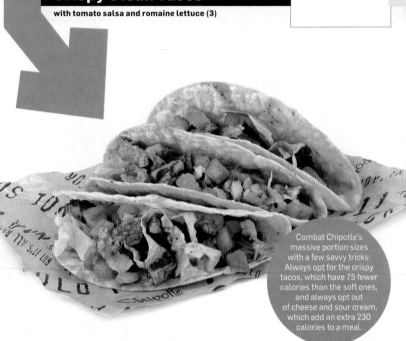

Combat Chipotle's massive portion sizes with a few savvy tricks: Always opt for the crispy tacos, which have 75 fewer calories than the soft ones, and always opt out of cheese and sour cream, which add an extra 230 calories to a meal.

Other Picks

Chicken Burrito with black beans, salsa verde, cheese, and romaine lettuce (½ burrito)

380 calories
13 g fat (5 g saturated)
913 mg sodium

Burrito Bowl
with pinto beans, carnitas, green salsa, and lettuce

368 calories
16 g fat (3 g saturated)
1,884 mg sodium

670 calories
25 g fat
(10.5 g saturated)
1,735 mg sodium

Not That!

Chicken Soft Tacos

with corn salsa, cheese, and romaine lettuce (3)

HIDDEN DANGER
Rice

This sorry excuse for a grain will spike your kid's blood sugar to the moon; there's not a single gram of fiber in a whole serving. Go riceless and rest easy.

160 calories,
4 g fat (0 g saturated)
330 mg sodium,
30 g carbohydrates

Genius
PARENT TRICK

Most people automatically assume steak is worse for you than chicken, but that's not always the case. At Chipotle, the chicken actually has 10 more calories than the steak. It's not much, but it's a good reminder that it's never safe to assume—especially with nutrition.

Teach your kids about the benefits of bowling—eating a burrito from a bowl instead of a tortilla. The white-flour tortilla adds 42 grams of carbohydrates, 670 milligrams of sodium, and 290 calories to your burrito. It's the nutritional equivalent of a gutter ball.

Other Passes

755 calories
36 g fat (12 g saturated)
2,453 mg sodium

Vegetarian Soft Tacos

with black beans, tomato salsa, guacamole, and cheese

775 calories
48 g fat (12 g saturated)
1,888 mg sodium

Chicken Salad

with black beans, cheese, and dressing

Chuck E. Cheese's

Unlike most big pizza chains, Chuck E. Cheese's has no thin crust option, which leaves you with the standard calorie- and carb-heavy slices. It redeems itself slightly by offering a handful of nonsoda drink options, as well as a salad bar. But beware: A kid left to run wild in a salad bar can do more harm than good.

SURVIVAL STRATEGY
Stick to the cheese, vegetable, and Hawaiian pizzas, and cap the slice consumption at two a kid. If they're still hungry, help them construct a salad from the bar.

HIDDEN DANGER
Hi-C
(12oz)

Hi-C® is not juice. In fact, it has more sugar per ounce than Coke®. And with Chuck's free refills flowing, the calories add up fast.

156 calories
42 g sugars

Eat This

Canadian Bacon and Pineapple Pizza

(1 medium slice) with 3 Buffalo wings and celery

410 calories
18 g fat
(5.5 g saturated)
1,028 mg sodium

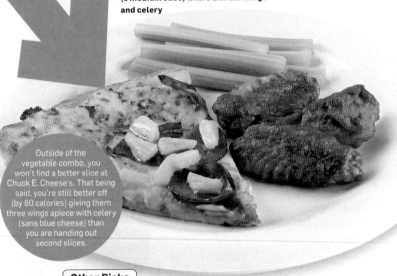

Outside of the vegetable combo, you won't find a better slice at Chuck E. Cheese's. That being said, you're still better off (by 80 calories) giving them three wings apiece with celery (sans blue cheese) than you are handing out second slices.

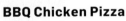

Other Picks

BBQ Chicken Pizza
(2 small slices)

428 calories
12 g fat (4 g saturated)
992 mg sodium

Hot Dog

170 calories
17 g fat (6 g saturated)
830 mg sodium

Apple Pie Pizza
(1 slice)

194 calories
2 g fat (0 g saturated)
24 g sugars

667 calories
27 g fat
(6 g saturated)
1,426 mg sodium

Not That!

Pepperoni and Sausage Pizza

(1 medium slice) with 2 Italian bread sticks

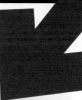

They've already got one oily bread product on their plate, why would they need another? Especially when each dense stick adds 193 calories and 11 grams of fat to your kid's meal.

Other Passes

454 calories
18 g fat (6 g saturated)
1,090 mg sodium

All Meat Combo Pizza
(2 small slices)

622 calories
28 g fat (7 g saturated)
2,296 mg sodium

Ham and Cheese

310 calories
13 g fat (4 g saturated)
29 g sugars

White Birthday Cake
(1 slice)

Genius
PARENT TRICK

"Where a kid can be a kid" is a motto you should follow. Load them up with tokens before the pizzas arrive and watch as the games keep them too distracted to overeat. It might cost you a couple of bucks, but you'll make it back on the extra pizza you don't have to buy.

UNHAPPY MEALS
Roasted Chicken Ciabatta

*652 calories,
31 g fat (9 g saturated),
1,936 mg sodium*

Roasted chicken anything seems like a universally safe bet, but Chuck sabotages this sandwich with a blanket of cheese and a thick coat of mayo. Beyond the high calorie and fat counts, this chicken sandwich sucks up your sodium allowance for an entire day.

Cold Stone Creamery

REPORT CARD
C

The average regular shake is nearly 900 calories, but the regular Like It™ size ice creams are almost all within the 300-calorie range. Factor that in with the creamery's real fruit toppings, light ice cream, and sorbet, and Cold Stone starts to compensate for its dangerous shakes and its more dubious ice cream add-ons.

SURVIVAL STRATEGY
Lace a Like It™ cup with light ice cream, fresh fruit, and maybe a touch of chocolate shavings or whipped cream for good measure.

SUGAR SP🔺KES

Dew Iced™ Smoothie (Like It™ size)

The Impact: 141 g sugars

Cold Stone likes to wave the healthy flag in celebration of its fruit smoothies, but then they tack this Mountain Dew® slush onto the menu. Instead of super-charging your child with sucrose, order a smoothie that sticks to the fruit-and-yogurt formula.

Eat This

Chocolate Light Ice Cream
with bananas, maraschino cherries, and Reddi Wip® (Like It™ size)

320 calories
8.5 g fat (5 g saturated)
40 g sugars

This version of a banana split gets the job done in spectacular fashion for one-third of the calories and one-fifth of the fat that normally goes into America's favorite sundae. Besides, if you're going to feed them ice cream, you may as well sneak some fruit in there, right?

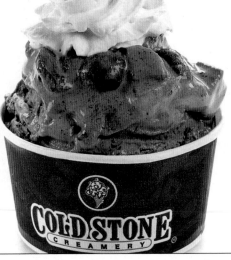

COLD STONE CREAMERY®

Other Picks

Raspberry Sorbet™
with raspberries and Nilla Wafers (Like It™ size)

255 calories
2.5 g fat (0 g saturated)
44 g sugars

Cake Batter Confetti™ Cake
6" round (1 slice)

350 calories
17 g fat (10 g saturated)
34 g sugars

Man-Go Bananas™ Yogurt Smoothie (Like It™ size)

360 calories
0 g fat
67 g sugars

60

520 calories
31 g fat
(17 g saturated)
47 g sugars

Not That!
Chocolate Ice Cream
with Reese's® Peanut Butter Cup (Like It™ size)

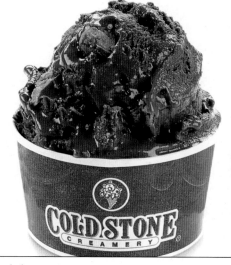

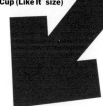

Reese's qualifies as the worst mix-in on the menu, beating out brownies and Oreo pie crust for the title. Get the same effect for fewer calories, less sugar, and more healthy fat by mixing chocolate ice cream with real peanut butter.

Other Passes

460 calories
25 g fat (14.5 g saturated)
38 g sugars

Raspberry Ice Cream
with graham cracker pie crust (Like It™ size)

510 calories
28 g fat (12 g saturated)
46 g sugars

Midnight Delight™ Cake
6" round (1 slice)

910 calories
42 g fat (30 g saturated)
96 g sugars

Very Vanilla™ Shake
(Like It™ size)

5,640

The jumping jacks a kid would have to do to burn off the 540 calories in a Love It™-size Oatmeal Cookie Batter Ice Cream.

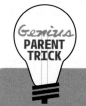

Genius
PARENT TRICK

Top your child's ice-cream cup with a big dash of ground cinnamon. By preventing the ice cream's sugar from passing through the stomach too quickly, cinnamon helps suppress the blood-sugar spike that follows a sweet dessert. Caloric cost: zero.

Così

Half of Così's kids' offerings cross the 500-calorie threshold, with the pepperoni pizza being one of the country's worst offenders with 911 calories. The adult sandwich section won't provide much relief, either, considering that almost everything Così squeezes between two loaves soars into the 600 to 900 calorie range.

SURVIVAL STRATEGY
Stick with the kids' turkey and tuna sandwiches and leave calorie-laden desserts and drinks behind the counter.

HIDDEN DANGER
Etruscan Whole Grain (1 slice)

Wonder why many Così sandwiches top 700 calories? Maybe because two slices of its whole grain bread have as many calories as a Big Mac.

270 calories
740 mg sodium
49 g carbohydrates

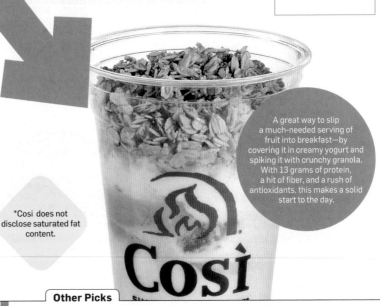

Eat This
Granola Peach Parfait

389 g calories
*6 g fat **
257 mg sodium

*Cosi does not disclose saturated fat content.

A great way to slip a much-needed serving of fruit into breakfast—by covering it in creamy yogurt and spiking it with crunchy granola. With 13 grams of protein, a hit of fiber, and a rush of antioxidants, this makes a solid start to the day.

Other Picks

Kids Gooey Grilled Cheese Sandwich

357 calories
*21 g fat**
759 mg sodium

Chocolate Croissant

370 calories
*18 g fat**
300 mg sodium

Three Bean Chili (cup)

159 calories
*1 g fat**
919 mg sodium

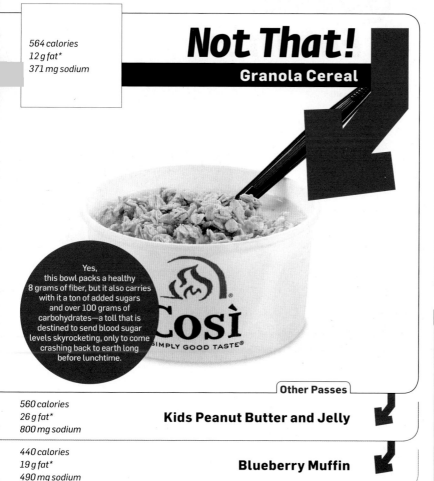

564 calories
12 g fat*
371 mg sodium

Not That!
Granola Cereal

Yes, this bowl packs a healthy 8 grams of fiber, but it also carries with it a ton of added sugars and over 100 grams of carbohydrates—a toll that is destined to send blood sugar levels skyrocketing, only to come crashing back to earth long before lunchtime.

COSÌ
SIMPLY GOOD TASTE®

Other Passes

560 calories
26 g fat*
800 mg sodium

Kids Peanut Butter and Jelly

440 calories
19 g fat*
490 mg sodium

Blueberry Muffin

374 calories
34 g fat*
987 mg sodium

Tomato Basil Aurora Soup
(10 oz cup)

STEALTH HEALTH FOOD

Moroccan Lentil Soup (10 oz cup)

*199 calories,
3 g fat,
1,159 mg sodium*

Lentils ought to be a regular food in every child's diet. They're lean and packed with protein and fiber, so your children will grow up tall with full bellies.

1,910◆

The average amount of sodium, in milligrams, that comes in each melt sandwich on Così's menu.

FOOD MYTH #2
Vegetarian meals are always healthy.

Many vegetarian meals are deceptively full of fattening oils and cheeses. With 824 calories, 51 grams of fat, and 2,929 milligrams of sodium, Così's Vegi Muffa-letta is the third most fattening sandwich on the menu, and it has 133 percent of your recommended daily sodium. For a *truly* healthy vegetarian option, try the Hummus and Fresh Veggies sandwich. It has just 8 grams of fat.

Dairy Queen

The lack of decent sides kills DQ's chances of serving a healthy kids' meal. Trans-fatty fries and onion rings are the only options, and you'll be lucky to get out of the building without a cold treat to take along for the ride. The child-size ice cream cone is a nice touch, but DQ's holy grail is the ubiquitous and often-mimicked Blizzard, which ought to be renamed the Avalanche.

SURVIVAL STRATEGY
Play solid defense: Skip sides entirely and offer your kid the choice between a soda or a child-size cone.

95

The number of minutes a child would have to spend jumping rope to burn off the 690 calories in a Chili & Cheese Foot Long Dog.

Eat This

Strawberry DQ® Sundae

(small)

260 calories
7 g fat
(4.5 g saturated)
36 g sugars

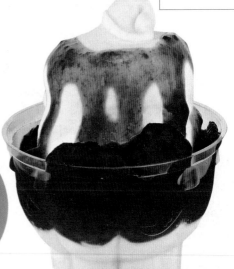

The DQ vanilla soft serve makes a reliably low-fat base for the sundae, with just 210 calories and 7 grams of fat. And the strawberry sauce's first ingredient is strawberries, which, sadly enough, can't be said for most fruit products.

Other Picks

Kid's Quesadilla Meal

350 calories
15 g fat (6 g saturated)
820 mg sodium

All-Beef Hot Dog

250 calories
14 g fat (5 g saturated)
770 mg sodium

DQ Sandwich

190 calories
5 g fat (2.5 g saturated)
18 g sugars

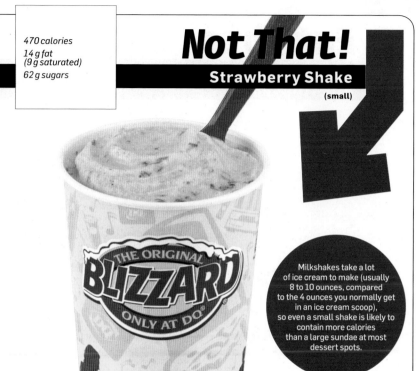

470 calories
14 g fat
(9 g saturated)
62 g sugars

Not That!
Strawberry Shake
(small)

Milkshakes take a lot of ice cream to make (usually 8 to 10 ounces, compared to the 4 ounces you normally get in an ice cream scoop), so even a small shake is likely to contain more calories than a large sundae at most dessert spots.

Other Passes

580 calories
26 g fat (10 g saturated)
1,300 mg sodium

Kid's Cheeseburger Meal

530 calories
29 g fat (4.5 g saturated, 3 g trans)
1,020 mg sodium

Crispy Chicken Sandwich

550 calories
22 g fat (10 g saturated, 2.5 g trans fat)
59 g sugars

Chocolate Coated
Waffle Cone with vanilla soft serve

UNHAPPY MEALS
Wild Buffalo Chicken Strip Basket
(4 pieces)

1,340 calories,
96 g fat
(18 g saturated, 11 g trans),
4,820 mg sodium,
120 g carbohydrates

This is what you call an abused chicken. The Wild Buffalo dipping sauce is a dubious combo of partially hydrogenated oil and hot sauce, and the fries that come in the basket are just as bad: Partially hydrogenated shortening is the most abundant ingredient besides potatoes.

HIDDEN DANGER
Trans Fats

Few chains can compete with the torrent of trans fats that soak the DQ menu board. Every year more than 500,000 people die of heart disease, and trans fats are among the leading causes. Since DQ is one of the few restaurants still frying in partially hydrogenated oil, anything that's touched the grease could be carrying a dangerous dose.

Denny's

Aside from a couple unhealthy invaders like the Little Dippers and the French Toastix™, Denny's asteroid inspired kids' menu is properly portioned for children. Its most impressive feat, however, is its choice offering of sides, which includes fruit medley, grapes, mashed potatoes, and applesauce. It's nice to see a variety of nonfried sides, especially when children so desperately need to increase their intakes of fruits and vegetables.

SURVIVAL STRATEGY
Pair a burger or pizza with a fruit side for an easy, kid-approved 400-calorie dinner.

SMART SIDES

Quaker Oatmeal (4 oz)

100 calories,
2 g fat (0 g saturated),
3 g fiber

The extra fiber in a little oatmeal will slow the kids' digestion to keep them feeling fuller, longer.

Eat This

Kid's D-Zone Smiley Alien Hotcakes

with meat

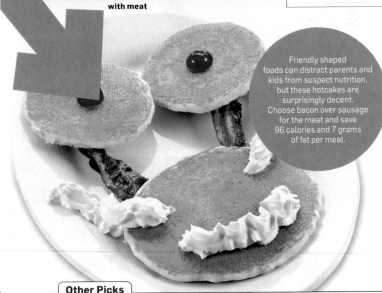

340 calories
12 g fat
(5 g saturated)
1,060 mg sodium

Friendly shaped foods can distract parents and kids from suspect nutrition, but these hotcakes are surprisingly decent. Choose bacon over sausage for the meat and save 96 calories and 7 grams of fat per meal.

Other Picks

Kid's D-Zone Cosmic Cheeseburger™

341 calories
20 g fat (6 g saturated,
1 g trans)
580 mg sodium

Sirloin Steak Dinner
with mashed potatoes and vegetable blend

450 calories
16.5 g fat (5.5 g saturated)
1,150 mg sodium

Root Beer Float

280 calories
10 g fat (6 g saturated)
47 g carbohydrates

770 calories
71 g fat
(13 g saturated)
1,094 mg sodium

Not That!

Kid's D-Zone Big Dipper French Toastix™

with syrup

Normally there isn't a huge nutritional discrepancy between pancakes and French toast, but clearly that doesn't hold true at Denny's. We suspect it's the heavy batter job they do on the bread and the amount of oil they use to fry up the toast that push these stix over the edge.

UNHAPPY MEALS
Western Burger with Fries

1,580 calories,
95 g fat (33 g saturated,
6 g trans),
2,780 mg sodium,
112 g carbohydrates

This meal might be a dream to your taste buds, but it's a nutritional nightmare to your belly. The beef is buried under a pile of onion rings, Swiss cheese, and sweetened steak sauce, and then it's dropped next to a heaping mound of French-fried potatoes. Our arteries are hardening at the thought.

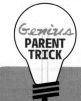

Genius
PARENT TRICK

Denny's will substitute Egg Beaters® for eggs at no extra charge. Just ask. Each one of these egg substitutes adds an additional 5 grams of protein while taking off 10 grams of fat.

Other Passes

566 calories
27 g fat (13 g saturated)
1,504 mg sodium

Kid's D-Zone Little Dipper Sampler
with applesauce and marinara sauce

983 calories
51 g fat (12 g saturated)
4,323 mg sodium

Lemon Pepper Tilapia
with vegetable rice pilaf

580 calories
29 g fat (15 g saturated)
72 g carbohydrates

Kids Oreo® Blender Blast Off

Domino's Pizza

Domino's suffers the same pitfalls of any other pizza purveyor: too much cheese, bread, and greasy toppings. If you don't know the pitfalls, you might bag your child a pizza with more than 350 calories per slice. To its credit, Domino's does keep the trans fat off the pizza and it also offers the lowest-calorie thin crust option out there.

SURVIVAL STRATEGY
Stick with the Crunchy Thin Crust pizzas sans sausage and pepperoni. Whenever possible, try to sneak on a vegetable or two per pie.

SMART SIDES

Buffalo Chicken Kickers™ (2)

90 calories, 4 g fat (0 g saturated), 320 mg sodium

Breadsticks are not the end-all of pizza sides. Two Kickers have about half the fat of a single breadstick and provide 8 grams of protein, making it a solid, belly-filling sidekick for a veggie pizza. Just be sure to keep the blue cheese out of dunking distance.

Eat This

Crunchy Thin Crust Cheese Pizza
12" (2 slices)

260 calories
17 g fat
(5 g saturated)
480 mg sodium

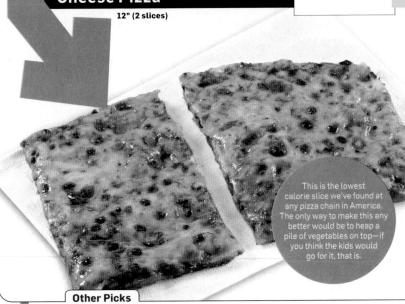

This is the lowest calorie slice we've found at any pizza chain in America. The only way to make this any better would be to heap a pile of vegetables on top—if you think the kids would go for it, that is.

Other Picks

Crunchy Thin Crust Philly Cheese Steak Pizza 12" (1 slice)

180 calories
10.5 g fat (5 g saturated)
375 mg sodium

Cheesy Bread Sticks
(2) with Marinara Dipping Sauce (1)

305 calories
14 g fat (5.5 g saturated)
540 mg sodium

Chicken Kickers™
(4)

180 calories
8 g fat (0 g saturated)
640 mg sodium

68

420 calories
16 g fat
(6 g saturated)
670 mg sodium

Not That!

Classic Hand-Tossed Cheese Pizza

12" (2 slices)

The only difference in these two slices is the crust: By making the switch from Domino's standard to their thin crust, you save 80 calories and 16 grams of carbohydrates a slice. It might not seem like much until you really consider how much pizza your family eats each year.

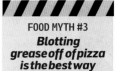

FOOD MYTH #3

Blotting grease off of pizza is the best way to make it healthy.

Obsessive blotting of a greasy pie may remove 3 or 4 grams of fat, but the decision to blot or not pales in comparison to the decisions concerning crust type and toppings. The best way to make a healthier pizza is to skip the thick crust, sausage, and pepperoni in favor of thin crusts strewn with vegetables and lean meats like ham and chicken.

DIPPING SAUCE DECODER (PER CONTAINER)

● **GARLIC:** 440 calories, 50 g fat (10 g saturated, 7 g trans)

● **SWEET ICING:** 250 calories, 3 g fat (2.5 g saturated), 55 g sugars

● **BLUE CHEESE:** 230 calories, 24 g fat (5 g saturated)

● **RANCH:** 200 calories, 21 g fat (3 g saturated)

● **HOT:** 120 calories, 12 g fat (2 g saturated)

● **MARINARA:** 25 calories, 0 g fat

Other Passes

300 calories
14 g fat (6 g saturated)
500 mg sodium

Hand-Tossed Crust Bacon Cheeseburger® Pizza 12" (1 slice)

700 calories
64 g fat (13 g saturated, 7 g trans)
570 mg sodium

Breadsticks
(2) with Garlic Dipping Sauce (1)

340 calories
18 g fat (6 g saturated)
1,000 mg sodium

Hot Buffalo Wings
(4)

69

Dunkin' Donuts

After years as a major trans-fat transgressor, Dunkin' has cleaned up its act and cut them almost entirely from the menu. Unfortunately, between deleterious donuts and bloated bagels, you're still left with a lesser-of-all-evils proposition.

SURVIVAL STRATEGY
Go for sandwiches made on English muffins for breakfast, flatbread sandwiches (preferably the Ham and Swiss) at all other times.

UNHAPPY MEALS
Sausage, Egg & Cheese Sandwich

800 calories,
52 g fat (24 g saturated),
1,960 mg sodium

This biscuit will make even the scrawniest kid's belly jiggle. With over 50 ingredients, including partially hydrogenated vegetable oil, this breakfast sandwich brings a host of unhealthy fats and nearly a day's worth of sodium to the start of the day.

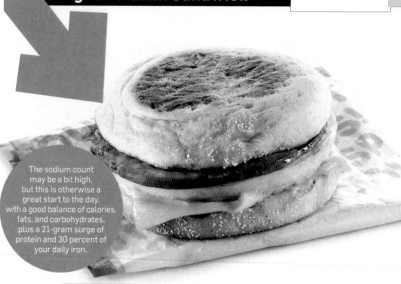

Eat This

Ham, Egg and Cheese English Muffin Sandwich

310 calories
10 g fat
(5 g saturated)
1,270 mg sodium

The sodium count may be a bit high, but this is otherwise a great start to the day, with a good balance of calories, fats, and carbohydrates, plus a 21-gram surge of protein and 30 percent of your daily iron.

Other Picks

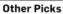

Sugar Raised Donut and French Cruller (1 of each)

360 calories
15 g fat (9.5 saturated fat)
425 mg sodium

Marble Frosted Donut

230 calories
11 g fat (4.5 g saturated)
13 g sugars

Ham and Swiss Flatbread Sandwich

350 calories
12 g fat (5 g saturated)
1,040 mg sodium

540 calories
25 g fat
(3.5 g saturated)
520 mg sodium

Not That!

Banana Walnut Muffin

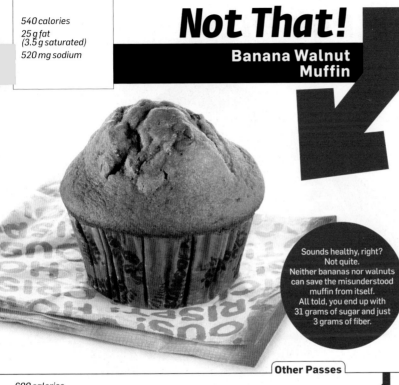

Sounds healthy, right?
Not quite.
Neither bananas nor walnuts
can save the misunderstood
muffin from itself.
All told, you end up with
31 grams of sugar and just
3 grams of fiber.

Other Passes

600 calories
25 g fat (11.5 g saturated)
760 mg sodium

Multigrain Bagel with Strawberry Cream Cheese (2 oz)

330 calories
18 g fat (9 g saturated)
18 g sugars

Glazed Cake Donut

460 calories
24 g fat (12 g saturated)
1,000 mg sodium

Three Cheese Flatbread Sandwich

77

The number of beds
a kid would have
to make to burn off
the 270 calories
from a Glazed Cake
Donut.

FOOD MYTH #4

**Smoothies are
a reliable
source of
fruit for children.**

With 104 grams, the
average smoothie at Dunkin'
Donuts is about 75 percent
sugar. The ensuing blood-
sugar spike activates fat-
storing mechanisms.

HIDDEN DANGER
**Multigrain
Bagel**

It sounds pretty healthy,
right? It's actually the most
caloric of all of Dunkin's
bagels and when spread
with cream cheese, contains
more calories than a Big Mac.

380 calories
650 mg sodium
68 g carbohydrates

Fazoli's

As long as you can keep the kids from ravishing the breadstick basket, this Italian-on-the-go chain is a sound choice. Most meals on the kids' menu fall below 300 calories, and the pasta toppers provide an additional nutritional boost. If only they added a whole-wheat noodle option, Fazoli's might take home an A.

SURVIVAL STRATEGY
Kids' pastas of any invention are fine, as long as they steer clear of fatty topping like meatballs and sausage.

UNHAPPY MEALS
Chocolate Chunk Cookie

590 calories,
28 g fat (12 g saturated),
45 g sugars

The most caloric cookie we've ever encountered, with more fat and calories than a Quarter Pounder® with Cheese at McDonald's® and as much sugar as two chocolate ice cream bars.

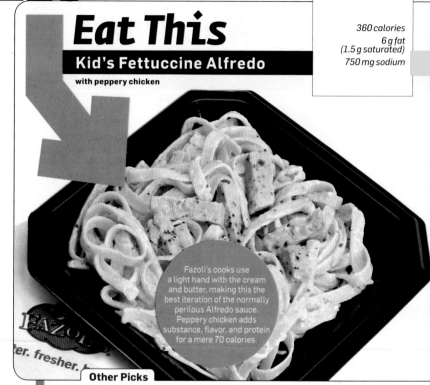

Eat This

Kid's Fettuccine Alfredo
with peppery chicken

360 calories
6 g fat
(1.5 g saturated)
750 mg sodium

Fazoli's cooks use a light hand with the cream and butter, making this the best iteration of the normally perilous Alfredo sauce. Peppery chicken adds substance, flavor, and protein for a mere 70 calories.

Other Picks

Kids Ziti with Meat Sauce

190 calories
6 g fat (2.5 g saturated)
710 mg sodium

Penne with Meat Sauce
(small)

500 calories
7 g fat (1.5 g saturated)
1,020 mg sodium

Original Lemon Ice
(regular)

180 calories
45 g sugars

430 calories
13.5 g fat
(2.5 g saturated)
830 mg sodium

Not That!

Kids' Spaghetti

with marinara and garlic shrimp

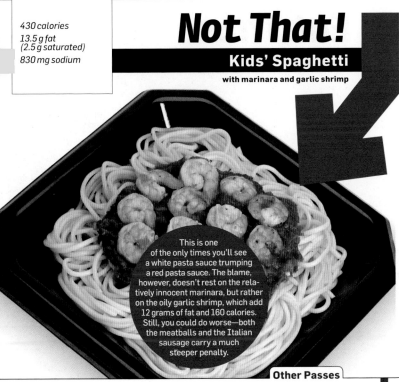

This is one of the only times you'll see a white pasta sauce trumping a red pasta sauce. The blame, however, doesn't rest on the relatively innocent marinara, but rather on the oily garlic shrimp, which add 12 grams of fat and 160 calories. Still, you could do worse—both the meatballs and the Italian sausage carry a much steeper penalty.

Other Passes

260 calories
13 g fat (6 g saturated)
880 mg sodium

Kids Meat Lasagna

620 calories
28 g fat (10 g saturated)
1,700 mg sodium

Pepperoni Pizza
(2 slices)

360 calories
90 g sugars

Pomegranate Lemon Ice

Genius
PARENT TRICK

There's no better way to coax a little green onto the plate than by mixing it in with noodles and marinara, so it's perfect that Fazoli's gives you the option to upgrade each dish with a helping of folate-rich broccoli. Broccoli's vitamin C will keep the kids' immune systems strong, and the extra fiber will compensate for the pasta's carbohydrates and help keep their bellies feeling full.

SUGAR SPIKES

Triple Berry Lemon Ice

The Impact:
91 g sugars

There's more than a brain freeze at stake here; it's nearly 100 percent sugar, with nary a trace of real fruit in this obscenely sweet slush. Let the kids' insulin rest and make some real lemonade when you get home.

IHOP

IHOP refuses to serve up nutritional information, but thanks to the New York City Board of Health, they were forced to publish calorie counts on their menus in April 2008. The big reveal shocked New York diners: 1,700-calorie cheeseburgers, 1,300-calorie omelets, and four salads with more than 1,000 calories. Because IHOP doesn't provide those numbers to the rest of the country, they still receive an automatic F.

SURVIVAL STRATEGY
Write letters, make phone calls, beg, scream, and plead for IHOP to provide nutritional information on all of their products.

SMART SIDES

Fresh Fruit Bowl
100 calories

Don't let the smell of sizzling butter and sausage patties lure you away from healthier side options. Set this bowl of cantaloupe, honeydew, watermelon, and grapes in the middle of your table to supplement a small order of flapjacks.

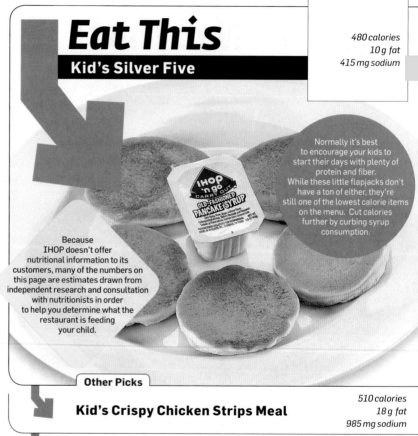

Eat This
Kid's Silver Five

480 calories
10 g fat
415 mg sodium

Normally it's best to encourage your kids to start their days with plenty of protein and fiber. While these little flapjacks don't have a ton of either, they're still one of the lowest calorie items on the menu. Cut calories further by curbing syrup consumption.

Because IHOP doesn't offer nutritional information to its customers, many of the numbers on this page are estimates drawn from independent research and consultation with nutritionists in order to help you determine what the restaurant is feeding your child.

Other Picks

Kid's Crispy Chicken Strips Meal

510 calories
18 g fat
985 mg sodium

Chocolate Chip Pancakes

630 calories
15 g fat
680 mg sodium

Grilled Ham

120 calories
8 g fat
510 mg sodium

790 calories
40 g fat
1,175 mg sodium

Not That!

Kid's Cheese Omelet

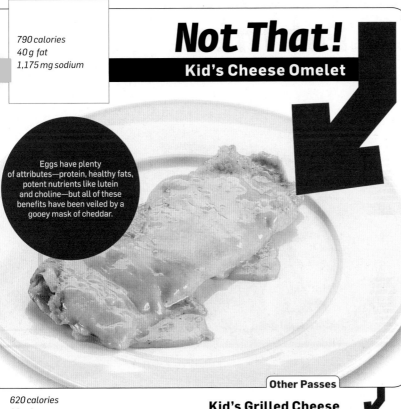

Eggs have plenty of attributes—protein, healthy fats, potent nutrients like lutein and choline—but all of these benefits have been veiled by a gooey mask of cheddar.

83,000

The approximate number of pancakes that IHOP serves every day of the year.

GUILTY PLEASURES

Belgian Waffle

390 calories, 19 g fat, 48 g carbs

It doesn't qualify as light fare, but with just 400 calories, it is significantly better than most IHOP breakfast options.

FOOD MYTH #5

Fruit condiments are healthy.

Sure, pure fruit preserves have a place on the breakfast table, but IHOP's fruit compote does not. Like so many other foods that invoke fruit in their names, this compote is sunk in a slurry of sugar and sweetened syrup. Ask for fresh strawberries instead.

Other Passes

620 calories
26 g fat
1,105 mg sodium

Kid's Grilled Cheese Sandwich Meal

790 calories
36 g fat (18 g saturated)
1,240 mg sodium

Harvest Grain 'N Nut® Pancakes

520 calories
22 g fat
525 mg sodium

Beef Sausage Links

75

Jack in the Box

No kid's entrée eclipses the 400-calorie mark, a rare feat among fast-food and sit-down purveyors. Stray far from the kids' menu, though, and you'll find trouble fast—particularly with the burgers, which can contain more than 1,100 calories. But the biggest reason Jack is stuck in the middle of the pack is trans fat. From the Curly Fries to the Chicken Strips, Jack's has the trans-fattiest menu in America.

SURVIVAL STRATEGY
Allow free rein of the kids' menu, but insist on a smart side like applesauce and a zero-calorie beverage.

GUILTY PLEASURES

Regular Beef Taco

*160 calories,
8 g fat
(3 g saturated, 1 g trans),
270 mg sodium*

Tacos from Jack's sounds like a bad idea, but two of these will weigh in under most of the burger and chicken options on the menu.

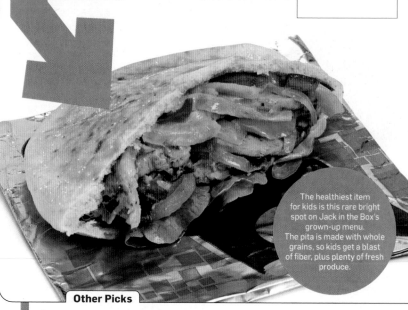

Eat This

Chicken Fajita Pita

*300 calories
9 g fat
(3.5 g saturated)
1,090 mg sodium*

The healthiest item for kids is this rare bright spot on Jack in the Box's grown-up menu. The pita is made with whole grains, so kids get a blast of fiber, plus plenty of fresh produce.

Other Picks

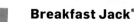

Breakfast Jack®
(American cheese, sliced ham, and grilled egg on a bun)

*290 calories
12 g fat (4.5 g saturated)
760 mg sodium*

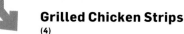

Grilled Chicken Strips
(4)

*180 calories
2 g fat (0.5 g saturated)
700 mg sodium*

Mozzarella Cheese Sticks
(3)

*240 calories
12 g fat (5 g saturated, 2 g trans)
420 mg sodium*

330 calories
15 g fat
(7 g saturated,
1 g trans)
770 mg sodium

Not That!

Kids Cheeseburger

Ounce for ounce, the burgers here are some of the worst in America. Even this tiny patty packs nearly half a day's worth of saturated fat between the buns. Add a small curly fries and you'll have a 600-calorie meal with 6 grams of trans fat—about three times the amount doctors say is safe to take in daily.

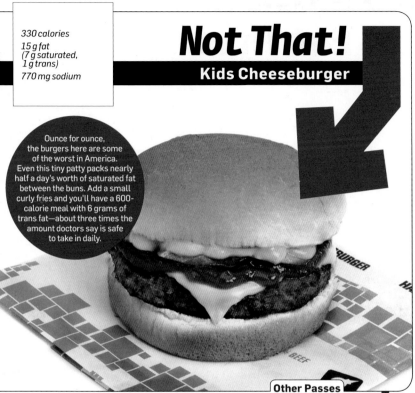

Other Passes

450 calories
20 g fat (4.5 g saturated, 4.5 g trans)
550 mg sodium

Blueberry French Toast Sticks
(4)

250 calories
12 g fat (3 g saturated, 3 g trans)
630 mg sodium

Kids Chicken Breast Strips
(2)

400 calories
19 g fat (6 g saturated, 3 g trans)
920 mg sodium

Egg Rolls
(3)

UNHAPPY MEALS
Bacon Cheddar Potato Wedges

720 calories,
48 g fat (15 g saturated,
12 g trans),
1,360 mg sodium,
48 g carbohydrates

For the record: bacon, cheese, and fried potatoes are not a healthful trio. What's worse, though, is that Jack in the Box cooks in trans-fatty vegetable shortening. The American Heart Association recommends limiting these fats to less than 1 percent of your diet—an allowance your child will surpass with just a couple bites of this side.

SUGAR SPIKES

Strawberry Ice Cream Shake (small)

The Impact:
77 g sugars

The shakes at Jack in the Box are loaded with sugar and cream, which contributes 35 grams of fat to this 730-calorie monster. If your kid simply must have something sweet, cheesecake is a surprisingly good choice. The swap will knock off 54 grams of sugar.

Jamba Juice

The lack of fresh fruit in kids' diets is a serious concern, and Jamba Juice offers a viable and tasty solution: Stick it all in a blender and let them slurp it up. Still, there are more than a few concoctions with concerning amounts of sugar and calories.

SURVIVAL STRATEGY
Stick with 16-ounce servings of the All Fruit selections and you can pack an extra few servings of fruit into your kid's diet. Skip over the Classics and the Creamy Indulgences—often built with sherbet and frozen yogurt.

STEALTH HEALTH FOOD

Omega-3 Oatmeal Cookie

*150 calories,
6 g fat (1.5 g saturated),
15 g sugars*

As nutritious as cookies can be. It's made with fiber-rich rolled oats, oat fiber, and ground flaxseed, the source of the heart-healthy omega-3s. And since it's seasoned with cinnamon, it creates a smoother ride for your kid's blood sugar.

Eat This

Strawberry Whirl™
(16 oz)

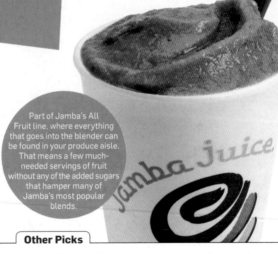

200 calories
0 g fat
42 g sugars

Part of Jamba's All Fruit line, where everything that goes into the blender can be found in your produce aisle. That means a few much-needed servings of fruit without any of the added sugars that hamper many of Jamba's most popular blends.

Other Picks

Mega Mango™
(16 oz)

220 calories
0.5 g fat
50 g sugars

Orange Mango Passion Juicies™
(24 oz)

280 calories
1 g fat
62 g sugars

Omega-3 Chocolate Brownie Cookie

150 calories
3.5 g fat
15 g sugars

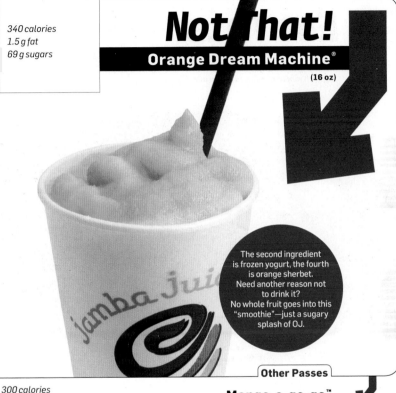

340 calories
1.5 g fat
69 g sugars

Not That!
Orange Dream Machine®
(16 oz)

The second ingredient is frozen yogurt, the fourth is orange sherbet. Need another reason not to drink it? No whole fruit goes into this "smoothie"—just a sugary splash of OJ.

Other Passes

300 calories
1.5 g fat
64 g sugars

Mango-a-go-go™
(16 oz)

330 calories
1.5 g fat
76 g sugars

Orange Juice
(24 oz)

380 calories
4 g fat
14 g sugars

Apple Cinnamon Pretzel

Genius
PARENT TRICK

If your kid isn't a big milk drinker, add a Calcium Boost to a Jamba smoothie. The supplement provides a full day's worth of calcium and vitamin D.

SUGAR SPIKES

Peanut Butter Moo'd® (30 oz)
*The Impact:
169 g sugars*

Peanut Butter Moo'd hardly qualifies as a smoothie. The mix of frozen yogurt, chocolate, banana, and peanut butter has more sugar than two pints of Ben & Jerry's® Butter Pecan™ Ice Cream.

132

The percentage by which Americans need to increase their fruit consumption in order to meet the recommended four ½-cup servings per day.

KFC

For a place with the word "fried" in its acronymic title, KFC manages to downplay the damage of their namesake goods by offering low-calorie Snacker sandwiches and a variety of relatively healthy vegetable sides.

SURVIVAL STRATEGY
Skip over the fried chicken—unless your family likes it skinless, in which case, have at it—and look instead to the Snackers and the Crispy Strips. Don't miss the opportunity to sneak a serving or two of vegetables into your kid's diet, assuming they don't come out of the fryer.

SUGAR SP KES

Teriyaki Wings (5)

The Impact:
30 g sugars

You probably wouldn't guess that the Teriyaki Wings have nearly three times as much sugar as the Sweet and Spicy Wings. You also probably wouldn't guess that they have more sugar than KFC's own Double Chocolate Chip Cake.

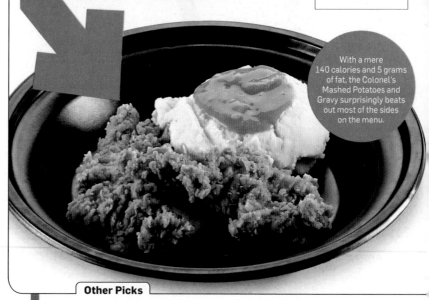

Eat This
Crispy Strips
(2) with mashed potatoes and gravy

380 calories
18 g fat
(3.5 g saturated)
1,360 mg sodium

With a mere 140 calories and 5 grams of fat, the Colonel's Mashed Potatoes and Gravy surprisingly beats out most of the sides on the menu.

Other Picks

Original Recipe Skinless Breast (2)

280 calories
4 g fat (0 g saturated)
1,040 mg sodium

KFC Buffalo Snacker®

260 calories
8 g fat (1.5 g saturated)
860 mg sodium

Lil' Bucket™ Strawberry Short Cake

210 calories
7 g fat (5 g saturated)
25 g sugars

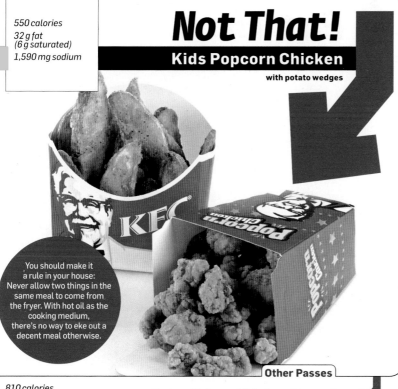

550 calories
32 g fat
(6 g saturated)
1,590 mg sodium

Not That!
Kids Popcorn Chicken
with potato wedges

You should make it a rule in your house: Never allow two things in the same meal to come from the fryer. With hot oil as the cooking medium, there's no way to eke out a decent meal otherwise.

Other Passes

810 calories *55 g fat (12 g saturated)* *1,820 mg sodium*	**Extra Crispy Chicken Breast** **and extra crispy thigh**
330 calories *15 g fat (3 g saturated)* *710 mg sodium*	**KFC Fish Snacker®**
410 calories *15 g fat (7 g saturated, 1.5 g trans)* *53 g sugars*	**Lil' Bucket™ Lemon Crème**

UNHAPPY MEALS
Chicken Pot Pie

770 calories,
40 grams fat
(15 grams saturated,
14 grams trans),
1,680 mg sodium,
70 g carbohydrates

Despite KFC's 2007 commitment to stop using trans fats in their cooking oil, the restaurant still allows this seriously hazardous meal to sneak onto the menu. In fact, every one of the (in)Famous Bowls™ still contains trans fats.

1,576

The number of stairs to the top of the Empire State Building. You'd have to make two trips to the top and back in order to burn off the calories in two pieces of Extra Crispy Chicken.

Krispy Kreme

What do you expect from a place that serves only doughnuts and corn-syrup–spiked drinks? The problem with Krispy Kreme isn't so much the fat and the calories of its staples (though they have plenty of both!), but rather the utter lack of any real nutritional takeaway to be found anywhere on its menu. There is but one bright spot for doughnut devotees: Krispy Kreme finally switched over to trans-fat–free frying oils in January 2008. (Collective sigh of relief.)

SURVIVAL STRATEGY
Unless they're running a marathon, stick to a single order of doughnut holes.

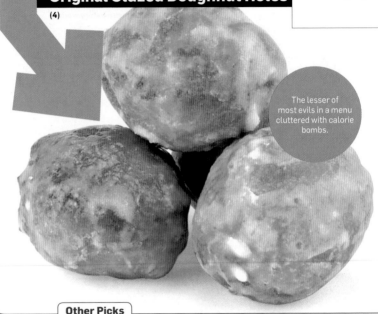

Eat This

Original Glazed Doughnut Holes
(4)

200 calories
11 g fat
(5 g saturated)
15 g sugars

The lesser of most evils in a menu cluttered with calorie bombs.

Other Picks

Glazed Cinnamon Doughnut

210 calories
12 g fat (6 g saturated)
12 g sugars

Glazed Chocolate Cake Doughnut Holes (4)

210 calories
10 g fat (4.5 g saturated)
17 g sugars

Very Berry Chiller (12 oz)

170 calories
0 g fat
43 g sugars

290 calories
14 g fat
(6 g saturated)
19 g sugars

Not That!
Powdered Cake Doughnut

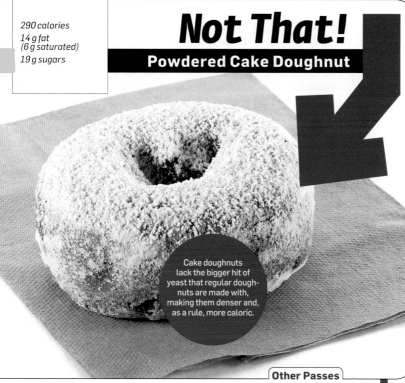

Cake doughnuts lack the bigger hit of yeast that regular doughnuts are made with, making them denser and, as a rule, more caloric.

Genius
PARENT TRICK

Choose a doughnut without decorations or embellishments. The difference between one Original Glazed and one topped-and-filled Caramel Kreme Crunch is 180 calories and 20 grams of sugar.

SUGAR SPIKES

Oranges & Kreme Chiller (small)

The Impact:
71 g sugars

Let your kid wash down a couple of doughnuts with this cloying beverage and you can expect a tantrum-inducing sugar crash in your near future. This is a dangerous amount of sugar, but the real *chiller* is the drink's 630 calories and 24 grams of saturated fat.

Other Passes

380 calories
20 g fat (10 g saturated)
24 g sugars

Apple Fritter

380 calories
19 g fat (9 g saturated)
30 g sugars

Caramel Kreme Crunch

620 calories
28 g fat (24 g saturated)
71 g sugars

Berries & Kreme Chiller
(12 oz)

5,200
The number of donuts Krispy Kreme makes every minute in North America.

83

McDonald's

REPORT CARD

B

Though not blessed with an abundance of healthy options for kids, Mickey D's isn't burdened with any major calorie bombs, either. Kid standards like McNuggets and cheeseburgers are both in the 300-calorie range.

SURVIVAL STRATEGY

Apple Dippers and 2% milk with a small entrée makes for a pretty decent meal-on-the-go. McDonald's quintessential Happy Meal® makes this possible—just beware the usual French fries and soda pitfalls.

UNHAPPY MEALS
Cheeseburger
with French fries
(small) and a Coca-Cola®
(small)

700 calories,
25 g fat
(8.5 g saturated fat),
915 mg sodium

The classic Happy Meal®
is a punishing blow to your
kid's diet, with more fat
and calories than an active
adult man, let alone a kid,
should take in from a
single meal.

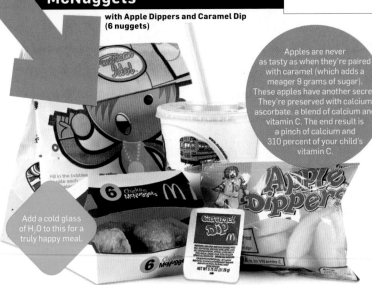

Eat This

Chicken McNuggets®

with Apple Dippers and Caramel Dip
(6 nuggets)

355 calories
15.5 g fat
(3 g saturated,
1.5 g trans)
705 mg sodium

Apples are never as tasty as when they're paired with caramel (which adds a meager 9 grams of sugar). These apples have another secret: They're preserved with calcium ascorbate, a blend of calcium and vitamin C. The end result is a pinch of calcium and 310 percent of your child's vitamin C.

Add a cold glass of H₂O to this for a truly happy meal.

Other Picks

Honey Mustard Snack Wrap®
grilled

260 calories
9 g fat (3.5 g saturated)
800 mg sodium

Egg McMuffin®

300 calories
12 g fat (5 g saturated)
820 mg sodium

Kiddie Cone

45 calories
1 g fat (0.5 g saturated)
6 g sugars

84

400 calories
23 g fat
(4 g saturated,
2 g trans)
1,000 mg sodium

Not That!

Chicken Selects Premium Breast Strips

(3)

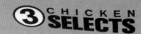

The only thing premium about these strips is the caloric price you pay to eat them. A thicker layer of crunchy breading puts each strip at 133 calories, compared to just 45 per McNugget.

HIDDEN DANGER
**Baked
Apple Pie**

This fruit pocket has more trans fats than anything else on the menu.
*270 calories,
12 g fat
(3.5 g saturated,
5 g trans)*

Other Passes

300 calories
12 g fat (6 g saturated, 0.5 g trans)
750 mg sodium

Cheeseburger

570 calories
13.5 g fat (3.5 g saturated)
665 mg sodium

Hotcakes
with syrup and margarine

250 calories
8 g fat (2 g saturated)
13 g sugars

McDonaldland® Cookies
(2 oz)

Olive Garden

There may be some pretty decent stuff on Olive Garden's menu, but you'll never know it—not as long as the country's largest sit-down Italian chain continues to make nutritional nondisclosure a policy.

SURVIVAL STRATEGY
The low-fat options on the Garden Fare® menu provide only sporadic chunks of information, and only a single option for kids: the 349-calorie Grilled Chicken entrée. Until they offer comprehensive data on all their dishes, as competitors Macaroni Grill and Fazoli's gladly do, proceed at your own risk.

Eat This

Kid's Spaghetti & Tomato Sauce

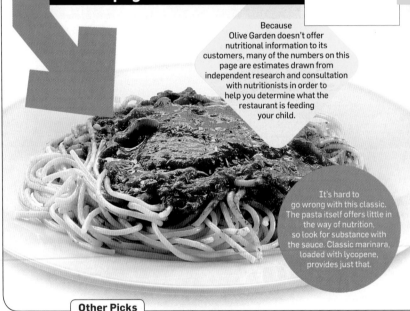

310 calories
6 g fat
770 sodium

Because Olive Garden doesn't offer nutritional information to its customers, many of the numbers on this page are estimates drawn from independent research and consultation with nutritionists in order to help you determine what the restaurant is feeding your child.

It's hard to go wrong with this classic. The pasta itself offers little in the way of nutrition, so look for substance with the sauce. Classic marinara, loaded with lycopene, provides just that.

Other Picks

Kids's Grilled Chicken with Pasta and Broccoli

350 calories
11 fat
485 mg sodium

Kid's Cheese Pizza

420 calories
18 fat
900 mg sodium

Torta di Chocolate

235 calories
7 g fat
20 g sugars

510 calories
18 g fat
940 sodium

Not That!
Macaroni & Cheese

A sauce based on cheese and cream could never compete with one made from simmered tomatoes.

Genius PARENT TRICK

Olive Garden will let you sub whole wheat linguine in place of regular white pasta. The exchange will add an extra 6 grams of fiber to your plate, making sure the meal's energy burns at a slow and steady pace.

Other Passes

560 calories
32 fat
500 mg sodium

Kid's Fettuccine Alfredo

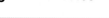

520 calories
25 fat
1,100 mg sodium

Kid's Chicken Fingers with Fries

450 calories
22 fat
45 g sugars

Kid's Sundae

UNHAPPY MEALS
Lasagna Classico

858 calories,
47 g fat,
1,403 mg sodium,
49 g carbohydrates

The combined power of four cheeses glosses these noodles with 75 percent of the day's fat allotment. Stick to cheese pizza if your kids want something gooey and saucy.

On The Border

On the Border's eagerness to please might be detrimental to your child's health. Each kids' meal entrée includes a drink, side, and kiddie sundae. Added together, most meals top 1,000 calories. The regular adult menu, with its 1,900-calorie fish tacos and quesadillas, offers little refuge.

SURVIVAL STRATEGY
As funny as it might sound, avoid all Mexican entrées on the kids' menu—every one is disastrous. Go with a burger or a corn dog, or carefully construct a Combo meal.

Genius PARENT TRICK

Order your child's meals with corn tortillas instead of flour. It will cut 130 calories, 4 grams of saturated fat, and 710 mg sodium per order.

Eat This

Kids Grilled Chicken

with black beans and sautéed vegetables

380 calories
13 g fat
(4 g saturated)
1,440 mg sodium

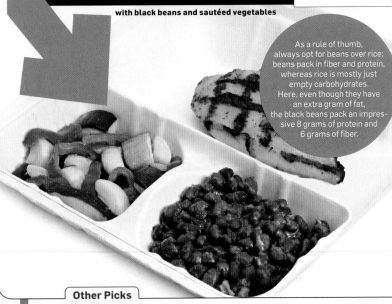

As a rule of thumb, always opt for beans over rice; beans pack in fiber and protein, whereas rice is mostly just empty carbohydrates. Here, even though they have an extra gram of fat, the black beans pack an impressive 8 grams of protein and 6 grams of fiber.

Other Picks

Hamburger
390 calories
23 g fat (7 g saturated)
290 mg sodium

Chicken Tortilla Soup
350 calories
22 g fat (9 g saturated)
1,540 mg sodium

Kids Corn Dog
320 calories
21 g fat (5 g saturated)
760 mg sodium

1,210 calories
56 g fat
(16 g saturated)
3,690 mg sodium

Not That!

Kids Chicken Crispy Taco Mexican Dinner

with Mexican rice and salad with chipotle honey mustard dressing

This is one of America's worst kids' meals. For taco lovers, the only tenable route is to order one or two chicken tacos off the Create Your Own Combo menu. Even then, you'll still have a meal with 500 calories and more than 20 grams of fat, so be extra careful when selecting sides.

Other Passes

---

710 calories
48 g fat (26 g saturated)
1,230 mg sodium

Kids Quesadilla

---

980 calories
57 g fat (29 g saturated)
1,850 mg sodium

Kids Bean & Cheese Nachos

---

630 calories
21 g fat (9 g saturated)
1,490 mg sodium

Kids Grilled Chicken Sandwich

900

The average number of calories in an On The Border salad without dressing. The average sodium content is 1,769 milligrams.

SMART SIDES

Sautéed Shrimp (4)

170 calories,
10 g fat (4 g saturated),
380 mg sodium

These crustaceans are supercharged with tryptophan, an amino acid that has the ability to increase serotonin levels in the brain. The payoff for child and parent alike is in regular sleeping patterns, appetite control, and improved mood.

GREAT GROWN-UP GRUB

Jalapeño-BBQ Salmon

590 calories,
21 g fat (6 g saturated),
1,220 mg sodium

This meal boasts 54 grams of protein, an astonishing 24 grams of fiber, and tons of healthy omega-3s.

Outback Steakhouse

For years we've pestered Outback to provide us with nutritional information. A spokesperson once told us: "Ninety percent of our meals are prepared by hand. Any analysis would be difficult to measure consistently." Yet no fewer than 50 national chain restaurants do just that.

SURVIVAL STRATEGY
Until they do what so many others are doing, we'll be forced to fail them and you'll be forced to trust that their food isn't too nutritionally deficient—which is quite a leap of faith.

Eat This

Joey Sirloin
with fresh steamed vegetables

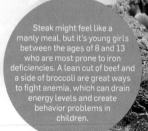

510 calories
20 g fat
900 mg sodium

Steak might feel like a manly meal, but it's young girls between the ages of 8 and 13 who are most prone to iron deficiencies. A lean cut of beef and a side of broccoli are great ways to fight anemia, which can drain energy levels and create behavior problems in children.

Because Outback Steakhouse doesn't offer nutritional information to its customers, many of the numbers on this page are estimates drawn from independent research and consultation with nutritionists in order to help you determine what the restaurant is feeding your child.

SMART SIDES

Sautéed Mushrooms
150 calories,
11 g fat, 12 g carbs

Mushrooms are a powerful force for bodily health, due largely to the sizeable dose of selenium. One serving of the fancy fungus contains half a day's value of this important mineral, which has antioxidant characteristics that have been shown to help ward off cancers, repair DNA, and decrease asthma and arthritis symptoms.

Other Picks

Kid's Grilled Chicken on the Barbie
with roasted garlic mashed potatoes

420 calories
18 g fat
825 mg sodium

Grilled Cheese
with fresh steamed green beans

500 calories
22 g fat
825 mg sodium

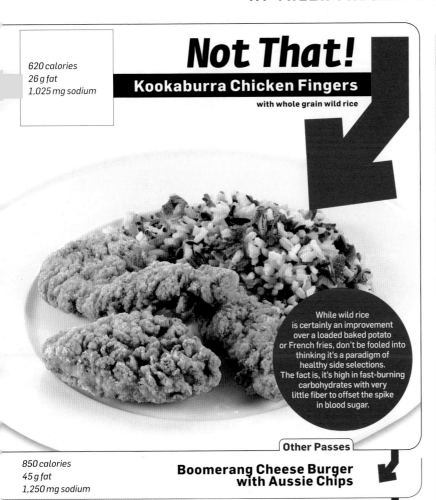

620 calories
26 g fat
1,025 mg sodium

Not That!
Kookaburra Chicken Fingers
with whole grain wild rice

While wild rice is certainly an improvement over a loaded baked potato or French fries, don't be fooled into thinking it's a paradigm of healthy side selections. The fact is, it's high in fast-burning carbohydrates with very little fiber to offset the spike in blood sugar.

Other Passes

850 calories
45 g fat
1,250 mg sodium

Boomerang Cheese Burger
with Aussie Chips

910 calories
48 g fat
1,005 mg sodium

Mac-A-Roo 'N Cheese
with dressed baked potato

93

The average amount of fat, in grams, ordered by kids at Outback, the worst-faring restaurant in a study that included 104 adolescents and 10 restaurants. At McDonald's, the meals ordered had 45 grams; at Wendy's and Taco Bell, the results were 34 and 32 grams, respectively.

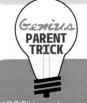

Genius
PARENT TRICK

"SOS" is restaurant speak for "sauce on the side," which is important at Outback, where cooks have a heavy hand with the fatty stuff. Try it out on your server and your kid won't even know.

Panera Bread

The kid-size sandwiches at Panera are appropriately portioned so that none tops 400 calories, but everything outside that safety zone is eligible for a red-flag warning, including adult sandwiches, Crispani® pizzas, and most breakfast offerings. Some of the more egregious selections sit close to 1,000 calories—enough to ruin an otherwise disciplined day of eating.

SURVIVAL STRATEGY
Push for a soup and half-sandwich combo. Most combinations will keep your kid under 500 calories and will provide a decent dose of nutrients.

MENU DECODER

● **WHITE WHOLE GRAIN WHEAT BREAD:** Made with flour milled from white whole wheat and malted barley, this loaf has all the fiber and nutritional breakdown of regular whole wheat bread, but with a milder taste.

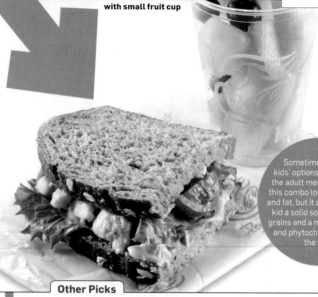

Eat This

Half Chicken Salad Sandwich on Whole Wheat

with small fruit cup

360 calories
13 g fat
(2.5 g saturated)
805 mg sodium

Sometimes the best kids' options are found on the adult menu. Not only is this combo lower in calories and fat, but it also offers your kid a solid source of whole grains and a mix of nutrients and phytochemicals from the fruit.

Other Picks

Egg & Cheese Breakfast Sandwich
380 calories
14 g fat (6 g saturated)
620 mg sodium

Turkey Chickpea Chili Soup
180 calories
5 g fat (1.5 g saturated)
800 mg sodium

Nutty Oatmeal Raisin Cookie
340 calories
14 g fat (6 g saturated)
21 g sugars

470 calories
17 g fat
(2 g saturated)
400 mg sodium

Not That!

Panera Kids™ PB&J

with strawberry yogurt tube

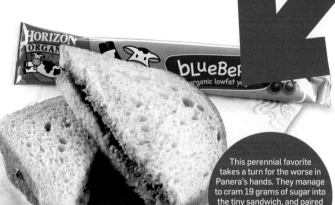

This perennial favorite takes a turn for the worse in Panera's hands. They manage to cram 19 grams of sugar into the tiny sandwich, and paired with the sweetened yogurt, it makes for a sucrose-saturated meal for your kid.

Other Passes

560 calories
21 g fat (14 g saturated)
740 mg sodium

Cinnamon Crunch Bagel
with reduced fat cream cheese

230 calories
14 g fat (9 g saturated)
720 mg sodium

Baked Potato Soup

430 calories
24 g fat (10 g saturated)
27 g sugars

Nutty Chocolate Chipper Cookie

HIDDEN DANGER
Hot Chocolate

Despite being a mere 11.5 ounces, this dubious beverage has more fat than any Panera Kids™ Deli Sandwich and more sugar than any of its saucer-size cookies.

410 calories,
17 g fat
(12 g saturated),
44 g sugars

GUILTY PLEASURES

Crispani Tomato and Fresh Basil Pizza (2 slices)

330 calories,
16 g fat (6 g saturated),
560 mg sodium

The antioxidant-rich tomatoes and the cracker-thin crust form the basis of a very reasonable pizza, but the often-overlooked basil is what takes it over the top. Like turmeric and cinnamon, basil is a natural anti-inflammatory, so it provides an all-around boost to your child's health.

Papa John's

Pizza joints suffer the curse of bad report cards because of their thick crusts, fat-speckled meats, and blankets of cheese. That said, Papa John's does have a few advantages over the competition: the absence of trans fats, the assortment of nonsoda beverage options, and the first whole wheat crust offered by a big US pizza chain.

SURVIVAL STRATEGY
Order Chicken Strips with Pizza Sauce to blunt the family's collective hunger. Follow with a slice of thin or wheat crust cheese or Spinach Alfredo.

13.4

Manhattan length, in miles. Johnny would have to walk it to burn off the 1,090 calories in two slices of Spicy Italian Pan Crust Pizza and small Coke®.

94

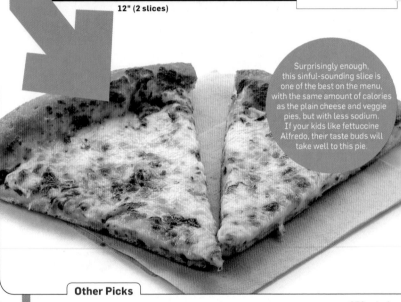

Eat This

Original Crust Spinach Alfredo Pizza

12" (2 slices)

400 calories
16 g fat
(6 g saturated)
900 mg sodium

Surprisingly enough, this sinful-sounding slice is one of the best on the menu, with the same amount of calories as the plain cheese and veggie pies, but with less sodium. If your kids like fettuccine Alfredo, their taste buds will take well to this pie.

Other Picks

Whole Wheat Crust Garden Fresh Pizza 14" (1 slice)

270 calories
9 g fat (2.5 g saturated)
660 mg sodium

Chickenstrips
with pizza sauce (2 strips)

180 calories
8 g fat (2 g saturated)
490 mg sodium

Apple Twist Sweetreat
(½ pie)

380 calories
16 g fat (4 g saturated)
23 g sugars

760 calories
44 g fat
(16 g saturated)
1,220 mg sodium

Not That!

Pan Crust Spinach Alfredo Pizza

12" (2 slices)

The dense, buttery pan crust adds to the overall calorie, fat, and sodium count, but doubles the damage by possessing the structural integrity to withstand unreasonable amounts of sauce, cheese, and toppings.

Genius PARENT TRICK

Don't get too fancy with the dipping sauce. Papa John's includes one of eight different sauces with each order, but some carry a hefty load of sodium, sugar, or fat. At only 20 calories per ounce, the standard Pizza Dipping Sauce is the safest bet.

UNHAPPY MEALS

Full Order of Wings (10)

1,000 calories, 70 g fat (20 g saturated), 4,200 mg sodium

As a meal, these wings gobble up nearly 2 days' worth of sodium and saturated fat. A side of blue cheese tacks on another 170 calories and 18 grams of fat.

Other Passes

300 calories
11 g fat (3.5 g saturated)
750 mg sodium

Original Crust Cheese Pizza
14" (1 slice)

520 calories
33 g fat (7.5 g saturated)
1,140 mg sodium

Cheesesticks
with Special Garlic Dip (2 sticks)

570 calories
15 g fat (3 g saturated)
33 g sugars

Cinnamon Sweetsticks
(4)

P.F. Chang's China Bistro

Give Chang's credit for offering options like "stock velveted" (which replaces oil with vegetable stock in the cooking process) and being flexible with substitutions. But without a designated Kids' Menu, young eaters are forced to fly blind with the grown-ups, where massive, 1,000-calorie entrées are hard to avoid.

SURVIVAL STRATEGY
Turn appetizers into entrées. Dumplings, lettuce wraps, and spring rolls are all healthy eats.

GREAT GROWN-UP GRUB

Oolong Marinated Sea Bass

*521 calories,
12 g fat (3 g saturated),
37 g carbohydrates*

This meal deserves a nutritional gold star. The sea bass is rich with omega-3s and contains 64 grams of protein, and the oolong-tea marinade is packed with antioxidants. The fish dish comes with spinach, one of the most nutrient-rich foods on the planet, and ginger-infused soy, which promotes digestive health.

Eat This

Chang's Chicken Lettuce Wraps

with special sauce

*432 calories
13 g fat
(3 g saturated)
44 g carbohydrates*

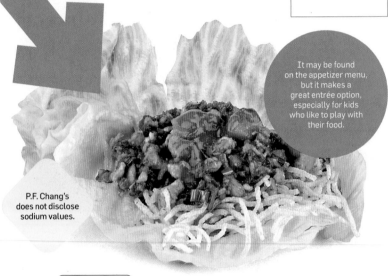

It may be found on the appetizer menu, but it makes a great entrée option, especially for kids who like to play with their food.

P.F. Chang's does not disclose sodium values.

Other Picks

Singapore Street Noodles

*572 calories
16 g fat (3 g saturated)
81 g carbohydrates*

Cantonese Shrimp

*330 calories
12 g fat (2 g saturated)
21 g carbohydrates*

Apple Pie Mini Dessert

*170 calories
4 g fat (2 g saturated)
34 g carbohydrates*

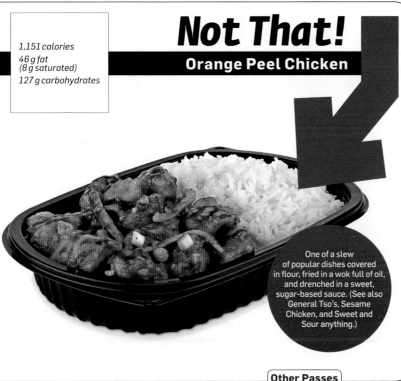

Not That!
Orange Peel Chicken

1,151 calories
46 g fat
(8 g saturated)
127 g carbohydrates

One of a slew of popular dishes covered in flour, fried in a wok full of oil, and drenched in a sweet, sugar-based sauce. (See also General Tso's, Sesame Chicken, and Sweet and Sour anything.)

Other Passes

1,198 calories
67 g fat (11 g saturated)
97 g carbohydrates

Chicken Lo Mein

977 calories
58 g fat (8 g saturated)
58 g carbohydrates

Kung Pao Shrimp

323 calories
12 g fat (7 g saturated)
50 g carbohydrates

S'Mores Mini Dessert

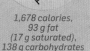

UNHAPPY MEALS
Tam's Noodle
with Savory Beef
and Shrimp

1,678 calories,
93 g fat
(17 g saturated),
138 g carbohydrates

If only the body had a warning system to protect us from unknowingly consuming massive doses of fat and carbohydrates. Even if you take half of this meal home in a to-go box, your child will still have eaten three-fourths of his or her daily fat.

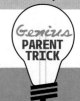

Genius
PARENT TRICK

Because diners are encouraged to order "family style" and pass dishes around the table, take charge of the ordering by telling your crew, "I know what's good here." Load up on the picks on this page and skip the passes and your family will be forced to eat healthy without ever knowing it.

Pizza Hut

Expect no surprises from this quintessential pizza parlor. The chain offers no kid-friendly beverage or side options, and with nothing else to choose from, a couple breadsticks and a soda tack hundreds of calories onto a pizza dinner. A thin-crust delivery can be a lifesaver in a pinch, but as for a buffet of nourishing options, Pizza Hut is an empty shack.

SURVIVAL STRATEGY
Avoid pepperoni at all costs. If the kids want meat, stick to ham and chicken, but try to add veggies whenever possible. The best possible scenario? Fit 'N Delicious Pizzas™. Any of them.

Eat This

Thin 'N Crispy Quartered Ham and Pineapple Pizza

12" (2 slices)

360 calories
12 g fat
(6 g saturated)
1,140 mg sodium

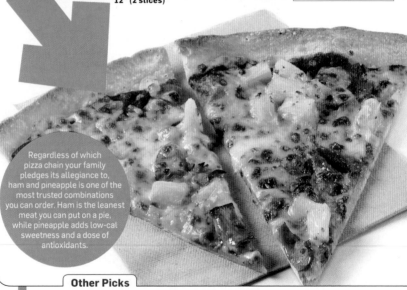

Regardless of which pizza chain your family pledges its allegiance to, ham and pineapple is one of the most trusted combinations you can order. Ham is the leanest meat you can put on a pie, while pineapple adds low-cal sweetness and a dose of antioxidants.

Other Picks

Thin 'N Crispy Pepperoni and Mushroom Pizza 12" (1 slice)

190 calories
8 g fat (3.5 g saturated)
560 mg sodium

Hand-Tossed Veggie Lover's Pizza 12" (1 slice)

210 calories
8 g fat (3.5 g saturated)
580 mg sodium

Fit 'N Delicious Diced Chicken, Red Onion & Green Pepper Pizza 12" (2 slices)

340 calories
9 g fat (4 g saturated)
1,040 mg sodium

400 calories
16 g fat
(9 g saturated)
1,140 mg sodium

Not That!

Thin 'N Crispy Cheese Pizza

12" (2 slices)

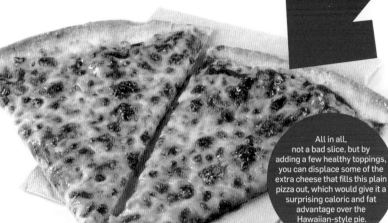

All in all, not a bad slice, but by adding a few healthy toppings, you can displace some of the extra cheese that fills this plain pizza out, which would give it a surprising caloric and fat advantage over the Hawaiian-style pie.

Other Passes

230 calories
11 g fat (4.5 g saturated)
620 mg sodium

Thin 'N Crispy Italian Sausage and Red Onion Pizza 12" (1 slice)

230 calories
10 g fat (4.5 g saturated)
620 mg sodium

Hand-Tossed Cheese Pizza
12" (1 slice)

420 calories
16 g fat (7 g saturated)
1,160 mg sodium

Hand-Tossed Veggie Lovers® Pizza
12" (2 slices)

Quizno's

Toasty or not, Quizno's offers some of America's worst sandwiches, including the 2,090-calorie large Tuna Melt. Cookies and fatty salads don't make matters any better. What does improve matters is Quizno's line of kid-size Sammies—the rare bright spot in an otherwise dark menu.

SURVIVAL STRATEGY

With a handful of Sammies at 200 calories, they make perfect meals for younger kids. You can double-up for the older eaters—even two of the healthier Sammies will be better than most small sandwiches.

GUILTY PLEASURES

Black Angus and Cheddar Breakfast Sandwich

390 calories, 17.5 g fat (9 g saturated), 1,040 mg sodium

Nothing beats Black Angus steak in the morning, and the 30-gram protein punch will help regulate blood sugar and keep your kid feeling strong through lunchtime.

Eat This

Roadhouse Steak Sammie

with dressing

*205 calories
4 g fat (1 g saturated)
565 mg sodium*

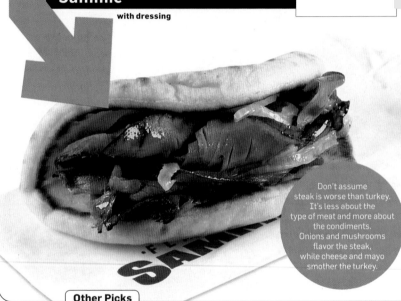

Don't assume steak is worse than turkey. It's less about the type of meat and more about the condiments. Onions and mushrooms flavor the steak, while cheese and mayo smother the turkey.

Other Picks

Small Honey Bourbon Chicken Sub

*310 calories
4 g fat (1 g saturated)
850 mg sodium*

Cantina Chicken Sammies
(2)

*410 calories
8 g fat (1 g saturated)
890 mg sodium*

Toasty® Turkey & Cheese with a Cup of Chili

*320 calories
11.5 g fat (3.5 g saturated)
1,235 mg sodium*

Not That!

Sonoma Turkey Flatbread Sammie

with cheese and dressing

300 calories
18 g fat
(4.5 g saturated)
815 mg sodium

Sammies are billed as low-price, low-calorie alternatives to Quizno's often disastrously caloric regular sandwiches, but clearly this little guy doesn't fit the bill.

Other Passes

500 calories
25 g fat (5 g saturated)
1,100 mg sodium

Honey Mustard Chicken with Bacon Sub (small)

620 calories
32 g fat (6 g saturated)
1,230 mg sodium

Alpine Chicken Sammies (2)

730 calories
22 g fat (7 g saturated)
1,680 mg sodium

Chili Bread Bowl

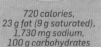

UNHAPPY MEALS
Country French Chicken Bread Bowl

720 calories,
23 g fat (9 g saturated),
1,730 mg sodium,
100 g carbohydrates

Soup is normally a safe route to go, but not when it comes served in a big pillowy bread bowl—which adds a totally unnecessary 400 calories to the meal. Need something to dunk? Try crackers.

FOOD MYTH #6

Salads are a low-fat, no-fail way to bring extra nutrition to your kid's diet.

Lettuce is healthy. Unfortunately, it's often relegated by restaurants to being a mere vehicle for a flurry of cheese, croutons, crumbled bacon, and fatty meats, making entrée-size salads consistently one of the worst things you can order from a menu. At Quizno's, the average salad with regular dressing and flatbread has 924 calories and 51 grams of fat. Nix the flatbread and sub in the balsamic vinaigrette to save up to 440 calories.

101

Red Lobster

Too bad Red Lobster makes it a policy not to disclose nutritional information—because we have a sneaking suspicion that they have some decent items on offer. But until they decide to show up to class and take the test, we'll be forced to fail them.

SURVIVAL STRATEGY
When it comes to seafood, the rule is pretty simple: Avoid anything that's been fried or covered in sauce.

SMART SIDES

Baked Potato with Pico de Gallo

*185 calories,
2 g fat,
37 carbohydrates*

Let your child enjoy the tasty health benefits of vitamin C and fiber found in potatoes—without decorating them with slabs and dollops of extra fat. The pico is made from carotenoid-rich tomatoes, and it only adds a measly 6 calories to the potato. That beats butter and sour cream any day.

Eat This

Snow Crab Legs
with seasoned broccoli and cocktail sauce

*318 calories
4.5 g fat
875 mg sodium*

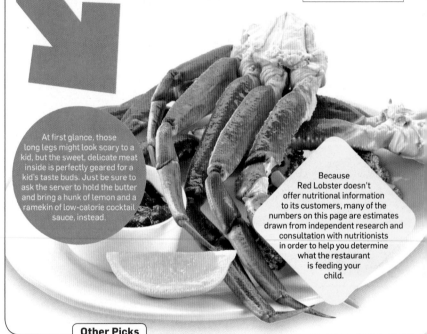

At first glance, those long legs might look scary to a kid, but the sweet, delicate meat inside is perfectly geared for a kid's taste buds. Just be sure to ask the server to hold the butter and bring a hunk of lemon and a ramekin of low-calorie cocktail sauce, instead.

Because Red Lobster doesn't offer nutritional information to its customers, many of the numbers on this page are estimates drawn from independent research and consultation with nutritionists in order to help you determine what the restaurant is feeding your child.

Other Picks

Garlic Grilled Jumbo Shrimp
and a baked potato with pico de gallo

*329 calories
5 g fat
670 mg sodium*

Kid's Popcorn Shrimp & Fries
with applesauce

*500 calories
22 g fat
970 mg sodium*

520 calories
28 g fat
1,110 mg sodium

Not That!

Grilled Chicken

with Caesar salad

It's not enough for the star of your plate to put on a good performance—you need some help from the supporting cast, too. Unfortunately, few players can muck up an otherwise worthy meal quite as quickly and thoroughly as a Caesar salad.

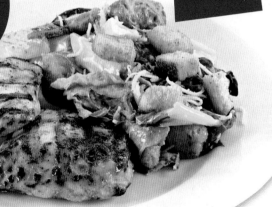

Genius PARENT TRICK

Pull your server aside quietly and ask him or her to limit your table to one round of biscuits. Seriously, each infamous Cheddar Bay Biscuit™ has 160 calories and 9 grams of fat.

DIP DECODER

● **LEMON JUICE:**
2 calories, 0 g fat

● **COCKTAIL SAUCE**
(large, 1/4 c): 87 calories, 2 g fat

● **TARTAR SAUCE** (1 oz):
100 calories, 10 g fat

● **MELTED BUTTER** (1 oz):
189 calories, 21 g fat

STEALTH HEALTH FOOD

Jumbo Shrimp Cocktail (10 shrimp)
228 calories, 4 g fat, 46 g protein

Aside from being a great source of lean protein, shrimp is packed with bone-strengthening vitamin D.

Other Passes

600 calories
35 g fat
985 mg sodium

Shrimp Linguine Alfredo
(half portion)

650 calories
38 g fat
1,560 mg sodium

Chicken Fingers & Fries
with veggies & ranch dip

Romano's Macaroni Grill

Romano's Macaroni Grill is home to a few of the worst kids' dishes in America and a menu that is more sodium-saturated than any we've ever come across. The only redeeming quality is that they allow diners to create their own pastas—which you should absolutely do.

SURVIVAL STRATEGY
Stick to kids' grilled chicken and spaghetti and meatballs, or an invented pasta made with wheat pasta with lots of veggies and red sauce.

HIDDEN DANGER
Roasted Chicken and Cheese Sandwich

This seemingly light lunch sandwich has more calories than a Burger King Triple Whopper® with cheese, mayonnaise, and medium fries.

1,630 calories,
91 g fat (23 g saturated),
2,520 mg sodium,
128 g carbohydrates

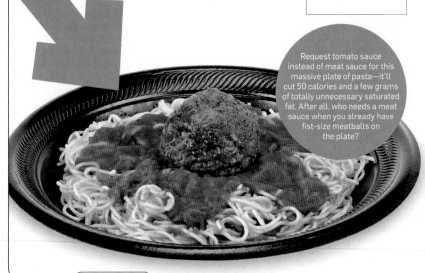

Eat This

Kids Spaghetti & Meatballs

with tomato sauce

500 calories
20 g fat
(8 g saturated)
1,520 mg sodium
22 g protein

Request tomato sauce instead of meat sauce for this massive plate of pasta—it'll cut 50 calories and a few grams of totally unnecessary saturated fat. After all, who needs a meat sauce when you already have fist-size meatballs on the plate?

Other Picks

Kids Grilled Chicken & Broccoli

390 calories
5 g fat (2 g saturated)
560 mg sodium

BBQ Chicken Pizza
(½ **adult pizza**)

485 calories
12 g fat (7 g saturated)
1,350 mg sodium

Italian Sorbetto with Biscotti

330 calories
4 g fat (2 g saturated)
80 mg sodium

Not That!

Kids Macaroni 'n' Cheese

600 calories
31 g fat
(20 g saturated)
1,720 mg sodium

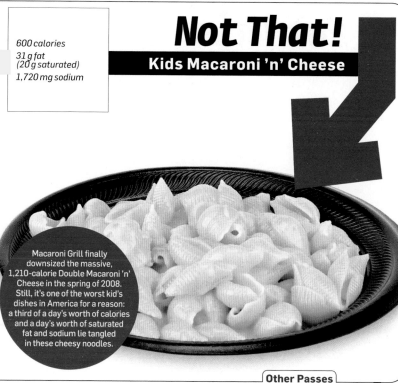

Macaroni Grill finally downsized the massive, 1,210-calorie Double Macaroni 'n' Cheese in the spring of 2008. Still, it's one of the worst kid's dishes in America for a reason: a third of a day's worth of calories and a day's worth of saturated fat and sodium lie tangled in these cheesy noodles.

Other Passes

730 calories
48 g fat (7 g saturated)
2,110 mg sodium

Kids Chicken Fingerias and Grilled Broccoli

920 calories
27 g fat (16 g saturated)
2,140 mg sodium

Kids Mona Lisa's Pepperoni Masterpizza

400 calories
23 g fat (14 g saturated)
100 mg sodium

Kid's Vanilla Ice Cream
with chocolate sauce

UNHAPPY MEALS
Twice Baked Lasagna with Meatballs

1,470 calories,
83 g fat
(41 g saturated),
4,420 mg sodium,
75 g carbohydrates

Garfield would really enjoy this lasagna meal, but that doesn't mean your kid should, and lucky for him, cartoons aren't real. In real life this meal would be better suited for four people. It provides the vast majority of the day's calories.

SMART SIDES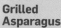

Grilled Asparagus

40 calories,
2 g fat (0 g saturated),
590 mg sodium

Asparagus can be a tough sell to a child, but you'll be the envy of every parent in the restaurant if you can pull it off. Asparagus is rich in inulin, a carbohydrate that humans don't digest. Instead, this carb fuels the growth of healthy, gut-protecting bacteria. Tell the kids they better feed the armies and fuel their war on evil bacteria.

Ruby Tuesday

No kids' menu is more polarized than Ruby Tuesday's, which serves up everything from a 276-calorie chicken breast to a 907-calorie plate of mini cheeseburgers. Ultimately, the few low-calorie options can't offset the fat bombs that lie scattered like landmines among Ruby Tuesday's kids' meals, but the numerous options for healthy sides help dampen the blow.

SURVIVAL STRATEGY
Stick to the Chicken Breast and Broccoli or Pasta with Marinara and your child can walk out unscathed.

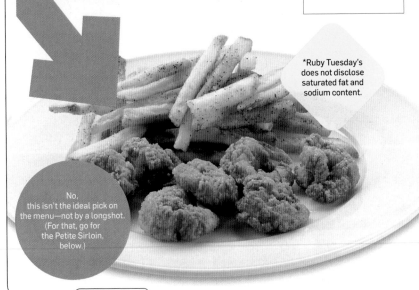

Eat This
Kid's Fried Shrimp & Fries

571 calories
21 g fat*
71 g carbohydrates

*Ruby Tuesday's does not disclose saturated fat and sodium content.

No, this isn't the ideal pick on the menu—not by a longshot. (For that, go for the Petite Sirloin, below.)

STEALTH HEALTH FOOD

White Bean Chicken Chili

*228 calories,
8 g fat,
26 g carbohydrates*

This chili is filled with navy beans and chicken, two low-fat foods with a protein punch. Add to that the fiber from the beans, and a cup of chili is likely to fill up a hungry kid better than a burger or a plate of French fries.

Other Picks

Chicken Oscar

469 calories
22 g fat*
7 g carbohydrates

Petite Sirloin
(7 oz) with creamy mashed cauliflower

359 calories
15 g fat*
16 g carbohydrates

Kids Pasta
with marinara

314 calories
4 g fat*
60 g carbohydrates

893 calories
47 g fat*
87 g carbohydrates

Not That!

Kids Turkey Minis & Fries

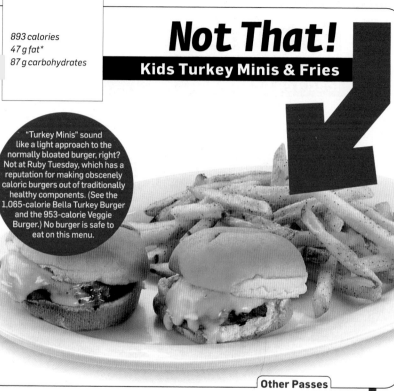

"Turkey Minis" sound like a light approach to the normally bloated burger, right? Not at Ruby Tuesday, which has a reputation for making obscenely caloric burgers out of traditionally healthy components. (See the 1,065-calorie Bella Turkey Burger and the 953-calorie Veggie Burger.) No burger is safe to eat on this menu.

SMART SIDES

Creamy Mashed Cauliflower

153 calories,
10 g fat,
14 g carbohydrates

This Southern recipe might be just what your children need to help them acquire a taste for cauliflower. The brainlike vegetable belongs to a family of vegetables called cruciferous vegetables. These vegetables— broccoli, cabbage, and Brussels sprouts, among others—might play a significant role in preventing cancer later in life.

HIDDEN DANGER
Parmesan Shrimp Pasta

Ordinarily you should nudge your kids toward the ocean waters, but not with this dish. The shrimp's leaner side is drowned out by 64 grams of cream-sauce fat.

1,216 calories,
64 g fat,
98 g carbohydrates

Other Passes

1,649 calories
95 g fat*
127 g carbohydrates

Parmesan Chicken Pasta

497 calories
35 g fat*
33 g carbohydrates

Kids Chop Steak & Mashed Potatoes

448 calories
24 g fat*
48 g carbohydrates

Kids Pasta
with butter

Starbucks

As any caffeine-addicted parent knows, there are few options for kids at a coffee shop. Starbucks is no exception. Whether due to an excess of sugar or a surge of caffeine (or both), nearly every drink here will have your kid treating your furniture like a trampoline. The food isn't any better; most snacks here are based on refined flour and sugar.

SURVIVAL STRATEGY
Get your kid hooked on lightly sweetened Tazo tea and you're golden. If not, skim milk with a shot of chocolate sauce is as safe as it gets.

GREAT GROWN-UP GRUB

Multigrain Bagel

360 calories,
5 g fat (0 g saturated),
420 mg sodium

This is one of the few things on the menu not too sweet for everyday consumption. It's packed with free-radical–fighting sunflower seeds. Couple that with 4 grams of fiber and 13 grams of protein, and your body might actually thank you for the trip.

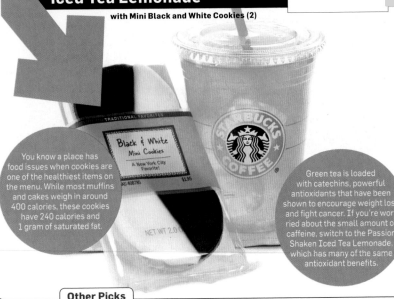

Eat This

Grande Tazo® Green Shaken Iced Tea Lemonade

with Mini Black and White Cookies (2)

370 calories
12 g fat
(1 g saturated)
55 g sugars

You know a place has food issues when cookies are one of the healthiest items on the menu. While most muffins and cakes weigh in around 400 calories, these cookies have 240 calories and 1 gram of saturated fat.

Green tea is loaded with catechins, powerful antioxidants that have been shown to encourage weight loss and fight cancer. If you're worried about the small amount of caffeine, switch to the Passion Shaken Iced Tea Lemonade, which has many of the same antioxidant benefits.

Other Picks

Grande Chocolate Milk
(nonfat milk with two shots of mocha syrup)

330 calories
3.5 g fat (0.5 g saturated)
54 g sugars

Cinnamon Raisin Bagel

330 calories
0 g fat
13 g sugars

Petite Vanilla Bean Scone

130 calories
5 g fat (3 g saturated)
9 g sugars

1,000 calories
52 g fat
(19 g saturated)
72 g sugars

Not That!

Grande White Hot Chocolate

(whole milk) with No Sugar Added Banana Nut Coffee Cake

Even with no sugar added, this cake still contains 420 calories and 28 grams of fat. Its sweetness comes from 36 grams of sugar alcohols, which, if ingested in excess, can create digestive problems.

Dark chocolate at least has antioxidants, but white chocolate isn't real chocolate at all. It's made from cocoa solids and corn syrup, and its role in this drink is deleterious: Combined with milk and whipped cream, it packs 520 calories and 61 grams of sugar.

Genius PARENT TRICK

Don't let the suits at Starbucks head-quarters dictate what your kids drink. Instead, help them customize their own beverages using any of the variety of flavored sugar-free syrups. At zero calories a pump, the price is right for a creative low-cal masterpiece.

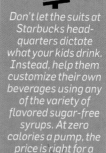

HIDDEN DANGER
Maple Oat Nut Scone

This little quick bread looks like a harmless snack, but it's actually a miniature nutritional nightmare. It has as much fat and calories as two slices of pepperoni pizza and more sugar than a pack of Reese's Peanut Butter Cups.

490 calories, 21 g fat (8 g saturated), 32 g sugar, 370 mg sodium

Other Passes

570 calories
15 g fat (9 g saturated)
83 g sugars

Grande Strawberries & Crème Frappuccino® Blended Crème

430 calories
18 g fat (2 g saturated)
26 g sugars

Walnut Bran Muffin

480 calories
22 g fat (12 g saturated)
24 g sugars

Blueberry Scone

Subway

A menu based on lean protein and vegetables is always going to score well in our book. With more than half a dozen kid-friendly sandwiches under 300 calories, plus a slew of soups and healthy sides to boot, Subway can satisfy even the pickiest eater without breaking the caloric bank. But, despite what Jared may want you to believe, Subway is not nutritionally infallible: Those rosy calorie counts posted on the menu boards include neither cheese nor mayo (add 160 calories per 6-inch sub) and some of the toasted subs, like the Meatball Marinara, contain hefty doses of calories, saturated fat, and sodium.

SURVIVAL STRATEGY
Cornell researchers have discovered a "health halo" at Subway, which refers to the tendency to reward yourself or your kid with chips, cookies, and large soft drinks because the entrée is healthy. Avoid the halo and all will be well.

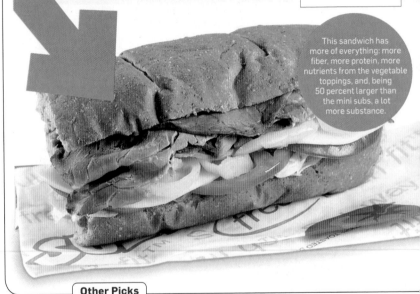

Eat This

Roast Beef Sub

6" with cheese on a wheat bun

340 calories
9.5 g fat
(4.5 g saturated)
930 mg sodium

This sandwich has more of everything: more fiber, more protein, more nutrients from the vegetable toppings, and, being 50 percent larger than the mini subs, a lot more substance.

Other Picks

Oven-Roasted Chicken Breast Sub
6"

310 calories
5 g fat (1.5 g saturated)
830 mg sodium

Steak & Cheese
6"

400 calories
12 g fat (6 g saturated)
1,110 mg sodium

Chili Con Carne

290 calories
8 g fat (3.5 g saturated)
990 mg sodium
12 g fiber

370 calories
22.5 g fat
(7 g saturated)
720 mg sodium

Not That!

Tuna Mini Sub

Approx. 4" with cheese on a white bun

Use the custom-sub shtick to your advantage. Load your kid up on veggies and you can easily knock out a couple servings for the day. Push for tomatoes, olives, sweet banana peppers, and spinach leaves.

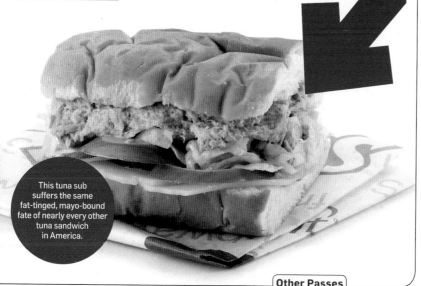

This tuna sub suffers the same fat-tinged, mayo-bound fate of nearly every other tuna sandwich in America.

SMART SIDES

Raisins
One little-known benefit of raisins is that they help fight cavities. Raisins contain oleanolic acid, a phytonutrient that kills the cavity-causing bacteria inside the mouth.

Other Passes

---

410 calories
10 g fat (3 g saturated)
1,070 mg sodium

Chicken Breast Wrap

---

560 calories
24 g fat (11 g saturated)
1,590 mg sodium

Meatball Marinara
6"

---

200 calories
12 g fat (5 g saturated)
1,180 mg sodium
2 g fiber

Golden Broccoli & Cheese Soup

SUGAR SPIKES

Sweet Onion Chicken Teriyaki Sandwich (6")

The Impact:
19 g sugars

Do you really want five teaspoons of sugar dumped on your sandwich—especially one that Subway considers a weight-loss option?

111

T.G.I. Friday's

We do applaud Friday's efforts to offer reduced portion sizes for high-calorie bombs, but we don't approve of their reluctance to provide hard data on any of their dishes. Between the array of deep-fried starters and mammoth sandwiches, it's clear they have something to hide.

SURVIVAL STRATEGY
The Lighter Side of Fridays contains five items with approximately "10 grams of fat and 500 calories." It's a sorry attempt at transparency, but until they offer real data, it's the best option.

Eat This

Half Rack of Ribs

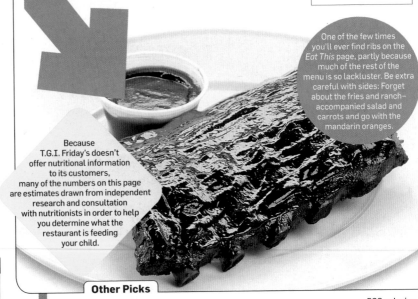

500 calories
18 g fat
650 mg sodium

One of the few times you'll ever find ribs on the *Eat This* page, partly because much of the rest of the menu is so lackluster. Be extra careful with sides: Forget about the fries and ranch–accompanied salad and carrots and go with the mandarin oranges.

Because T.G.I. Friday's doesn't offer nutritional information to its customers, many of the numbers on this page are estimates drawn from independent research and consultation with nutritionists in order to help you determine what the restaurant is feeding your child.

Other Picks

Dragonfire Chicken

500 calories
10 g fat
825 mg sodium

Kid's Mac & Cheese

240 calories
7 g fat
770 mg sodium

Kid's Sherbet

150 calories
0 g fat
22 g sugars

1,430 calories
82 g fat
1,450 mg sodium

Not That!

Loaded Potato Skins

(½ order)

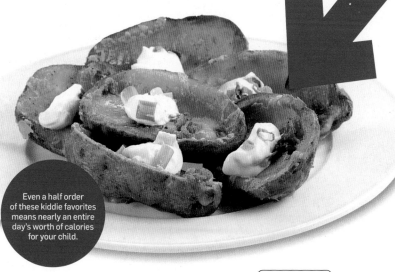

Even a half order of these kiddie favorites means nearly an entire day's worth of calories for your child.

Other Passes

1,360 calories 78 g fat 1,890 mg sodium	**Friday's Chicken Sandwich**
600 calories 20 g fat 1,100 mg sodium	**Kid's Spaghetti**
310 calories 14 g fat 28 g sugars	**Kid's Ice Cream**

76

The percentage of 300 chefs recently surveyed who felt that they were serving regular-size portions of steak and pasta. In reality, the average serving was 2 to 4 times bigger than the government-recommended portion size!

UNHAPPY MEALS
Peruvian Herb Roasted Chicken

1,320 calories

In real life, roasted chicken is a reliably nutritious meal for busy parents the world over, but whichever Friday's chef crossed the equator to drag back this monstrous bird should lose his job. The restaurant manages to turn a reliably nutritious meal into the caloric equivalent of six scoops of ice cream.

Taco Bell

Diners live and die by the mix-and-match opportunities Taco Bell presents, where any two items can either be a reasonable 400-calorie meal or a 900-calorie saturated-fat fest.

SURVIVAL STRATEGY
Cut out the big-ticket items like Mexican Pizzas and Nachos and direct your kid's attention to the crunchy tacos, bean burritos, and anything on the Fresco menu.

HIDDEN DANGER
Fiesta Taco Salad

Hearing that your kid actually wants to eat salad might sound exciting at first, but not when that salad packs as much fat as 15 slices of bacon. Here's a no-fail rule to establish in your family: Nothing is to be eaten out of oversize fried tortilla bowls.

840 calories,
45 g fat
(11 g saturated,
1.5 g trans),
1,780 mg sodium

Eat This

Fresco Crunchy Beef Tacos
(2)

300 calories
16 g fat
(5 g saturated)
740 mg sodium

Choose crunchy over soft tacos when you run for the border—you'll save 30 calories and 280 milligrams of sodium per taco.

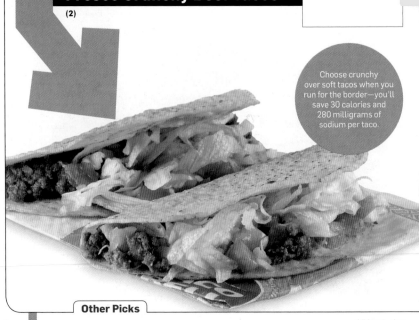

Other Picks

Steak Gordita
Nacho Cheese

270 calories
12 g fat (2 g saturated, 1 g trans)
680 mg sodium

Chicken Grilled Taquitos

310 calories
11 g fat (4.5 g saturated)
980 mg sodium

Pintos 'n Cheese

160 calories
6 g fat (3 g saturated)
670 mg sodium

540 calories
28 g fat
(8 g saturated)
1,640 mg sodium

Not That!

Ranchero Chicken Soft Tacos

(2)

These tacos may seem similar, but with the soft tacos you're getting nearly twice the calories, 75 percent more fat, and more than double the sodium.

Other Passes

340 calories
19 g fat (3.5 g saturated, 2.5 g trans)
670 mg sodium

Steak Chalupa
Nacho Cheese

520 calories
28 g fat (12 g saturated)
1,420 mg sodium

Chicken Quesadilla

290 calories
17 g fat (4 g saturated)
830 mg sodium

Cheesy Fiesta Potatoes

Genius
PARENT TRICK

Defang this cheesy, saucy menu by ordering everything Fresco style. This simple, free designation substitutes the cheese and sauce for Fiesta Salsa—a blend of diced tomatoes, onions, and cilantro. Most items outside the Fresco Menu can still be ordered this way.

UNHAPPY MEALS
Grilled Beef Stuft Burrito

680 calories,
30 g fat (10 g saturated,
1 g trans),
2,120 mg sodium

This burrito earns its big figures on sheer size; it's more than twice as big as a chalupa. When it comes to feeding your kids on the fly, remember to stick with the rational rations.

Uno Chicago Grill

The fact that Uno invented deep-dish pizza, one of the most fat- and calorie-dense foods on the planet, merits an automatic F, but we'll look past that to the more reasonable flat-bread pizzas and the handful of redeeming entrées, like the Kid's Grilled Chicken and the Kid's Pasta.

SURVIVAL STRATEGY
Do not, under any circumstances, order deep-dish pizza—a single "individual" pizza can house up to 2,300 calories. Instead, split a couple of flatbread pies and large house salads with the family.

SUGAR SP KES

Uno Deep Dish Sundae (½)

The Impact: 68 g sugars

This dessert slaps a load of sugar onto the end of the meal, not to mention 700 calories and 18 grams of saturated fat. If you plan to order indulgences like this, split them with as many people as you can wrangle over to the table.

Eat This

Cheese & Tomato Flatbread Pizza

(½) and House Side Salad with fat-free vinaigrette

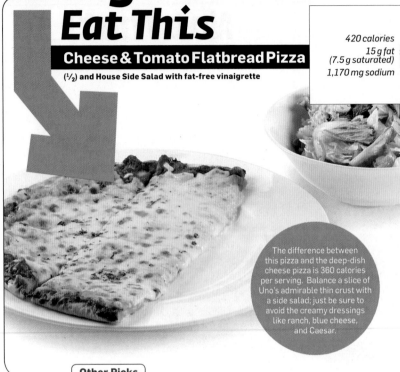

420 calories
15 g fat
(7.5 g saturated)
1,170 mg sodium

The difference between this pizza and the deep-dish cheese pizza is 360 calories per serving. Balance a slice of Uno's admirable thin crust with a side salad; just be sure to avoid the creamy dressings like ranch, blue cheese, and Caesar.

Other Picks

Grilled & Skewered BBQ Shrimp
and brown rice with Craisins® and mango

430 calories
7 g fat (0.5 g saturated)
1,085 mg sodium

Kid's Grilled Chicken

180 calories
6 g fat (0 g saturated)
840 mg sodium

Kid's Slush

140 calories
0 g fat
32 g sugars

700 calories
26 g fat
(12 g saturated)
1,640 mg sodium

Not That!
Kid's Cheese Pizza

The thick, doughy crust and a glut of cheese make this a perilous pizza to feed your kid. The only redeeming quality? It's 100 calories and 420 milligrams of sodium lighter than the kids' pepperoni pizza.

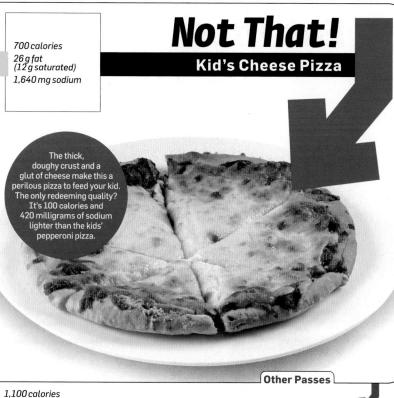

1.8

The number of times around the world Uno Chicago Grill could wrap the pasta it sells each year.

MENU DECODER

● **PHASE:** A mix of partially hydrogenated soybean oil and artificial flavoring that Uno uses to season the Kid's Corn. If they go for the corn, ask for the corn Phase-free.

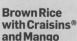

SMART ● SIDES
Brown Rice with Craisins® and Mango

170 calories, 5 g fat (0.5 g saturated), 30 g carbohydrates

Whole grains are the foundation of good nutrition, and this brown-rice dish makes whole grains taste delicious. It's sweetened with real fruit, and a splash of olive oil gives it a rich flavor and a healthy dose of omega-3s.

Other Passes

1,100 calories
62 g fat (24 g saturated)
1,640 mg sodium

Shrimp Scampi

320 calories
20 g fat (4 g saturated)
780 mg sodium

Kid's Chicken Caesar Salad

840 calories
36 g fat (18 g saturated)
98 g sugars

Kid's Sundae

117

Wendy's

Wendy's official kid's menu may be a tiny concession to the little ones, but it is free of the belly-busters that hamper most menus. Plus, the rest of the menu offers ample options for a growing kid; a cup of chili and a baked potato, chicken salad, even a burger with a cup of mandarin oranges all qualify as nutritionally commendable meals.

SURVIVAL STRATEGY
The Super Value Menu® is full of solid choices, as long as you avoid the 480-calorie add-on of fries and a regular soft drink.

SUGAR SPIKES

Vanilla Frosty™ Float with Coca-Cola®

The Impact:
69 g sugars

This is a cloying combination of two hyper-sweetened drinks, so you can't expect the outcome to be good. Settle for a junior Frosty and cut two-thirds of the sugar. If your kid wants dessert, stick to the classic chocolate Frosty, junior-size, for 160 calories and 21 grams of sugar.

Eat This

Single Burger with Everything

430 calories
20 g fat
7 g saturated)
870 mg sodium

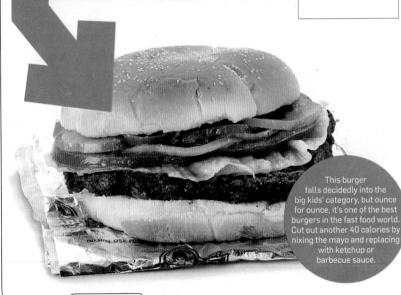

This burger falls decidedly into the big kids' category, but ounce for ounce, it's one of the best burgers in the fast food world. Cut out another 40 calories by nixing the mayo and replacing with ketchup or barbecue sauce.

Other Picks

Small Chili
with a broccoli and cheese baked potato

540 calories
8 g fat (3.5 g saturated)
1,240 mg sodium

Crispy Chicken Sandwich

330 calories
14 g fat (2.5 g saturated)
670 mg sodium

Jr. Cheeseburger

270 calories
11 g fat (5 g saturated)
690 mg sodium

540 calories
25 g fat
(8 g saturated)
1,360 mg sodium

Not That!
Chicken Club Sandwich

Chicken doesn't always trump beef, especially when it's dressed with bacon and cheese. At 320 calories, the Ultimate Chicken Grill sandwich is the best chicken sandwich on the menu.

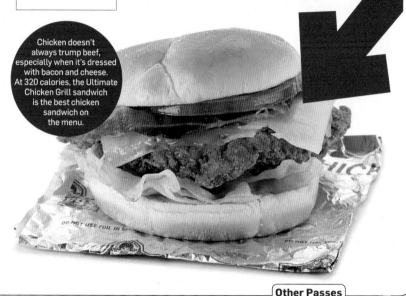

Other Passes

670 calories
39 g fat (16.5 g saturated, 1.5 g trans)
1,530 mg sodium

Southwest Taco Salad
with reduced fat sour cream

360 calories
27 g fat (5 g saturated)
740 mg sodium

Crispy Chicken Nuggets
(5 pieces) with Honey Mustard Nuggets Sauce

320 calories
16 g fat (4.5 g saturated)
860 mg sodium

Homestyle Chicken Go Wrap

Genius
PARENT TRICK

If your kid insists on a dip, think outside the sauce. Some locations carry reduced-fat ranch and honey mustard salad dressings, which can be substituted in place of the nugget sauce. This sleight of hand will make up to 80 calories and 13 grams of fat disappear from your child's meal.

SAUCE DECODER
(1 OZ EACH)

● **ZESTY ONION:** 150 calories, 15 g fat (2.5 g saturated)

● **RANCH:** 140 calories, 15 g fat (2.5 g saturated)

● **HONEY MUSTARD:** 90 calories, 6 g fat (1 g saturated)

● **BUFFALO:** 80 calories, 8 g fat (1.5 g saturated)

● **SWEET & SOUR:** 45 calories, 0 g fat

● **BARBECUE:** 40 calories, 0 g fat

EAT
THIS
NOT
THAT!

FOR
KIDS!

Your Ticket to Eat Anywhere

Maybe your family doesn't eat out at chain restaurants, or maybe you're fortunate enough to live in a city where your eating options extend beyond the world of Big Macs and Bloomin' Onions. Or maybe you just like to balance your Taco Bell with tuna rolls. Either way, parents need to know exactly what they're getting into when they decide to eat out, whether the restaurant of choice is a mom-and-pop pizza parlor or a neighborhood sushi joint.

We know what you're thinking: There's no way my kid's going to eat at a sushi restaurant. While she might not be ready for the raw sea urchin nigiri or the fugu-tasting menu, there are a surprising number of great options at sushi restaurants, each perfectly suited to a young eater's taste buds. Same goes for Indian, Spanish, Thai, and all of the other great cuisines you tend to ignore when a chicken nugget-craving crew of youngsters is in tow.

These cuisines—increasingly available everywhere from suburban strip malls to the far-flung corners of this country—are built around a variety of vegetables, lean proteins, and antioxidant-packed spices and flavor agents that make them a pleasure to eat and a boon to your kid's overall health.

It would be a shame to miss out on the melting pot of menus this country has to offer. Take a chance from time to time. That way, your kids get to explore and appreciate new foods from an early age, reaping the culinary and nutritional benefits of a well-rounded eater. And you get a break from the stovetop and the drive-thru window. Everybody wins.

In this chapter, we'll show you how to navigate a world of cuisine and become master of your children's nutritional universe.

Learn how to eat well and shed pounds at your favorite neighborhood restaurants with the Ultimate Menu Decoder interactive tool at **eatthis.com**

5 Ways to Win Over a Picky Eater

Exasperated moms and dads will try anything to win over a finicky eater: begging, bribing, even sneaking new foods into their kids' diets in hopes of a breakthrough at the dinner table. Thwarted and dejected, they form support groups and commiserate over chicken-finger lust and mac-and-cheese mania.

But it doesn't have to be this way. True, kids aren't born with an innate desire to devour lima beans and Dover sole, but parents have tools for teasing out their kids' more sophisticated taste buds. Follow these five simple rules and you'll be well on your way to raising an adventurous eater.

1. **START YOUNG.** Let your child cruise through his early years with nary a vegetable on his fork and you'll have raised a picky eater for life.

2. **HONE THE TASTE BUDS AT HOME.** Kids are more likely to try new foods in a familiar setting. Once they've seen or tasted something mom or dad has cooked for them, they'll be more willing to seek it out on a restaurant menu.

3. **BUILD OFF OF FAMILIAR FOODS.** Barbecued chicken is a staple in most American homes, so use that as a jumping-off point for exploring new cuisines. Indians have tandoori chicken, Thais have chicken satay, and the Japanese have chicken teriyaki—all twists on that comfortable kid-favorite with hints of exotic flavors. By accustoming their taste buds to foreign flavors with familiar vehicles, you'll slowly open up new doors.

4. **PLAY "FIRST BITE, LAST BITE."** In his book *The Parking Lot Rules and 75 Other Ideas for Raising Children*, author Tom Sturges suggests this simple strategy: To get a child to try a new food, promise him he can have the last bite of your dessert if he tries a first bite of a new food. Whether it's poached salmon or simply a strange new fruit, he doesn't need to eat the whole thing, he just needs to try the first bite. Maybe he'll hate it, but who knows? Maybe he'll discover something new, healthy, and delicious!

5. **DON'T INSULT THEIR TASTE BUDS.** It's true, kids have sensitive palates, and it's important to avoid excess spice on your way to introducing them to new flavors. But that doesn't mean food should be boring. A splash of soy sauce, a touch of Tabasco, or a bit of balsamic vinegar could be the difference between outright rejection and love at first bite.

Breakfast Diner

HOME FRIES

The equivalent of starting your day with a big plate of French fries. Stick with the grits, or sub in fresh fruit instead —many diners will do it free of charge.

TOAST

Insist that all toast brought to the table be of the wheat variety. One of the main nutrients you and your kids need for breakfast is belly-filling fiber, and making the simple switch from white to wheat will give you a much-needed 5-gram fiber boost.

FRENCH TOAST, PANCAKES, AND WAFFLES

Each of these three breakfast favorites makes for a less-than-ideal start to your kid's day. That's because all are based on refined flour, and all eventually get covered in sugary syrup. The surge of quick-burning carbohydrates spikes blood sugar and signals the body to start storing fat. And when the blood sugar levels come crashing down, so do your kid's energy levels and attention span.

BACON OR SAUSAGE

This might seem like an insignificant decision, since most people consider both of these breakfast meats to be equally treacherous. The truth is, two sausage links have about 160 calories and 12 grams of fat, whereas two strips of bacon contain 80 calories and 8 grams of fat.

BREAKFAST SPECIALS

Our value-oriented breakfast specials come with your choice coffee or tea and a small juice.

MT. AIRY
TWO EGGS, ANY STYLE, with your choice of breakfast meat, home fries, grits or white cheddar grits. White, wheat or rye toast. 7.95
Add Bagel or English muffin for .... $.50.

WAYNE JUNCTION
CLASSIC EGGS BENEDICT Grilled Canadian bacon served under poached eggs and rich Hollandaise neatly stacked on a toasted English muffin. Comes with your choice of home fries, grits or white cheddar grits. 8.95

WYNDMOOR
THICK-CUT SLICES OF CINNAMON-RAISIN CHALLAH FRENCH TOAST with your choice of breakfast meat. Served dusted with powdered sugar. 7.95

GRAVERS
THREE FLUFFY BUTTERMILK PANCAKES with your choice of breakfast meat....... 7.45
Add bananas, blueberries or strawberries 1.00

UPSAL
GOLDEN MALTED BELGIAN WAFFLE with your choice of breakfast meat. 7.45
Add bananas, blueberries or strawberries and whipped cream 1.00

MARTIN'S
HONEY-BUCKWHEAT PANCAKES with bananas and served with your choice of breakfast meat. 8.50
blueberries or chocolate chips 1.00

FRENCH TOAST, PANCAKES, WAFFLES

cooked on our griddle and served with butter and syrup.
Top your griddles with bananas, blueberries, chocolate chips or strawberry topping for 1.00

PANCAKES
STACK (3)
SHORT STACK (2)
BUTTERMILK PANCAKES
Stack 4.25
Short Stack 3.75
HONEY BUCKWHEAT PANCAKES
Stack 5.50
Short Stack 4.75
WHOLE GRAIN PANCAKES
Stack 5.50
Short Stack 4.75

FRENCH TOAST
TEXAS STYLE FRENCH TOAST
Full Stack 3.50
Short Stack 2 .... 2.75

BELGIAN WAFFLE
BELGIAN WAFFLE 3.50

EGG COMBOS

All carefully prepared 3-egg omelettes come with your choice of home fries, cheese grits and white or wheat toast

3 EGG OMELETTES

CHEESE OMELETTE 4.75
HAM OR BACON OMELETTE 4.95
SPINACH & FETA OMELETTE 4.75
VEGGIE OMELETTE 4.95
Mushroom, Onion, Pepper & Tomato
WESTERN OMELETTE 4.95
Ham, Onion & Pepper
PEASANT OMELETTE 4.75
Sausage, Potatoes & Onion
LOX & ONION OMELETTE 6.25
SUBSTITUTE EGG WHITES for .. 1.00
ADDITIONAL OMELETTE ITEMS ..... .50¢
EACH
Ham, Bacon, Sausage, Potato, Peppers,
Broccoli, Onions, Spinach, Mushrooms,
Tomato, Cheese (American, Swiss,
Mozzarella or Cheddar)

FARM FRESH EGGS

served with home fries or grits & toast
ONE EGG, Any Style, with Toast .. 1...
TWO EGGS, Any Style, with Toast 2.25
with Home Fries & Toast 3.75
STEAK & EGGS 6 oz. Center Cut Strip
Steak with Two Eggs prepared Any Style,
served with your choice of Home Fries or
Grits and toast 12.95
FISH & GRITS Cornmeal-dusted Catfish
lightly fried and served with Grits or
Cheese Grits 6.95
with Two Eggs 8.45

CONTINENTAL CHOICES

BREADS & MUFFINS

TOAST 1.00
ENGLISH MUFFIN 1.00
ASSORTED MUFFINS 1.35
choice of blueberry, bran, apple or corn
BAGEL 1.00
choice of plain, sesame seed, poppy or
everything
with Cream Cheese 1.50
DANISH 1.25

SIDE ORDERS

HOME FRIES 1.50
BACON, SAUSAGE, SCRAPPLE .. 1.85
CORNED BEEF HASH 2.25

CEREALS & FRUITS

CEREAL with Milk ....
with choice of fruit ....
KETTLE OATS ....
with choice of fruit ....
GRITS .... 1.
with Cheese .... 2.
FRESH FRUIT SALAD 3.2-
with Cottage Cheese 4.25

BEVERAGES

CHILLED JUICES
Orange, Apple, Grapefruit, or Tomato ...
1.50
BOTTOMLESS COFFEE 1.50
HOT TEA 1.00
ICE COLD MILK 1.50

ALL DAY BREAKFAST

Served from 3:00 p.m. to closing Monday-Saturday 3:30 p.m. to closing Sunday
We feature 100% homemade breads.
Choice of breakfast meat includes: Bacon, sausage links and scrapple.
Home fries can be prepared with fried onions at no additional charge.
An 18% gratuity will be added to parties of six or more.

EGGS, ANY STYLE

Despite vilification by the food police, eggs are one of the healthiest foods on the planet. A large raw egg contains 75 calories and 5 grams of fat—much of that healthy, unsaturated fat, including omega-3 fatty acids. Plus, eggs are rich in choline, a nutrient essential to brain and memory function. Any style of preparation will do, but the absolutely healthiest choice here is poaching, a slow-boiling method that produces creamy whites and yolks without the addition of cooking fat.

OATMEAL

The best choice on the menu. Oats are low in fat and sodium and contain plenty of soluble fiber, which helps lower bad cholesterol and regulate blood sugar levels.

GRITS

The southern version of Cream of Wheat®, made with yellow or white cornmeal. At 175 calories for a side, it outshines any breakfast potato that might be offered on the menu.

FRESHLY SQUEEZED OJ

Yes, it might constitute a serving of fruit for your child, but that serving comes with as much as 150 calories and 35 grams of sugar. That much sugar that early in the morning might provide an initial surge of energy but it eventually gives way to a good old-fashioned sugar crash.

Pizzeria

BREADSTICKS

Skip 'em. First of all, you're already eating pizza, so what's the need for another version of oil-soaked bread? On top of that, the tub of garlic sauce the pizza places so thoughtfully provide for dipping is really just a slurry of trans fat–bearing partially hydrogenated oils. That one tub has as many calories as two slices of pizza. Which would you prefer?

MOZZARELLA STICKS

Few things on this planet are worse for you than breaded and fried cheese. They might be a kid favorite, but at 125 calories and a heap of saturated fat per small stick, they are a parent's nightmare. Curb the cheese craving with an 80-calorie string cheese.

CALZONE

These football-size dough pockets hold an ungodly amount of cheese and toppings; even a small hunk of calzone could run up to 500 calories and 25 grams of fat. If it's cheese and sauce you seek, stick to pizza.

KIDS' PIZZA

It's almost always better to give your kids a slice or two from a large pizza than it is to order the kids' pizza. That's because kids' portions are often the same exact serving as a personal pizza that any adult might order on his or her own—and those pack anywhere between 550 and 750 calories.

APPETIZERS & SIDES

Breadsticks A 12" roll covered with fresh garlic. Served with garlic dipping sauce. 2.99

French Fries A large order of our delicious golden fries. 3.29

Onion Rings A large order of our golden battered onion rings. 3.99

Mozzarella Sticks Six lightly seasoned breaded mozzarella sticks served with marinara sauce. 8.99

Cheese Fries A large order of fries, smothered in cheese sauce 3.79

Buffalo Wings Tender Chicken wings, golden fried, then tossed in buffalo sauce. Served with blue cheese dressing. (24) 12.49

OUR SPECIALS

Red or White Pie Red, Our version of the traditional Neapolitan, cheese pizza. White, A delicious blend of fresh garlic, oregano, Romano, Mozzarella, and our special white herb sauce! 9.59

Calzone Traditional style with pepperoni, sausage, meatballs, peppers, onions, fresh garlic, Romano and Mozzarella all wrapped up in our homemade pizza dough! 11.59

KIDS MENU

Mac 'n' Cheese Just like Mom makes. 4.99

Kids Pizza A 5" thin crust cheese pizza with your choice of dipping sauce. 5.99

Chicken Fingers Breaded chicken breast tenderloins, fried to golden brown perfection. Served with your choice of dipping sauce. 4.99 with French Fries 5.99

Burger and Fries A quarter-pound meat patty and cheddar cheese served with French Fries 5.99

OUR PIZZA PIES

3 Cheese Pizza Mozzarella, Romano, and Gruyere with our marinara

Pizza Marinara No cheese, Vegan option! 8.59

Veggie Lovers Pizza A mountain of fresh vegetables piled high onto ou

Meat Lovers Pizza 5 toppings - Bacon, Beef, Ham, Pepperoni, and Sausage

The Cheese Steak Pizza with Fresh Grilled Rib Eye Steak, Cheese, Mushrooms a Onions 15.59

Sicilian Pizza with tomatoes, onion, sausage, anchovies, parmesan and herbs 15.99

Hawaiian Style Pizza A red pie topped with tender diced ham & juicy pineapple chunks 12.99

Buffalo Chicken A red pie topped with tender cooked chicken breast, marinated in our own special buffalo sauce. 13.59

Thick Crust American A combination of ground beef, Cheddar cheese, tomatoes, onions and peppers with sauce on top 11.59

OLD WORLD SALADS

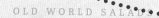

House Salad Fresh chopped Romaine lettuce, red onions, black olives & tomatoes. with blue cheese, ranch or red wine vinaigrette 5.50

Caesar Salad Fresh chopped Romaine lettuce, croutons, black olives, and shredded parmesan cheese with Caesar dressing served on the side 6.50

Antipasto Salad Quality Italian meats & cheese over a bed of romaine lettuce topped with olives, onions, roasted peppers, shredded parmesan & red wine vinaigrette 8.50

Chicken and Veggie Salad our house salad with broccoli, carrots, celery, cucumbers topped with seasoned, grilled chicken breast. 8.50

Buffalo Chicken Salad Breaded chicken tenderloin strips, tossed in buffalo sauce, on top of our house salad. 8.50

VEGGIE PIZZA

Consider this a vegetable-eaters starter kit, complete with enough cheese and sauce to make those veggies go down easier. Seriously, considering the lack of vegetables in most kids' diets, you need to take advantage of any opportunity to slip in a serving of produce.

SICILIAN PIZZA

Don't be fooled by the authentic-sounding place of origin: This is just a code word for a thick, oily crust with little of the stuff—marinara, vegetables—that your kid actually needs.

THICK CRUST

Not only does the extra dough mean a 75-calorie premium on every slice, it also lends the pizza the structural integrity to withstand a heavier bombardment of toppings. In total, figure double the calories for thick over thin crust.

CHICKEN AND BROCCOLI

Broccoli contains sulforaphane and chicken is packed with selenium. While both have been shown to be potent cancer- and disease-fighters on their own, studies show that eating the two together may multiply their beneficial effects by as much as 13 times.

Family Restaurant

SECRET SAUCE

There's no secret here: Nearly every mysterious sauce across this great land consists of 80 percent mayonnaise and 20 percent ketchup, usually with a smattering of chopped pickles thrown in. Replace it with decidedly less-secretive barbecue sauce and save 100 calories.

FRENCH DIP

We have no idea what makes this sandwich French—it was invented in Los Angeles—but it's a surprisingly safe choice. Roast beef is nearly every bit as lean as roast turkey, and the beef stock dipping sauce only adds about 25 calories to the total.

CHICKEN SANDWICH

Not always as safe as it seems. An array of variables can make this either the healthiest choice on the menu or one of the most deceptively bad. Here's the quick checklist: Is it fried? Is there mayo or ranch? Does it come with cheese? Answer yes to more than one of these questions, and your kid may as well eat a cheeseburger.

OMELETTES

OMELETTES ARE OUR SPECIALTY. MAKE YOUR CHOICE OF 3 OR 4 FARM FRESH EGGS

THE STANDARD *2 or 3 eggs any style, hash browns, choice of meat, toast and jelly*

VEGGIE *green pepper, onion, mushrooms, tomatoes, broccoli and cheese*

GREEK *gyro meat, feta cheese, tomatoes and onion*

SOUTHERN *green pepper, onion and ham, smothered in sausage gravy*

MEXICAN *homemade chili, tomatoes, onion and cheese*

MUSHROOM *mushrooms and cheese*

FETA CHEESE *imported Greek feta cheese and tomatoes*

CHEESE

HAM AND CHEESE *generous portions of ham and cheese*

WESTERN *green pepper, onion and ham*

FARMERS *our most popular omelette, ham, green pepper, onion, potatoes and cheese*

CLOVELEAF *corned beef, potatoes and eggs*

2 OR 3 EGGS, *Any Style, Choice of Meat, Toast and Jelly*

SANDWICHES

HAMBURGER *served with onions, lettuce, tomatoes, pickles and our secret sauce on a bun*
$3.49

GYROS *served with tomatoes, onions and our on special sauce on pita bread*
$4.89

CHICKEN GYRO *sliced chicken breast served with tomatoes, onion and special sauce on pita bread*
$5.49

CLOVERLEAF CLUB *bacon, lettuce, tomato with Turkey, Swiss and American cheeses*
$5.69

GRILLED CHICKEN *marinated in olive oil with oregano, garlic, salt and pepper*
$4.89

TRIPLE DECKER *ham or Turkey and 3 slices of Swiss or American cheese*
$4.59

PATTY MELT *1/4 lb. burger cooked to order with grilled onion and Swiss on rye*
$3.89

RIBEYE STEAK HOAGIE *grilled with onions, green peppers and mushrooms, topped with Swiss cheese*
$5.99

FRENCH DIP *served hot with thinly sliced roast beef on a baguette and a side of au jus*
$5.99

TUNA FISH SANDWICH
$3.69

HOT DOG
$1.89

CHILI DOG
$1.99

BLT
$3.59

FISH SANDWICH *breaded and deep fried served with tartar sauce and cole slaw*
$4.69

SIDES

When it comes to eating at American-style family restaurants, nutritional battles are won and lost on the "sides" front. As a rule, starches—including rice, pasta, and potato dishes—are losers, packed full of quick-burning carbohydrates that spike blood sugar and do little to fill your kids up. Steamed, roasted, or grilled vegetables; fresh fruit; or even applesauce are the winners in the bunch.

CHEESE FRIES

Pretty much the worst thing anyone— kid or parent—can put in his or her body. A single appetizer-size order with a side of ranch is the caloric equivalent of 14 Taco Bell® beef tacos. Even if you split an order among four people, you're still looking at nearly 700 calories and 40 grams of fat per serving.

BAKED POTATO

Loaded baked potatoes are too caloric to be considered a healthy side, but a jacket stuffed with steamed broccoli and a bit of melted cheese makes a filling, nutritious, 400-calorie meal for a kid.

CHICKEN FINGERS

The perennial favorite might be an easy way to get your child to eat his dinner, but it's a nutritional cul-de-sac. Even if it's not on the menu, most kitchens will cook up grilled chicken fingers, which are still perfect for dunking but carry half the calories and only 25 percent of the fat.

DINNERS

ALL DINNERS INCLUDE CHOICE OF POTAOES, COLE SLAW OR SALAD, AND FRENCH OR GARLIC BREAD

FRIED CHICKEN *half chicken, fried to a golden brown*
$7.99

GROUND ROUND *half lb ground beef, smothered in sauteed onions and beef gravy*
$7.79

BATTER DIPPED COD *3 pieces of batter dipped cod, fried to a golden brown*
$7.59

SHRIMP *battered-dipped and fried to a golden brown*
$7.69

PORK CHOPS *two large chops marinated and grilled to perfection*
$8.69

GYROS DINNER *delicious beef and lamb served on pita bread with homemade sauce*
$7.19

2 GRILLED CHICKEN BREAST DINNER *marinated in olive oil, garlic, oregano, salt and pepper*
$9.29

CHICKEN CORDON BLEU DINNER *2 grilled chicken breasts, topped with ham and Swiss cheese*
$9.49

RIBEYE STEAK HOAGIE *grilled with onions, green peppers and mushrooms, topped with Swiss cheese*
$8.1

SIDES

BISCUITS
w/sausage gravy
$2.99

FRENCH FRIES
$1.99

CHEESE FRIES
$3.59

CHILI CHEESE FRIES
$4.59

VEGETABLE MEDLEY
$2.99

COLE SLAW
$1.99

FRUIT MEDLEY
$3.99

BAKED POTATO
$2.59

MASHED POTATO
w/gravy
$3.59

KID'S CORNER

HOT DOG AND FRENCH FRIES
$4.29

GRILLED CHEESE AND FRENCH FRIES
$4.99

CHICKEN FINGERS
$4.99

Chinese Takeout

Noodle Corner

HOURS OF OPERATION
11:00AM-12:00 MIDNIGHT
FREE OUTGOING DELIVERY

TEL 245-58*

APPETIZERS

A1.	PuPu Platter (for 2)	$7.25
	Egg Rolls, Chicken Fingers, Spareribs, Teriyaki Beef, Chicken Wings, Crab Rangoon	
A10.	Chicken Fingers	$7.25
A2.	Mini Pu Pu Platter	$9.95
	Teriyaki Beef (2), Boneless Spare Ribs, Chicken Wings (2), Crab Rangoon (2), Chicken Teriyaki (2)	
A11.	Dumplings (Pork or Vegetable) (6)	$3.95
A3.	Beef Teriyaki (6)	
A12.	Crab Rangoon (6)	$7.55
A4.	Egg Roll (2)	$4.25
A13.	Dim Sim Siu Mi (6)	$3.75
A5.	Shanghai Spring Rolls (2)	$4.75
A14.	Chicken Teriyaki	$3.95
A15.	Vegetable Egg Rolls(2)	$7.55
A7.	Chicken Wings (7)	$3.95
A8.	Fried Shrimps (6)	$5.95
A17.	Scallion Pancake	$7.55
A9.	Spareribs	$3.95
A18.	Boneless Spareribs	$7.55
		$7.25

SOUP

	n Soup	$2.05
	d Sour Soup	$2.05
	op Soup	$1.65
	se Vegetable Soup	$2.05
	se Special Soup	$7.55

BEEF

B1.	Beef with Green Peppers	$9.55
B10.	Beef with Mushrooms	$10.25
	Beef with Broccoli	$9.55
	Beef in Szechuan Sauce	$9.55
	Beef with Pea Pods	$9.55
	Spicy Beef with Peanuts and Peppers	$9.55
	Crispy Beef with Pea Pods	$9.55
	Spicy Shredded Beef in Garlic Sauce	$9.55

B5.	Beef with Pea Pods and Bamboo Shoots	
B14.*	Hunan Spiced Beef	$10.25
B6.	Mongolian Barbecued Beef	$9.55
B15.*	Beef with Black Bean Sauce	$10.25
B7.	Beef with Scallions	$9.55
B16.*	Orange Flavored Beef	$9.55
B8.	Beef with Chinese Vegetables	$10.55
B17.*	House Special Lamb	$9.55
B9.	Sesame Beef	$11.95
		$10.95

PORK

P1.	Pork with Pea Pods	$8.95
P5.*	Spicy Double Cooked Pork	$8.95
P2.	Pork with Broccoli	$8.95
P6.*	Spicy Shredded Pork in Garlic Sauce	$8.95
P3.	Pork with Scallions	$8.95
P7.*	Hunan Pork	$8.95
P4.	Three Delights with Pork, Shrimp, or Chicken	$9.55

POULTRY

C1.	Chicken with Cashews	$9.05
C12.	Kung Pao Chicken	$9.05
	Chicken with Pea Pods	$9.05
C2.	Tender Chicken w/Black Bean Sauce	$9.05
C13.*		
C8.	Moo Goo Gai Pan	$9.05
C14.*	Orange Flavor Chicken	$9.75
C4.	Eight Treasure Chicken	$9.05
C15.*	Curried Chicken	$9.05
C5.	Chicken with Broccoli	$9.05
C16.*	Jordan Chicken (General Gau's Chicken)	$9.75
C17.*	Chef's Chicken Delight with Spicy Sesame	$9.95
C6.	Chicken with Pineapple	$9.05
C18.*	Sesame Crispy Chicken	$9.95
C7.*	Spicy Szechuan Chicken with Peanuts	$9.05
C19.*	Fresh String Beans with Chicken and Beef	$9.05

LUNCHEON SPECIALS

Served daily 11:30 a.m. to 2:30 p.m. (except Sunday & Holidays). Served with choice of Pork Fried Rice or choice of Hot and Sour Soup, Egg Drop Soup or Wonton Soup. (Soup not included with Take-Out or

1. Chicken Wings (3), Egg Roll $5.25
12.* Spicy Chicken with Peanuts, Spareribs $6.55
2. Teriyaki Beef (2), Chicken Wings (2), Egg Roll .. $5.95
13. Eight Treasure Chicken, Teriyaki Beef $6.75
3. Boneless Spareribs (4), Egg Roll $5.95
14. Chicken with Pea Pods, Chicken Fingers (3) .. $6.25
4. Teriyaki Beef (2), Spareribs (2), Shrimp (2) $6.95
15. General Tso's Chicken, Egg Roll $7.25
5. Chicken Fingers (4), Chicken Wings (2) $5.55
16. Combo Lo Mein, Boneless Spareribs $5.75
6. Sweet and Sour Pork, Egg Roll $5.25
17.* Shrimp with Garlic Sauce, Egg Roll $7.25

7. Sweet and Sour Chicken, Egg Roll $5.25
18. Shrimp with Lobster Sauce, Egg Roll $7.25
8. Beef with Green Pepper, Egg Roll $6.25
19.*
9. Beef with Broccoli ....
20. Vegetarian's Delight, Egg Roll ....
10.* Spicy Double Cooked Pork, Egg Roll ....
21.* Meatless Chow Mein, Egg Roll ....
(Or choice of Chicken, Shrimp, Beef or Pork Chow Mein) ....
11. Pork with Broccoli, Egg Roll $5.75
22.* Shredded Beef Szechuan Style (Or choice of Chicken, Shrimp, or Pork ....

WEIGHT WATCHERS

All Weight-Watchers' orders are steamed. There is no seasoning or corn/starch used in cooking.

W1. Mixed Vegetables $5.95
W2. Mixed Vegetables (Choice of Pork, Chicken, Beef or Shrimp) $8.95
W3. Broccoli or Snow Pea Pods or Asparagus $5.95

MOO-SHI

Moo-Shi is a very popular mandarin dish which contains mushrooms, cabbage, fungus, dried lily flower, eggs and meat served with 8 pancakes and Hoi Sin Sauce

M1. Moo-Shi (Chicken, Beef, Pork, Shrimp, or Vegetables) $7.95
M2. Moo-Shi Peking Style (Spicy) $8.05

VEGETABLES

Vegetarian's Delight $6.55
Stir Fried Pea Pods $6.55
* Spicy Eggplant in Garlic Sauce $6.25
Snow Pea Pods with Water Chestnuts .. $6.55
* Spicy Broccoli $6.25
Brocoli in Oyster Sauce $6.55
String Beans, Szechuan Style (Meatless) $6.25

SWEET SOU...

SW1. Sweet and Sour Pork ......
SW3. Sweet and Sour Shrimp ......
SW2. Sweet and Sour Chicken ......
SW4. Sweet and Sour Combo ......

NOODLES

L1. Lo Mein (Choice of Pork, Chicken, B... Shrimp)
L2. Combo Lo Mein ......
L4. Shanghai Noodles ......
L6. Shanghai Noodles (Meatless) ......
L7. Cold Noodles in Sesame Sauce ......

RICE

R1. Steamed Rice ......
R2. Fried Rice (Choice of Pork, Chicken, B... $5.95
R3. Combo Fried Rice ......
R6. Brown Rice ......

"LIGHT ON THE SAUCE"

You won't see this phrase anywhere on the menu, but it's one you should rely on when ordering Chinese food. Real Chinese food comes lightly sauced, not drowning in a gloppy tide of sugary goo. Employ this phrase for a touch of authenticity and a savings of hundreds of calories for your family.

BEEF AND BROCCOLI

Not the healthy dish it pretends to be. That's because the thick brown sauce brings a dangerous amount of saturated fat and sodium to the plate.

STEAMED MIXED VEGETABLES

Expect broccoli, carrots, and snow peas, a potent mix of nutrient-dense vegetables. Make a simple rule in your house: Every time you eat Chinese, everyone (including you) must eat at least one portion of this healthy side.

RICE

The most seemingly innocent part of the meal is actually one of the most problematic. A single scoop could add 300 calories to a meal, and all of those calories come from fast-burning carbohydrates. If you can't imagine a Chinese meal without rice, try a small scoop of brown rice, which at least brings some fiber to the table.

Genius PARENT TRICK

Make your kids use chopsticks. It takes 20 minutes for our stomachs to convey to our brains that we're full, so working a bit for their food (while refining fine motor skills) is a good way to prevent the overeating.

Italian

BRUSCHETTA

Loaded with chopped tomatoes, garlic, and fresh basil, these crunchy hunks of grilled bread are the Italian take on chips and salsa. At less than 200 calories a serving, it's a solid starter for the table. Sell it to your kid by calling it "fresh tomato pizza."

PASTA E FAGIOLI

Soup is always a good idea (assuming we're not talking about chowder or a soup with cheese in the title) because it provides low-calorie padding for the belly before the unhealthier entrées arrive. This particular soup, found throughout Italy and rich with tomatoes, pasta, and fiber-packed beans, is like a high-octane, more-satisfying version of SpaghettiOs®.

MACARONI AND CHEESE

There is absolutely nothing Italian about macaroni and cheese. So for the sake of authenticity—and your kid's waistline—institute a "No-Mac" policy at Italian restaurants.

CHEESE RAVIOLI

A substantial improvement over the normal macaroni and cheese for two reasons: First, the pasta is stuffed with ricotta, a naturally low-calorie and low-sodium cheese that trounces Cheddar, and second, it's sauced with marinara, the nutritional standard-bearer of the Italian menu.

Appetizers

Homemade Mozzarella with roasted peppers & fresh tomatoes 7.95
Bruschetta with marinated tomatoes, fresh basil and garlic crostini 7.95
Fried Fresh Calamari 8.95
Fried Mozzarella Sticks 8.95
Sautéed Mussels in marinara or fra diavolo sauce 8.95
Combination Platter fried calamari, mozzarella sticks and eggplant parmigiana 14.95

Soups and Salads

Pasta E Fagioli 7.95
Minestra d'Aglio 6.95
House Salad mixed greens with fresh tomatoes 6.95
Insalata Caprese with mozzarella di bufala campana, plum tomatoes, fresh basil and extra virgin olive oil 7.95
Arugula Salad with goat cheese, roasted pepper, red onions and tomatoes in a citrus vinaigrette 8.95

Pasta

Macaroni and Cheese 9.95
Capellini al Pesto, angel hair pasta in tomato and basil pesto 12.95
Cheese Ravioli, stuffed with ricotta cheese and smothered in marinara 12.95
Lasagna marinara, lasagna sheets and ricotta cheese topped with mozzarella and baked to perfection 11.95

Meat

Bistecca Fiorentina 24.95

Homemade Sausage
with Sweet Peppers 16.95

Neapolitan Beef Ragu 14.95

Neapolitan Meatballs 15.95

Pork Chops 19.95

Seafood

Shrimp & Scallops in
fra diavolo or marinara sauce 19.95

Grilled Prawns in Lemon 19.95

Baked Branzino 23.95

Tuna and Ricotta Fritters 17.95

Grilled Lobsters 25.95

Chicken

Grilled Double Breast Of Chicken with fresh rosemary
and herbs over arugula 11.95

Pizzaiola sautéed in marinara with mushrooms and peppers 13.95

Chicken Marsala sautéed in marsala wine with
shallots and mushrooms 13.95

Chicken Balsamic sautéed with onions, mushrooms
and fresh tomatoes in a sweet balsamic sauce 1

Chicken Francaise lightly dipped in egg and delic
sautéed in a butter lemon sauce 13.95

Dolce

Gelato in various flavors 4.95

Panna Cotta topped with wild berries 5.95

Cannoli topped with Nutella 4.95

Tiramisu delicately layered with a hint of coffee

INSALATA CAPRESE

The fresh mozzarella cheese used in this
tricolored salad is naturally low in fat
and sodium, and the tomatoes and basil
add a nice antioxidant hit. This beats
out Caesar salad any day of the week.

PIZZAIOLA

It's like chicken Parmesan,
minus all the excess calories.
This preparation combines a grilled
or sautéed meat—usually chicken or
veal—with a marinara sauce spiked
with peppers and mushrooms.
Not only does the pizzaiola
treatment save Parm-devotees
a few hundred calories, but it
also packs a few servings of
vegetables into
a single dish.

GELATO

Unlike most
American ice
creams, which are
made with heavy
cream, gelato is
made with milk,
making a scoop
a relatively low-
impact indulgence.

TIRAMISU

Delicious, yes, but this ubiquitous Italian
dessert is made from ladyfingers, egg yolks,
mascarpone cheese, and chocolate, a dubious
combination that leaves even a tiny
slice with 450 calories and
25 grams of fat.

SAUCE DECODER

LISTED FROM BEST TO ABSOLUTE WORST:

Marinara
This is virtually fat-free, plus it delivers
at least one serving of fruit in the form of
antioxidant-packed tomatoes.

Pesto
It's high in fat, but most of that is healthy monounsaturated fat from olive oil. Plus basil and garlic
both contain strong cancer-fighting compounds.

Butter and Parmesan
The food of choice for half of this country's
young eaters, this simple combination might
seem fairly innocent. The problem is, it offers no
viable nutrition for your kids—just fat from the
sauce and quick-burning carbs from the pasta.

Alfredo
The same as Butter and Parmesan (above), only
with the addition of heavy cream. Avoid at all costs.

Sushi

MISO SOUP

Every bit as comforting and approachable as a bowl of chicken noodle soup, but with just 80 calories a bowl. So rich and familiar is the taste of a good miso soup that the kids won't even notice that those little green strands floating about in the clouded broth are seaweed!

YAKITORI

Skewers of lean meat, usually chicken, grilled over an open flame. Lightly sauced, low in calories, and high in quality protein, these are perfectly tailored for the little ones. Plus, what kid can resist food on a stick?

TERIYAKI

This reduction of soy, sweet wine, and sugar comes painted on a variety of meats and vegetables at Japanese restaurants. The sweet-salty sauce makes nearly anything it touches palatable, so why not encourage your kids to try it on salmon? The monster dose of omega-3s is critical for brain development as well as a dozen other bodily functions.

TEMPURA

Japanese chefs use a lighter batter than that reserved for more familiar fried foods, making the shrimp, asparagus, carrots, and other foods they coat and fry less-oil soaked than the onion rings and fried mozzarella sticks most kids crave. Even so, it's still food cooked in boiling fat, so split an order for the whole table.

KRAB

Krab with a K (also called "crab sticks" on menus) refers to imitation crab made from surimi, finely chopped white fish—usually hake or pollock—pressed into logs that resemble crab legs. While it is highly processed, it still contains many of the same health benefits as fish, but without any of the fishy smell or taste that scares most kids away.

appetizers

Miso Soup

House Salad

Roll Appetizer (3pcs California roll, 3pcs crab salad roll, 3pcs takka maki, 3pcs negi hamachi)

Sashimi Appetizer Combo (tuna, white fish & octopus)

Sushi Appetizer Combo (nigiri: tuna, white fish, shrimp, crabstick & 2 pcs tekka maki)

Yakitori (choice of chicken, or roasted with special sauce)

teriyaki

Chicken Teriyaki	Tofu Teriyaki
Steak Teriyaki	Shrimp Teriyaki
Pork Teriyaki	Scallop Teriyaki
Salmon Teriyaki	Tuna Teriyaki

tempura

Vegetable
15 pieces vegetable

Chicken
7 pieces chicken & vegetable

Shrimp
7 pieces shrimp & vegetable

Salmon
7 pieces salmon & vegetable

Tempura Combo
3 pieces shrimp, 3 pieces salmon, 3 pieces chicken & vegetable

nigiri-sushi
One serving consists of two pieces

Alaska King Crab	Kanpachi (wild yellowtail)
Amaebi (sweet shrimp)	Saba (spanish mackeral)
Blue Fin Tuna	Shake (fresh salmon)
Ebi (boiled shrimp)	Shake (smoked salmon)
Escolar (seared fatty white tuna)	Spicy Tuna (original or jalapeno)
Hamachi (yellowtail)	Suzuki (bass)
Hirame (fluke)	Tai (red snapper)
Hotategai (scallop)	Tako (boiled octopus)
Ika (squid)	Tobiko (flying fish roe)
Ikura (salmon roe)	Unagi (fresh water eel)
Kanikama (crab stick)	Uni (sea urchin)

sushi combinations
Served with Miso Soup & Salad

Matsu Sushi Dinner
California roll, spicy tekka maki, 5pcs nigiri sushi consisting of: tuna, shrimp, white fish, tamago and smoked salmon

Traditional Sushi & Sashimi Dinner Traditional Sushi Dinner plus sashimi appetizer

Traditional Sushi Dinner
Nigiri sushi consisting of: tuna, white fish, mackerel, smoked salmon, yellowtail, shrimp, octopus, crab stick, tamago, crab roe & tekka maki

specialty rolls

Black & White (white fish tempura, scallions, black sesame seeds)

Tuna Cubed (blue fin tuna and escolar topped with fatty tuna & wasabi tobiko)

Grand Canyon (unagi, avocado & cucumber topped with broiled escolar, masago & silver sauce)

Green Dragon (Alaska king crab, unagi topped with avocado and tempura crunch)

Hawaiian (spicy salmon, tempura crunch & cucumber topped with avocado & tuna)

Jumbo (crab stick, cucumber, hamachi, unagi & masago)

Fire Island (California roll topped with spicy tuna, scallions and tempura crunch)

Fuji Volcano (shrimp tempura and avocado topped with unagi & spicy masago sauce)

Matsu (unagi, avocado, crabstick, tamago & masago)

maki sushi

One serving consists of 6 pieces unless noted

Alaska Roll (smoked salmon, cream cheese & masago)
California Roll (crab stick & cucumber)
Futomaki 4 pcs (crab stick, shrimp, tamago, pickle & cucumber)
Gobo Maki (pickled burdock)
Ikura Maki (salmon roe)
Kappa Maki
Mexican Roll (boiled shrimp & avocado)
Negi Hamachi Maki (yellowtail & scallions)
Natto Maki (fermented soybeans)
Philadelphia Roll (smoked salmon, cream cheese & masago)
Shrimp Tempura Maki 4pcs (shrimp tempura, cucumber & crab roe)
Spicy Tekka Maki (spicy tuna original or jalapeno)
Spider Maki 4 pcs (soft shell crab roll & masago)
Unagi Maki (fresh water eel)

SOY SAUCE
While Japanese meals are lean, low-fat, high-protein affairs, one real danger comes from excessive sodium intake. A single tablespoon of soy sauce has over 1,000 milligrams of sodium—half the recommended maximum for a day. Luckily, most sushi places now offer the low-sodium variety, which cuts the sky-high count in half.

TUNA ROLL
Consumption of tuna sushi has recently been linked to high levels of mercury intake, which can negatively affect language, visual-spatial skills, and brain development in young kids. Children under the age of 6 and pregnant women are the most susceptible to mercury's ill effects, so limit your kid to one or two pieces of tuna-based sushi per visit, or just cut it out entirely.

CALIFORNIA ROLL
A mix of sweet (crab), creamy (avocado), and crunchy (cucumber), this popular Americanized roll is the perfect fit for a kid's tastes. Plus, at 300 calories for eight vegetable-stuffed pieces, this might be one of the healthiest kids' meals in America. No, the crab is not likely to be real, but for a kid, that might be a good thing.

PHILADELPHIA ROLL
It's not the healthiest item on the menu, but it's a great beginner roll for kids. The salmon is smoked, so that solves the raw issue most kids might have, plus the avocado and cream cheese give it a nice richness. At 350 calories for 8 pieces, it makes a perfect meal.

Indian

APPETIZERS

If there's one area where normally healthy Indian cuisine hits a nutritional pothole, it's with the starting dishes. From potato-stuffed samosas to the crispy fritters called *pakora*, a vast majority of the appetizers make a pit stop in boiling oil on the way to your plate. That means that they also pick up an unnecessary dose of calories and saturated fat in transit.

NAAN AND ROTI

Both are hot flatbreads baked up soft and pillowy in the tandoori oven, and both are absolutely addictive. Stick to a single basket, but make it roti instead of naan—roti is made with whole-wheat flour, giving it an extra dose of fiber.

VINDALOO

Proceed with caution: Many versions of this fragrant chicken stew come with a serious dose of dried chiles, and the heat may be overwhelming to a sensitive palate.

CURRY

Many kids are turned off by the pervasive smell, but Indian curry contains turmeric, a miracle spice known to fight cancer and cardiovascular disease, slow mental decline, and boost insulin resistance. If they won't do curry, Indian yellow rice and tandoori chicken also contain turmeric.

APPETIZERS

VEGETABLE SAMOSA *Two crisp turnovers, stuffed with spiced potatoes, peas, and herbs.* $2.50
VEGETABLE PAKORA *Assorted vegetable fritters gently seasoned and deep fried.* $2.50
CHICKEN PAKORA *Chicken fritters.* $3.25
SHRIMP PAKORA *Shrimp dipped in spiced batter, deep fried.* $6.95
HOUSE SPECIAL PLATTER *A fine presentation of our choice appetizers, recommended for two.* $6.95
VEGETARIAN PLATTER *Assorted vegetable appetizers, recommended for two.* $5.95
PANEER PAKORA *Pieces of homemade cheese, dipped in chickpea flour and fried.* $3.25

SOUPS AND SALADS

VEGETABLE SOUP *Soup made from fresh vegetable, lentils, spices and delicate herbs.* $2.50
MULLIGATAWNY SOUP *A traditional chicken soup with lentils and spices.* $2.50
RAITA *Homemade whipped yoghurt with cucumbers, potatoes and fresh mint.* $2.50
GREEN SALAD *Lettuce, tomatoes, green peppers, and onions.* $2.50

BREADS

NAAN *Leavened bread, soft and fluffy.* $2.25
ROTI *Whole wheat bread* $1.50
ALOO PARATHA *Whole wheat bread, stuffed with potatoes* $2.50
PANEER KULCHA *Naan stuffed with homemade cheese, spices, and herbs* $2.50

RICE SPECIALTIES

CHICKEN BIRYANI *Classic mulgai dish of curried rice with chicken, dried fruits and nuts* $9.95
LAMB BIRYANI *Curried rice with lamb, dried fruits and nuts* $10.95
HOUSE SPECIAL BIRYANI *Our special biryani cooked with chicken, lamb, shrimp, vegetables, dried fruits and nuts* $13.95
PEAS PULLAO *Rice cooked with peas, raisins and nuts* $3.95

OUR CHEF RECOMMENDS

SEAFOOD FANTASY *Start with tandoori fish and tandoori shrimp, followed by your choice of shrimp masala or shrimp cury, dal, naan, pullao and green salad.* $19.95
THALI HOUSE VEGETARIAN *A traditional Indian meal served on a silver platter with dal, chana masala, mattar paneer, rice, poori or roti, raita and gulab jamun.* $12.95
VEGETABLE SEEKHAM *Fresh carrots, cauliflower, green peas, homemade cheese, pineapple chunks cooked with spices, sauce and nuts.* $9.95
LAMB DANSHIK *Tender lamb and chick peas lentils cooked with pineapple and herbs.* $11.95
LAMB KASHMIRI *Lamb cooked in an onion, ginger, garlic and peach sauce.* $11.95
CHICKEN LA-JAWAB *Tender boneless chicken pieces and apple chunks cooked in ginger, garlic sauce and nuts.* $11.95

CHICKEN

CHICKEN MAKHANI *The legendary tandoori chicken cooked in tomato and garlic sauce* $10.95
CHICKEN VINDALOO *Boneless chicken and potatoes in a highly spiced sauce* $9.95
CHICKEN SHAHI KORMA *Tender chicken cooked in a rich sauce with nuts and cream* $9.95
CHICKEN SAAGWALA *Boneless chicken cooked with creamed spinach* $9.95
CHICKEN TIKKA MUGLAI *Tandoori chicken and mushrooms cooked in tomato and garlic* $10.95
CHICKEN TIKKA BHUNA *Chicken tikka cooked dry with onions, tomato and bell peppers* $9.95
CHICKEN TIKKA MASALA *Tandoori roasted chicken tikka in a tomato and butter sauce* $10.95
CHICKEN CURRY *The original cooked in onions, garlic, ginger, yoghurt, and spices* $9.95
CHICKEN JALFEREZI *Tender, boneless chicken cooked with onions, tomato and bell peppers* $9.95
CHICKEN DILRUBA *Chicken cooked with mushrooms* $9.95
CHICKEN ASPARAGUS *Chicken cooked with asparagus and fresh spices sauce* $10.95
CHICKEN ACHAR *Chicken cooked in tomato, onion gravy with pickled spices* $9.95
CHICKEN CHILLY *Tendar boneless chicken pieces onions, tomatoes, bell peppers cooked in sweet and sour sauce, mint flavored* $10.95

LAMB

LAMB SHAHI KORMA *Tender lamb, in a rich sauce with nuts and cream $10.95*

LAMB SAAGWALA *Chunks of lamb in creamed spinach $10.95*

LAMB BHUNA *Pan-broiled lamb, cooked in specially prepared herbs and spices with a touch of ginger and garlic $10.95*

LAMB VINDALOO *Lamb and potatoes cooked in a sharply spiced tangy sauce $10.95*

KEEMA MATTAR *Ground lamb cooked with peas and herbs $10.95*

BOTI KABAB MASALA *Tandoor broiled lamb sauteed in our special exquisite curry to gastronomic satisfaction $11.95*

LAMB ACHAR *Tender lamb cooked in tomato, onion, gravy with pickled spices $10.95*

LAMB ASPARAGUS *Lamb and asparagus cooked in a special ginger, garlic and onion sauce $11.95*

VEGETABLE

NAVRATAN CURRY *Nine assorted garden fresh vegetables sauced in a traditional onion and tomato sauce $8.95*

DAL MAKHANI *Black lentils and beans, cooked in onions, with tomatoes and cream $8.95*

SAAG PANEER *Chunks of homemade cheese in creamed spinach and fresh spices $8.95*

ALOO SAAG *Spinach and potatoes with fresh spices $8.95*

ALOO GOBHI MASALA *Fresh cauliflower and potatoes, cooked dry in onions, tomatoes and herbs $8.95*

MATTAR PANEER *Fresh homemade cheese, cooked with tender garden peas and fresh spices $8.95*

ALOO MATTAR *Garden fresh green peas and potatoes with fresh spices $8.95*

MATTAR MUSHROOMS *Garden fresh peas and mushroms cooked with garlic, ginger, and onions $8.95*

BAIGAN BHARTHA *Roasted eggplant sauteed in onion, tomatoes and green peas $8.95*

MALAI KOFTA KASHMIRI *Garden fresh vegetables and homemade cheeseballs cooked in a rich sauce with nuts and cream $9.95*

CHANNA MASALA PUNJABI *A North Indian specialty, subtly flavored chick peas, tempered with ginger $8.95*

KADI PAKORA SINDHI *Dumpling of mixed vegetables, cooked in chick peas flour, yoghurt and mustard sauce $8.95*

PANEER SHAHI KORMA *Tender chunks of homemade cheese, cooked with nuts and a touch of cream in fresh herbs and spices $9.95*

PANEER MASALA *Tender chunks of homemade cheese, cooked with tomato and butter $9.95*

PANEER ACHAR *Homemade cheese cooked in tomato onion gravy with pickled spices $9.95*

PANEER CHILLY *Homemade cheese, onions, tomatoes, bell peppers cooked in sweet and sour sauce, mint flavored $9.95*

TANDOORI

TANDOORI CHICKEN *Chicken marinated in yoghurt and freshly ground spices, then broiled in the tandoor (half) $9.95*

TANDOORI FISH *Swordfish marinated in an exotic recipe of exciting spices and herbs, broiled on charcoal $13.95*

TANDOORI SHRIMP *Jumbo shrimp seasoned with spices and herbs, baked in the tandoor $14.95*

CHICKEN TIKKA *Boneless, tender chicken, gently broiled $9.95*

RESHMI KABAB *Mild, tender, pieces of chicken breast, marinated in a very mild sauce barbecued on a skewer in the tandoor $10.95*

BOTI KABAB *Juicy cubes from leg of lamb, broiled to perfection in the tandoor $10.95*

SEEK KABAB *Finger rolls of ground lamb, spiced with fresh ginger $10.95*

DRINK SPECIALTIES

LASSI SWEET $2.75

MANGO LASSI $2.75

MANGO JUICE $2.00

STRAWBERRY LASSI *seasonal* $2.75

SODAS $1.25

KESAR PISTA SHAKE *seasonal* $2.75

ACCOMPANIMENTS

MANGO CHUTNEY *spicy, sweet & sour relish* 4.00

PICKLES *mango, lemon, chili* 3.00

PAPADUM *thin bean wafer* 3.00

RAITA *tomato and cucumber in a yogurt sauce* 3.00

DAL

Lentils stewed with a variety of flavorful Indian spices. Packed full of fiber, protein, and antioxidants, you'd be hard-pressed to find a better dish to feed your family in the restaurant world.

TANDOORI

The perfect place to find approachable food for a youngster. Tandoori dishes have been roasted at high heat in a tandoor —a scorching clay oven. Chicken is the obvious choice for this healthy treatment, but shrimp and fish make for an even healthier dinner.

CHICKEN TIKKA

Lean chicken marinated in yogurt and spices, then roasted tandoori-style. Not only is this the most kid-friendly dish on the menu, it's also one of the healthiest. A single serving weighs in at a svelte 250 calories.

LASSI

Blended fruit drinks made with yogurt, milk, and just a touch of sugar. The most popular is blended with mango and makes for a great low-calorie dessert that kids will beg for once they get a taste. Go ahead, let 'em have one.

CONDIMENTS

While sauces and condiments can be the most destructive parts of American-style meals, the table sauces that come with Indian food are one of the healthiest parts of the meal. Both raita, a cool yogurt and cucumber sauce, and chutney, a salsa-like condiment made with mango or fresh mint, are perfectly suited for a kid's appetite and should be used with reckless abandon.

Deli

OIL AND VINEGAR

Seems like a harmless splash to lubricate the sandwich and make it all go down easier, right? Not exactly. The vinegar is harmless, but the oil used in most sub shops is of the low-grade soy variety, carrying a 100-calorie penalty for every few inches of sandwich.

BLT

Probably not as bad as you think. With four strips of bacon and a light coating of mayo, this sandwich still manages to hover right around the 400-calorie mark.

WRAP

Beware the healthy foods that aren't! The tortilla this comes wrapped in packs up to 300 calories on its own and provides ample surface area for a surplus of cheese and dressing. All told, the average chicken wrap weighs in at 600 calories—about 50 percent more than the average grilled chicken sandwich.

ITALIAN HERO

This popular combo order combines a mountain of the fattiest, saltiest meats around: pepperoni, salami, capicolla. Add to that Italian dressing and sodium-laden provolone cheese, and even a small sandwich will top 600 calories and approach 2,000 milligrams of sodium.

Sandwich Delights

CHICKEN CLUB with smoked bacon, brie cheese, plum tomatoes & ranch dressing

TURKEY BREAST with lettuce, cranberry sauce, and stuffing on wheat $6.25

ROAST BEEF & TURKEY BREAST with lettuce, gree▢ pepper, tomato and a splash of oil and vinegar ....$▢

TARRAGON CHICKEN SALAD with fresh herbs, l▢tuce, tomato, red onion, and Maitre Tarragon mu▢ dressing on wheat..........................$6.25

BACON CHICKEN SALAD blended with real ba▢ red onion, fresh herbs, served with lettuce an▢ on wheat...........................$6.25

BLT with mayonnaise on toasted wheat brea▢

CUCUMBER AND HERB CHEESE SPREAD ▢ lettuce, tomato, red onion and a splash of ▢ vinegar $5.25

VEGETABLE HUMMUS WRAP with cucu▢ peppers, red onions, lettuce tomato and ▢ roasted garlic hummus in a wheat wra▢

GREEK WRAP marinated chicken cub▢ cucumber, tomato, red onion, olives, ▢ feta cheese, Greek dressing in a wra▢

CITY DELI CLUB 3 layers of turkey▢ cheddar cheese, tomato & lettuce

CAPRI SMOKED TURKEY & PEP▢ ▢ne cheese, cherry peppers & h▢

ITALIAN HERO COMBO prosci▢ provolone, pepperoncini peppe▢ Italian vinaigrette on Italian b▢

DELIGHT FULL HONEY GLA▢ cheese with cole slaw & hor▢

Hot Sandwiches

...RNED BEEF or PASTRAMI with melted swiss
, red onion, sauerkraut, and honeycup mustard
.............$6.25

...ADELPHIA CHEESESTEAK with onion & green
...per, topped with melted jack cheese and served on
...ench roll $9.25

...T ROAST BEEF AND GRAVY with herb cheese
...bread on a bulky roll.................$6.25

...HOT GARDENBURGER with melted Swiss cheese, lettuce, tomato, red onion in a wheat wrap with roasted
garlic hummus.................$6.25

Gourmet Salads Sandwiches

**All Platters Served With Tossed Salad & Choice
Of Coleslaw, Potato Salad Or Macaroni Salad.**

Sandwich/ Platters

Chicken Salad 4.99
Classic Tuna Salad 4.95
Seafood Salad 4.50
Egg Salad 4.95

Italian Tuna 4.95
Italian Seafood 4.95
Dill Chicken Salad .4.95
Shrimp Salad 5.50

Build-Your-Own

SERVED WITH LETTUCE, TOMATO AND ONION.
BREAD: Jewish Rye - Wheat - Bulky Roll - White -
Wheat - Wraps (Wheat - White)
CHEESE: American - Swiss - Provolone - Cheddar $.75
EXTRA: Roasted Garlic Hummus - Bacon $.75 EXTRA
Cucumbers - Green Peppers - Black Olives $.50 EXTRA

Boiled Ham 3.99
Turkey Breast 3.99
Roast Beef 4.50
Pastrami 3.99
Corned Beef 3.99
Genoa Salami 3.99
Hard Salami 3.99

Smoked Turkey 3.99
Virginia Ham 3.99
Cappicola Ham 3.99
Prosciutto 3.50
Liverwurst .... 3.
Bologna ....
Spiced Ham ....
Black Forest Ham . 3.9

$6.25

...ocado,
...99

...th provo-
...rd

...lla, salami,
...tomatoes,
............$8.25

...EY with swiss
...............$6.25

...east with ham,
...dressing.....$8.99

...nion, lettuce,
...9.25

HOT SANDWICHES
Stay away! Calories at delis rise in direct proportion to the temperature of the sandwich being made. Among the worst offenders in the hot sandwich department: hot pastrami and Swiss, meatball, sausage and peppers, and, of course, the disastrous cheesesteak.

TUNA SALAD
Tuna and salad may each be perfectly healthy on their own, but when smashed together they become one of the most consistently bad orders in a sandwich shop. "Salad" in this case is a euphemism for a bucket of mayo, making a small scoop of this menu item three times as caloric as a serving of turkey or ham.

CHEESE
Choose Swiss and mozzarella over Cheddar and provolone. Not only are they lower in fat and calories, but Swiss in particular has only a fraction of the sodium.

YOUR CHOICE OF HAM, TURKEY, OR ROAST BEEF
Surprisingly, there is only a marginal caloric and fat discrepancy among these three ubiquitous cuts. All contribute about 100 calories and 8 grams of fat to a small sandwich. One warning: Watch out for smoked ham and turkey, which tend to have precariously high sodium levels.

Mexican

CHIPS AND SALSA

Salsa is the world's greatest condiment, with only 15 calories and 0 grams of fat in a generous scoop, plus a ton of lycopene from the tomatoes. Problem is, a basket of chips will cost you at least 600 calories, and when they're complimentary, those calories can pile up quickly. Limit the family to one basket and save any leftover salsa to lavish generously on your entrées.

TORTILLAS

No, not all tortillas are created equally. In fact, the wrong tortilla can be your worst enemy at a Mexican restaurant, packing up to 400 calories on its own. To dampen the damage, have all tacos and fajitas made with corn tortillas; they're lower in calories and higher in fiber than standard flour tortillas.

FAJITAS

The sizzling skillet has a magical way of making onions and peppers more appealing to veggie-phobic kids. Because the serving size is so massive, it's a great dish to split between two kids, which cuts the 900-calorie entrée into a reasonable 450-calorie portion for each. You can knock off another 150 calories each if you ask the server to hold the cheese and sour cream.

Appetizers

CHIPS AND SALSA Made fresh daily in our kitchen

TAQUITOS (2) Corn Tortilla or (2) Flour Tortilla
Your choice of any meats, garnished with Guacamole 4.25

FLAUTAS (2) Corn Tortilla or (2) Flour Tortilla
Your choice of any meats, garnished with Guacamole 4.25

NACHOS 1/2 SIZE Felipe's Beans, served over a bed of Chips, topped with Melted
Cheese and Guacamole   Plain 5.00   Meat 6.00

QUESO FUNDIDO (Cheese Fondue) Melted Cheese with your choice of meat,
garnished with Avacado & Green Onion.
Served with Tortillas.   Plain 5.75   Meat 6.75

CHIPOTLE CHICKEN WINGS (Felipe's Favorite) Wings simmered and sautéed in
Alma's Chipotle Sauce. Has a Kick To It! 7.95

CABICHE COCKTAIL Fish marinated in Felipe's Homade Cocktail Sauce & Limes.
Garnished with Cilantro, Tomatoes, Onions, and Avocados.
Want it Spicy? Just ask. 7.50

ANTOJITOS PLATTER A combination of Taquitos, Flautas, Mini Tacos,
Quesadillas, Chicken Wings, Tostaditas and Nachos. 10.50

Entrees

Want it spicier? Just ask! All Mexican Dishes available with your choice of two of
any of the following: rice, beans, refried beans, salad or pico de gallo

CARNITAS The best carnitas in town! Pork simmered for hours with spices to
create a tender succulent taste

ASADA Steak marinated with Felipe's special seasoning and grilled to order

POLLO Skinless and boneless chicken marinated with Felipe's achiote seasonings

CHILE VERDE Diced pork cooked in tomatilo sauce

PESCADO Fish grilled with garlic butter and salsa mexicana

ENSENADA Fish lightly battered

ENCHIPOTLE Grilled shrimp sauteed in Felipe's chipotle sauce. Very spicy.

MACHACA Sautéed strips of pork, eggs, bell peppers, tomatoes, onions

CARNE DESHEBRADA Shredded beef simmered with a touch of wine and Felipe's spice

FAJITAS ASADA Combination of strips of steak, bell peppers, tomatoes and onions

FAJITAS POLLO Combination of chicken, bell peppers, tomatoes and onions

PICADILLO Ground beef simmered with diced tomatoes and onions

VEGETARIANO A combination of grilled vegetables lightly seasoned

CHORIZO CON PAPAS Mexican sausage grilled to order with potatoes and onions
(eggs by request)

NOPALES Strips of cactus grilled to order with diced tomatoes and onions

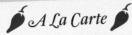

A La Carte

TACOS

All tacos are served on a soft flour tortilla with cheese and lettuce. Hard shell or corn tortilla by request.

Taco filled with...
- *Asada, Fajitas Asada 3.50*
- *Carne Desbrada, Carne Desbrada, Carnitas, Pollo, Picadillo, Fajitas Pollo, Chorizo con Papas, Nopales, Machacha, Chile Verde 3.25*
- *Ensenada or Pescado 3.50*

TACO SALAD

Lettuce, rice, beans, jack and cheddar cheese, fresh salsa, guacamole, sour cream served with or without crisp shell.

BURRITOS

A meal in itself that starts with a large flour tortilla and your choice of any meat, then we add rice, beans and cheese all wrapped inside. Frijoles de la olla by request.

Burrito filled with...
- *Fajitas Asada, Chile Relleno 8.00*
- *Carne Desbrada, Carnitas, Pollo, Picadillo, Fajitas Pollo, Vegetariano, Chorizo con Papas,*
- *Nopales, Machaca, Chile Verde 7.25*
- *Ensenada or Pescado 8.50*

TOSTADAS

A crisp corn tortilla spread with beans, your choice of entree, topped with fresh lettuce, guacamole and cheese.

Tostadas with...
- *Asada, Fajitas Asada 8.00*
- *Carne Desbrada, Carnitas, Pollo, Picadillo,*
- *Fajitas Pollo, Vegetariano 7.25*

NACHOS

First we start with a good portion of fresh chips, add beans, your favorite meat and cover it with melted cheese and garnished with guacamole.

Nachos with...
- *Asada, Fajitas Asada 8.50*
- *Carne Desbrada, Carnitas, Pollo, Picadillo 7.5*

QUESADILLAS

Your choice of meat and melted cheese in between two flour tortillas, garnished with guacamole.

Quesadillas with...
- *Asada 8.00*
- *Carne Desbrada, Carnitas, Pollo, Picadillo 7.45*

ENCHILADAS

A soft corn tortilla, stuffed with cheese or meat, and smothered with enchilada sauce or tomatillo sauce then topped with melted cheese and lettuce.

Enchiladas with...
- *Carne Desbrada, Carnitas, Pollo 4.25*
- *Cheese 4.25*

EMPANADAS

Corn pastry filled with cheese and your choice of meat and vegetable.

Empanadas with...
- *Carne Desbrada, Carnitas, Pollo 4.25*
- *Cheese 4.25*

CHILE RELLENO

A Chile Poblano stuffed with cheese and topped with special sauce.

QUESADILLAS

Mexico's thin, crispy answer to that American kid favorite, grilled cheese, has nothing even closely resembling nutrition to offer your loved ones. Whereas a homemade quesadilla might contain $\frac{1}{2}$ cup of shredded cheese on a small tortilla, the restaurant equivalent is a hubcap-size wrap housing up to 2 cups of Cheddar and Jack cheeses. The damage? 700 calories and 40 grams of fat.

GUACAMOLE

Yes, avocados are loaded with heart-healthy fats, but they're also stuffed full of belly-expanding calories, making a small bowl of guacamole a 400-calorie proposition. Go ahead and order the guac—just make sure it's shared with the rest of the table, okay?

EMPANADAS

This South American staple has migrated onto many a Mexican menu in this country. Which is rather unfortunate, considering that it's a fried meat-and-cheese filled pastry. Ouch.

REFRIED BEANS

Don't be scared by the name: While this popular Mexican staple carries a bit of fat with each serving, refried beans also come with a big dose of protein, fiber, and antioxidants. (Yes, refried beans pack quite an antioxidant punch.) All of these factors make the beans considerably better for you than the rice they're served with.

Seafood

SHRIMP COCKTAIL

There are few better ways to start any meal in the restaurant world. Shrimp are virtually fat-free and are loaded with protein, which is a vital component of satiety. Studies show that starting a meal with lean protein makes you less likely to overeat come entrée and dessert time.

CLAM CHOWDER

The cream-based New England variety might be the better-known chowder, but nutritionally, it can't hold a candle to tomato-based Manhattan-style chowder.

CRAB LEGS

Young boys might be tempted to try to scare their sisters with these giant claws, but trapped inside is a sweet, nonfishy, lean meat that is pitch-perfect for a young eater's taste buds.

MELTED BUTTER

It might look like a small ramekin, but those 2 tablespoons of melted butter contain over 200 calories and a full day's worth of saturated fat, all but erasing any benefits your family is getting from eating seafood.

GREAT STARTERS

OYSTERS ON THE HALF SHELL Six market oysters served with a shallot and vinegar mignonette or cocktail sauce **$7.99**

SHRIMP COCKTAIL 8 of our butterfly shrimp served with our homemade cocktail sauce **$5.99**

MOZZARELLA STICKS Mozzarella cheese lightly breaded and golded fried. Served with marinara **$5.99**

SAUTEED MUSHROOMS Broiled in lemon, white wine and butter **$5.99**

CIAPPINO Variety of fresh seafood in a rich spicy tomato broth **$5.99**

APPETIZER SAMPLER A sharable platter of Harbor House favorites. Shrimp cocktail, sautéed mushrooms and popcorn shrimp **$7.99**

BROCCOLI BITES Tender broccoli and creamy American cheese double dipped in a light batter and fried **$5.99**

SOUP

New England clam chowder **Cup $2.99   Bowl $3.99**
Seafood gumbo **Cup $2.99   Bowl $3.99**

SEAFOOD BUFFET

Features snow crab legs, steamed shrimp, steamed mussels, steamed clams, crawfish, fresh fish, hot and cold pasta dishes, seafood gumbo, fresh fruit, salad bar, and much more **$24.99**

SPECIALTY DISHES

The following served with one trip salad bar and choice of baked potato or fries. Add .50 for sweet potato.

TURF 9 oz. USDA choice ribeye grilled on open flame and one whole steamed lobster served with lemon and melted butter **MP**

RIBEYE STEAK Top quality black angus ribeye steak grilled on open flame to your specifications **$21.99**

LOBSTER THERMIDOR Baked in a rich cream sauce with a touch of Sherry **$27.95**

OVEN BROILED SEAFOOD

BROILED FISH — Choose from Alaskan whitefish, Flounder or Catfish. Seasoned and grilled over an open flame. Served over rice pilaf **$10.99**

SWORDFISH — a thick steak covered in herb butter and broiled. Served over rice pilaf **$12.99**

BROILED ATLANTIC SALMON — An 8 oz. portion of delicious pink salmon broiled in our special seasonings. Served over rice pilaf **$10.99**

BUTTERFLY SHRIMP — 12 pieces of shrimp basted in our unique mixture of seasonings, then broiled. Served over rice pilaf **$1**

SCALLOPS — Fresh sea scallops perfectly seasoned and broiled. Served over rice pilaf **$15.99**

BLACKENED AHI TUNA — with ginger-citrus sticky rice, sesame sugar snaps and wasabi **$22.99**

STUFFED LOBSTER — Whole lobster oven broiled and stuffed with crab mea dressing **$36.95**

FRIED PLATTERS

Served with slaw, hushpuppies and tartar sauce.

Popcorn Shrimp 7.99
Fish & Popcorn Shrimp 10.49
Clam Strips 7.99
Sea Scallops 13.99
Oysters 13.99
Butterfly Shrimp 12.99
Fish & Chips 7.99
Skinless, Boneless Flounder 7.99
Farm Raised Catfish Filets 7.99

CATFISH

A great introductory fish for finicky eaters who refuse to try anything but fried shrimp at seafood restaurants. The flaky white flesh is relatively low in fat, which means that it's low in the fishy flavor that repels many a young diner.

BROILED SALMON

When it comes to fish, conventional nutritional wisdom is turned on its head: The fattier the fish, the better. That's because most of the fat is of the omega-3 variety, the kind proven to aid in the fight against everything from diabetes to asthma. Fatty salmon leads the way in omega-3s.

BLACKENED

The best flavor masker in the kitchen, this combination of dried spices such as paprika, onion powder, and cayenne can make a mild white fish like snapper, tilapia, or catfish taste like something close to chicken. Bonus: The spices in the blackening blend are calorie-free and loaded with antioxidants.

POPCORN SHRIMP

It's too bad that 75 percent of kids eating at seafood spots opt for these crunchy morsels. Even though they're tiny, they still weigh in at a hefty 500 calories.

FISH AND CHIPS

The biggest calorie bomb on the menu by an unhealthy measure. Add tartar sauce to the mix and you're looking at three-quarters of an 8-year-old's calorie allotment for the day. Yikes.

BBQ

PORK CHOP

In the world of barbecued meats, this is a relatively lean choice. At about 300 calories for a 4-ounce chop, this weighs in considerably lighter than the fat-speckled ribs and brisket.

SMOKED CHICKEN

Even with the skin on and slathered in barbecue sauce, this takes the prize for best entrée on the menu. Either white or dark meat will do, though the breast will save your kid about 75 calories over the leg.

SWEET TEA

The drink of choice at most 'cue shacks across the South, but would you put 9 spoonfuls of sugar in your cup of tea if you were making it at home? Well, then you shouldn't let your kids order it here, because ounce for ounce, true sweet tea has nearly as much sugar as a Mountain Dew®.

OUR MEATS

NORTH CAROLINA PULLED PORK	6.29
KANSAS CITY BURNT ENDS	6.29
TEXAS SLICED BEEF BRISKET	6.29
BARBECUED PORK CHOP	6.29
RED HOT SMOKED SAUSAGE	6.29

MEMPHIS DRY-RUBBED BARBECUED RIBS

Lone Bone (one rib)	2.75
Rib Sandwich (2 ribs)	6.29
1/3 Slab (3-4 ribs)	11.95
1/2 Slab (5-6 ribs)	13.95
Full Slab (12 Ribs)	21.95

SMOKED CHICKEN

1/4 Chicken	5.95
1/2 Chicken	9.95
Whole Chicken	16.95

BARBECUED BURRITO 5.29
Large flour tortilla stuffed with rice & ... cheese, cabbage, salsa, sour ... and cilantro

... d pork, chicken, or burnt ends
6.29

OUR MEALS

OUR $60 VALUE

(1) Slab of Ribs

(1) Pint of Pulled Pork, Burnt Ends, Beef Brisket, Pulled Chicken, or Hot Sausage

(1) Barbecued or Jamaican Jerk Half Chicken

(1) Pint each, Baked Beans & Cole Slaw

(4) Biscuits

(2) Quarts of Lemonade or Iced Sweet Tea

Half-pints of BBQ sauces

OUR $90 VALUE

(2) Slabs of Ribs

(2) Pints of Pulled Pork, Burnt Ends, Beef Brisket, Pulled Chicken, or Hot Sausage

(2) Barbecued or Jamaican Jerk Half Chickens

(1) Quart each, Baked Beans, Collard Greens, Black-eyed Corn & Cole Slaw

(6) Biscuits

(2) Quarts of Lemonade or Iced Sweet Tea

Half-pints of BBQ sauces

See our BAR MENU for specialty drinks and beers on tap. Also serving homeade Lemonade and Iced Sweet Tea.

144

OUR OTHERS

BIG GREEN SALAD WITH CORNBREAD 4.75
Choice of or Italian
With pulled chicken or spicy chicken salad 6.29

HOT OPEN-FACED BRISKET SANDWICH 8.95
With mashed potatoes, pan gravy, collard greens and cornbread

FRIED CATFISH 10.75
Cornmeal crusted and served with cole slaw, hush puppies and mash potatoes

BLACKENED CATFISH 10.75
Grilled in spices and served with cole slaw, mash potatoes and black-eyed corn

PEEL 'N' EAT SHRIMP 12.95

POTLIKKER WITH BISCUITS 1.95
Ask and we'll tell ya

OUR SWEETS

PIE 2.95

KEY LIME PIE 2.95

FRUIT COBBLER WITH WHIPPED CREAM 2.95

DREAM BAR 1.95

OUR SIDES

BAKED BEANS 1.95 cup
3.95 pint
6.95 quart

HUSH PUPPIES $.95
1.95
3.95

BLACK-EYED CORN 3.95
6.95 q

HOMEMADE PICKLES 1.95 half pint

PAN GRAVY 3.95

COLE SLAW 3.95
6.95

BISCUITS $.

GREEN BEANS 3.95
6.95

MASH POTATOES 3.95
6.95

COLLARD GREENS 1.95 cup
3.95 pint
6.95 quart

RICE & BEANS 1.95 cup
3.95 pint
6.95 quart

ALL PLATTERS
served with choice of two sides, hush puppies and a biscuit.

HUSH PUPPIES

Fried balls of cornbread, often dipped by eager Southerners into tubs of whipped butter. If your kid gets one taste of these little weapons of mass destruction, a dangerous addiction will be born.

PEEL 'N' EAT SHRIMP

A superfood for growing boys and girls. Shrimp are high in vitamin B_{12} and vitamin D, which work together to help build strong, dense bones. And this low-calorie, protein-rich finger food is just messy enough to make it fun to eat.

BISCUITS

Though most restaurants have found a way to swap out the partially hydrogenated frying oils that used to saturate French fries and chicken nuggets in trans fats, no one seems to know how to make a trans fat–free biscuit. Restaurants rely on lard and semisolid fats to make biscuits flaky, and until a suitable replacement is made available, biscuits—with up to three times the amount of trans fats one should consume in a day—should be avoided at all costs.

COLLARD GREENS

The best side on this menu, and any menu, for that matter. Even if they're stewed with a ham hock, these bitter greens have an obscenely high level of vitamins A, C, and K, plus a punch of phytochemicals.

Thai

APPETIZERS

SPRING ROLLS Vegetables $5.95

VIETNAMESE SUMMER ROLLS Shrimp or tofu $6.95

FRIED WONTON Chicken $6.95

STEAMED DUMPLING Chicken or vegetables $5.95

FRIED TOFU
Deep-Fried Fresh Tofu. Served with sweet sauce topped with crushed peanuts $4.50

PEAK GAI YANG
Special Thai B.B.Q. Wings marinated with Thai sauce $5.95

CHICKEN SATAY
Skewered chicken breast with peanut sauce dressing $7.95

PLA MUOK TOD
Deep fried squid served with sweet Chili sauce $6.95

MEE GROB
The most famous Thai crispy noodle with tomato-Tamarind sauce tofu, bean sprouts $4.50

KA-NA-NAM-MAN-HOI
Steamed broccoli with oyster sauce, sesame oil and fried onion $4.50

SALADS

CUCUMBER SALAD
With sweet and sour sauce $4.00

THAI SALAD
Green salad, bean curd, cucumber, carrot with peanut sauce dressing $4.50

THAI CHICKEN SALAD
With chicken breast and peanut sauce dressing $8.95

TOFU SALAD
Steamed tofu tossed with spicy lime dressing $8.95

GREEN PAPAYA SALAD
Lime juice, string beans, tomato, crushed peanuts $4.50

YUM WOON SEN
Glass noodle with chicken tossed with spicy lime dressing $8

YUM YAI
Boiled chicken, egg, and shrimp over a bed of lettuce topped fresh peanuts and sweet & sour sauce $9.95

SPICY BBQ BEEF SALAD
Tossed with spicy lime dressing $9.95

VEGETABLES & TOFU

SAUTEED SPINACH $10.95

SZECHWAN STRING BEANS $10.95

GARLIC EGGPLANT $10.95

ORANGE TOFU .$10.95

SPRING ROLLS

A healthy dose of carrots, cucumbers, and fresh herbs await inside, but Thai rolls come in two seasons: spring rolls, which are deep fried, and summer rolls, which are not. Now choose accordingly.

GREEN PAPAYA SALAD

It might sound strange to your kid, but the mix of shredded fruit, tomatoes, lime juice, peanuts, and a touch of palm sugar make for a perfectly refreshing and healthy starter. No offense, Mom, but it's 10 times more exciting than the iceberg salad you serve at home.

CHICKEN SATAY

This classic Thai street food combines two kid-favorite—chicken and peanuts—on a stick. Considering that an entrée portion contains less than 300 calories, mostly from lean protein, there's nothing not to love about satay.

TOFU

It might have the reputation as a low-calorie source of protein, but the soybean slab also serves as an edible sponge, so any treatment that involves oil—especially deep frying—will carry with it a few hundred calories of extra baggage.

146

SPECIALTIES

THAI BBQ CHICKEN .$10.95

BBQ PORK RIBS. $10.95

ORANGE CHICKEN $11.95

TERIYAKI CHICKEN $10.95

HONEY DUCK
Topped with house honey and hoisin sauce $12.95

GARLIC SCALLOPS $12.95

FISH WITH BLACK BEAN SAUCE $12.95

THAI CHILLI FISH
Lightly fried and topped with thai chilli sauce... $12.95

PLA LARD PRIK
Crispy snapper with chili, garlic and tamarind $12.95

NOODLE

PAD THAI

Stir-fried Thai noodles with shrimp, chicken, or vegetable, crushed peanuts, beansprouts & scallions. $7.95

PAD SEE YU

A traditional Thai broad noodles stir fried with broccoli, egg sweet soy sauce. (chicken or beef) $7.95

LAD NARD

Stir- fried broad noodles sweet soy sauce topped with gravy bean oyster and broccoli, carrot. (chicken or beef) $7.95

MEE GROB LAD NARD

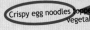
Crispy egg noodles topped with brown gravy sauce, mushrooms, vegetables and chicken $7.95

BA MEE

Egg noodle topped with ground chicken, lime juice, ground peanut, and bean sprouts $7.95

PAD WOON SEN

Stir-fried glass noodle with shrimp, mushroom, egg, onion, tomato & cabbage in soy bean sauce $7.95

RICE

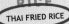
THAI FRIED RICE

With onion, carrot, pineapple, choice of chicken or beef $7.95

SPICY BASIL FRIED RICE

With chili, onion, and fresh basil. (chicken or beef) $7.95

VEGETABLES FRIED RICE $7.95

MANGO STICKY RICE $2 .50

RICE $1.00

PAD THAI

The perfect dish for all the spaghetti-loving boys and girls out there. Glass noodles are tossed with eggs, peanuts, cilantro, fresh lime juice—and often chicken, shrimp, or tofu. A kid-size portion has 450 calories, with only a small amount of (healthy) fat from the peanuts.

CRISPY NOODLES

There's only one way for noodles to end up crispy: a sizzling bath in hot oil. Expect dishes containing them to outpace stir-fried noodle dishes by 200 calories and 10 grams of fat.

THAI FRIED RICE

The only thing that keeps this rice from sticking to the giant woks chefs fry it in is a small pond of oil, most of which ends up in the dish.

MANGO STICKY RICE

Don't be fooled by the fruit: This dessert is a carb catastrophe. Go for the mango sorbet, instead.

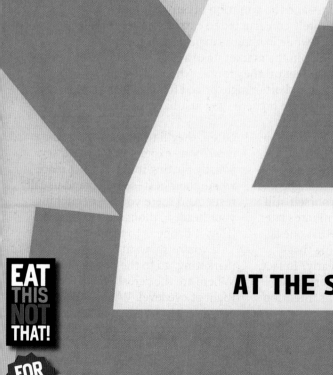

4

AT THE SUPERMARKET

Win the Supermarket Sweepstakes

It is a place as colorful as a park in July, as full of wonder as a Disneyland vacation—and as dangerous to our children's health as a minefield with a play set in the middle of it. I'm talking, of course, about the American supermarket, that dazzling monstrosity of concrete and cinder block where food marketers compete for our attention—and the attention of our children.

Supermarkets are intricately constructed to extract the maximum amount of money from your pocket while loading as many cheap calories into your cart as possible. Next time you're in the market, take a look—literally—at what's on offer, specifically about 5 feet off the ground, where your eyes fall. You'll see lots of appealing, unhealthy, and often high-priced foods placed there, while the more healthful stuff is a little higher—you just have to search a bit for it.

Indeed, searching the shelves in a state of confusion is a common experience. Have you ever gone into the market for what you thought was a quick stop and found yourself still trapped in the aisles 45 minutes later, frantically searching for that one last item—and maybe thinking that memory loss has set in early? In fact, it's not you, it's your supermarket— many grocery store chains intention- ally switch around the placement of their products from time to time to cause shoppers confusion, because more time spent in the market means, in most cases, more money spent.

Often, they'll try to get you to try a new, more-expensive brand of, say, jam, by putting it in the exact place where their best-selling brand usually rests. And there you are, scratching your head, as though it's your fault. (Hey, it happens to me, too!)

If you really want a lesson in food marketing, go to the cereal aisle. Where are the cereals targeted to you? Right at eye level. Where are the cereals with the dancing leprechauns, chocolaty vampires, and cuddly honey bears? At about hip level, right where kids can spot them. Oh, and here's the rub: Where's the candy? In most markets, the candy aisle is directly across from the cereal aisle—because all parents with kids need cereal, and all kids love candy, and . . .

You get the gist. Now, where can you find the milk, the eggs, the butter—the stuff every shopper needs? Invariably, they're all the way at the back of the store, so even a quick pop-in to get one of these staples with the kids in tow means that they'll be exposed to as many swaggering pirates, smiling clowns, and cereal-chowing sports heroes as possible.

Instead of falling victim to modern marketing, use these tricks to protect your children—and your paycheck.

STICK TO THE EDGE. Think of the grocery store as a battleground, and the edges of the store—where the produce, dairy, and meat are sold—as your green zone. Keep your kids there, and make only strategic, solo incursions into the middle aisles to snag beans and whole-grain cereals—lest your little ones be abducted by cartoon pitchmen hawking sugar.

CHOOSE REAL FRUIT. Believe it or not, 51 percent of children's food products have pictures of fruit on the package, but no actual fruit inside.

Even fruit juices can be deceiving—most are just flavored sugar water. So stick to the fresh stuff. You can get all the vitamin C you need in one day from just one orange—with only half the calories of a glass of OJ.

KNOW YOUR GRAINS. If the label says, "Made with whole grain," that doesn't mean it's healthy—just pick up a box of Franken Berry and you'll see what we mean. A product only needs to be made of 51 percent whole grain ingredients in order to carry this label. To make sure, check that the word "whole" is next to every flour listed in the ingredients.

DON'T GO AU NATURAL. The phrase *all natural* has no specific FDA definition, and there is no legislation or standards for it. Just about anything can be called "all natural."

BANISH TECHNOSUGAR. Sugar shows up in so many products, and under so many different names, that you may not even know that it's there. Look for these aliases: maltose, sorghum, sorbitol, dextrose, lactose, fructose, high-fructose corn syrup (HFCS), and glucose. And then there are the healthy-sounding versions: molasses, brown rice sugar, fruit juice, turbinado, barley malt, honey, and organic cane juice. All sugars spike insulin levels and affect the body in the same way. A good rule of thumb is to skip any product that lists sugar as one of its first four ingredients.

SKIP THE COCKTAILS. Stay away from beverages containing the words "drink," "cocktail," "punch," "beverage," or "-ade." Unless something is called "100 percent fruit juice," it's not. Even 100 percent fruit juices provide minimal nutritional value and contain as many or more calories as soft drinks. That being said, fruit juice can be a healthier alternative to soda. Mix 100 percent fruit juices with seltzer water to make a fruit spritzer, which is carbonated like soda, but has fewer calories.

KICK THE RABBIT. A cartoon character pitching food is always a bad sign. Case in point: Trix yogurt, which touts itself as "the most fun and colorful yogurt" (this is the yogurt of choice in some elementary school cafeterias). For the best nutritional value, opt for unsweetened yogurt and add your own fruit.

DON'T BE FRESH. The idea of "fresh" fruits and vegetables is great, but unless you're buying strawberries in June or tomatoes in August, that produce was probably picked unripe, trucked thousands of miles, and set to ripen under the loving, all-natural fluorescent lighting of your supermarket chain. Frozen produce, on the other hand, is usually allowed to ripen on the vine and is then frozen immediately, so it often contains more nutrients—and flavor. If you want fresh, only buy it if you're going to eat it within 3 or 4 days.

TRICK THEM WITH FRUIT. Canned pineapple, mandarin oranges, and peaches are a genius way of satisfying a kid's sweet tooth without giving them actual sweets. Just avoid the ones packed in sweetened syrup.

LEAN ON BEANS. Think of beans— which are packed with protein, fiber, and nutrients—as miniature weight-loss pills. Buy them in cans and add them to pastas, soups, salad, dips, and burritos—wherever you can disguise them.

ADD RAISINS. Raisins are packed with vitamins and minerals, but most commercial cereals coat their raisins with sugar. Be smart—buy straight-up bran and add your own, far health-ier, raisins.

DON'T GET BITTEN. Frostbite sets in after 3 to 4 months in the freezer. Don't buy big economy bags of foodstuffs and think you'll save money by storing them; you'll just wind up throwing a lot out.

SNACK BEFORE SHOPPING. One of the sneakiest supermarket tricks isn't played on your eyes or your ears, it's played on your nose. Even super-markets that don't bake bread on premises—and most don't—seem to smell like a bakery because they often pull baked goods from the freezer and nuke them to create a "lovin'-from-the-oven" scent. Whole Foods Markets are geniuses at the "scents-make-sense" game: Note the chocolate-making stations and the chicken rotisseries at the fronts of the stores. To keep your nose from triggering your salivary glands—which are, by the way, directly tied to your wallet—make sure you and your kids are fed before you shop. (Sugar-free gum or other smart ways to keep their mouths

working can also cut down on the "screaming-bloody-murder-until-you-buy-me-that" tantrums.)

HOW TO USE THIS SECTION
As any parent knows, kids have very specific tastes, which is why this section focuses on comparisons between similar foods (peanut butter cookies vs. peanut butter cookies; apple juice vs. apple juice)—so that you can find the healthiest versions of all of the foods they love most. The boxes are color-coded to help you find the relevant comparisons. Happy shopping!

Check out even more great grocery store pics, along with the 125 best foods for you and your family, at **eatthis.com**

What You Can Learn from Labels

Nutrition Facts

Serving Size 1 Cup (32g/1.1 oz.)
Servings Per Container About 10

Amount Per Serving	Cereal	Cereal with ½ Cup Vitamins A&D Fat Free Milk
Calories	120	160
Calories from Fat	10	10

	% Daily Value**	
Total Fat 1g*	2%	2%
Saturated Fat 0.5g	3%	3%
Trans Fat 0g		
Cholesterol 0mg	0%	0%
Sodium 150mg	6%	9%
Potassium 35mg	1%	7%
Total Carbohydrate 28g	9%	11%
Dietary Fiber 1g	4%	4%
Sugars 15g		
Other Carbohydrate 12g		
Protein 1g		

Vitamin A	10%	15%
Vitamin C	25%	25%
Calcium	0%	15%
Iron	25%	25%
Vitamin D	10%	25%
Thiamin	25%	30%
Riboflavin	25%	35%
Niacin	25%	25%
Vitamin B6	25%	25%
Folic Acid	25%	25%
Vitamin B12	25%	35%
Phosphorus	2%	15%
Zinc	10%	15%

Amount in cereal. One half cup of fat free milk contributes an additional 40 calories, 65mg sodium, 6g total carbohydrates (6g sugars), and 4g protein.

**Percent Daily Values are based on a 2,000 calorie diet. Your daily values may be higher or lower depending on your calorie needs:

	Calories	2,000	2,500
Total Fat	Less than	65g	80g
Saturated Fat	Less than	20g	25g
Cholesterol	Less than	300mg	300mg
Sodium	Less than	2,400mg	2,400mg
Potassium		3,500mg	3,500mg
Total Carbohydrate		300g	375g
Dietary Fiber		25g	30g

Calories per gram: Fat 9 • Carbohydrate 4 • Protein 4

INGREDIENTS: SUGAR; CORN FLOUR; WHEAT FLOUR; OAT FLOUR; PARTIALLY HYDROGENATED VEGETABLE OIL (ONE OR MORE OF: COCONUT, COTTONSEED, AND SOYBEAN); SALT; SODIUM ASCORBATE AND ASCORBIC ACID (VITAMIN C); NIACINAMIDE; REDUCED IRON; NATURAL ORANGE, LEMON, CHERRY, RASPBERRY, BLUEBERRY, LIME, AND OTHER NATURAL FLAVORS; RED #40; BLUE #2; ZINC OXIDE; YELLOW #6; TURMERIC COLOR; PYRIDOXINE HYDROCHLORIDE (VITAMIN B6); BLUE #1; RIBOFLAVIN (VITAMIN B2); THIAMIN HYDROCHLORIDE (VITA-...

The Food and Drug Administration requires all manufacturers to provide accurate and comprehensive information on ingredients and nutritional content on the back labels of packaged products. But all those random numbers and eight-syllable words can be daunting even for nutritionists, so to make matters easy on you, we've concocted a super simple four-step plan for choosing the healthiest product in every supermarket category. Start with number 1 and start eliminating products.

1 CALORIES After all, they're the largest contributor to obesity and the cluster of serious maladies—diabetes, heart disease—that come with it. If two similar products have servings within 25 calories of each other, move on to 2.

2 UNHEALTHY FATS If it contains trans fat (look for partially hydrogenated oils), or if "interesterified" oils or "stearate-rich" appear in the ingredients, find another product. Safe? Move on to 3.

3 SUGARS Always choose the food with the least amount. If sugars are within 3 grams, go on to 4.

4 FIBER The more, the better. Still a close call? Check out the tiebreaker.

THE TIEBREAKER NUMBER OF INGREDIENTS The product that has the least wins.

Food manufacturers will put anything on their packages in hopes of persuading a busy mom to fill up her cart with their goods—no matter how dubious they might be. Unfortunately, the FDA does little to regulate the vagaries that clutter the fronts of cookie boxes and juice containers. As a result, most of these health claims have, at best, a tenuous relationship with the truth.

We've picked out four products with glitzy front labels that tell one tale and back labels that tell quite another. There are hundreds of other products cluttering the aisles guilty of the same offense, so spot the tricks on these labels and use your exaggeration detector on everything else in the supermarket.

Lunchables

Be skeptical of packages adorned with cartoon characters, Hollywood heroes, or promises of toys inside. Studies show that products marketed directly to children are often poorer in terms of nutrition than regular packaged goods.

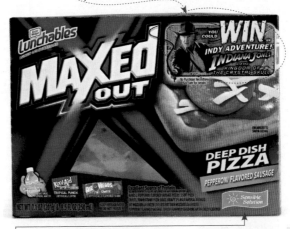

This isn't "sensible"—it's a science project gone awry. The ingredient list takes the better part of an afternoon to read through and requires a chemistry book even to begin to understand. All told, there are no fewer than 70 ingredients on the list, from the undesirable (partially hydrogenated soybean oil, high-fructose corn syrup, sodium nitrite) to the unpronounceable (acesulfame potassium, sodium stearoyl lactylate).

■ According to Kraft, "The Sensible Solution green flag on package labels is an easy way to identify better-for-you choices from among many food and beverage products. Sensible Solution criteria require that ALL qualifying products contain limited amounts of calories, fat (including saturated and trans fat), sodium, and sugar." A panel of Kraft nutritionists use US Dietary Guidelines in determining which of their products are worthy of recognition. Despite the seemingly strict standards this green flag is meant to represent, the Maxed Out Deep Dish pizza contains 510 calories and 36 g sugars.

Smart Start Cereal

■ The front of the cereal box is dominated by a slew of vague terms that hit on current "healthy" buzz words in the packaged food industry, but ultimately deliver scarcely little substance.

"Strong Heart": With no formal definition from the FDA, it's difficult to discern what it actually refers to. Perhaps the 5 grams of fiber, which *have* been shown to help stabilize cholesterol levels? Or maybe the 38 items that clutter the ingredients list, which include a barrage of preservatives, synthetic sweeteners, and artificial flavorings?

"Antioxidants": Most cereals can make the same claim, since most are fortified with a near-standard mix of minerals and antioxidant-carrying vitamins like A, C, and E.

"Smart Start": The most misleading term of them all. A real smart start would mean a cereal high in fiber, low in sugar, and with a relatively short ingredient list. Unfortunately, this cereal only meets one of the criteria.

This cereal is anything but "lightly sweetened." In fact, each flake is battered with a barrage of sweeteners, including sugar, molasses, honey, corn syrup, and high-fructose corn syrup.

All told, there are eight references to sweeteners in the ingredients list, more than any other cereal we've found in the supermarket aisles.

The resulting 17 grams of sugar make Smart Start one of the sweetest cereals on the market—just 3 grams of sugar shy of a Haagen Dazs Vanilla and Almond Ice Cream bar.

Among the many sweetened kids' cereals with less sugar per serving than Smart Start: Lucky Charms, Frosted Flakes, Trix, Froot Loops, Cocoa Pebbles.

Whole grain, yes, but wholesome? Hardly. These oats are covered in an unsavory mix of "sugar, canola oil with TBHQ and citric acid to preserve freshness, molasses, honey, BHT for freshness, soy lecithin." Try to avoid ingredients with their own acronyms.

The FDA defines "low sodium" as anything under 140 milligrams, which is exactly what this cereal has. Most cereals can claim the same, though, since it's a sugar- (not salt-) driven product.

SMART START®
Maple Brown Sugar

Nutrition Facts
Serving Size 1¼ Cups (60g/2.1 oz.)
Servings Per Container About 7

Amount Per Serving	Cereal	Cereal with ½ Cup Vitamins A&D Fat Free Milk
Calories	220	260
Calories from Fat	20	20

	% Daily Value**	
Total Fat 2.5g	4%	4%
Saturated Fat 0.5g	3%	3%
Trans Fat 0g		
Cholesterol 0mg	0%	0%
Sodium 140mg	6%	8%
Potassium 380mg	11%	17%
Total Carbohydrate 47g	16%	18%
Dietary Fiber 5g	19%	19%
Soluble Fiber 2g		
Insoluble Fiber 3g		
Sugars 17g		
Other Carbohydrate 25g		
Protein 6g		

Vitamin A (10% as beta carotene)	25%	30%
Vitamin C	25%	25%
Calcium	2%	15%
Iron	25%	25%
Vitamin D	10%	25%
Vitamin E	100%	100%
Thiamin	25%	30%
Riboflavin	25%	35%
Niacin	25%	25%
Vitamin B₆	25%	25%
Folic Acid	25%	25%
Vitamin B₁₂	25%	35%
Pantothenate	25%	35%
Phosphorus	25%	35%
Magnesium	20%	20%
Zinc	25%	25%

*Amount in cereal. One half cup of fat free milk contributes an additional 40 calories, 65mg sodium, 6g total carbohydrates (6g sugars), and 4g protein.

**Percent Daily Values are based on a 2,000 calorie diet. Your daily values may be higher or lower depending on your calorie needs.

	Calories:	2,000	2,500
Total Fat	Less than	65g	80g
Sat. Fat	Less than	20g	25g
Cholesterol	Less than	300mg	300mg
Sodium	Less than	2,400mg	2,400mg
Potassium		3,500mg	3,500mg
Total Carbohydrate		300g	375g
Dietary Fiber		25g	30g

Calories per gram: Fat 9 • Carbohydrate 4 • Protein 4

INGREDIENTS: OAT BLEND (WHOLE OATS, OAT BRAN, RICE, SUGAR, MAPLE AND BROWN SUGAR FLAVORED OAT CLUSTERS (SUGAR, TOASTED OATS [ROLLED WHOLE OATS, SUGAR, CANOLA OIL WITH TBHQ AND CITRIC ACID TO PRESERVE FRESHNESS, MOLASSES, HONEY, BHT FOR FRESHNESS, SOY LECITHIN], WHEAT FLAKES, CRISP RICE [RICE, SUGAR, SALT], CORN SYRUP, POLYDEXTROSE, HONEY, NATURAL AND ARTIFICIAL FLAVORS, CINNAMON, BHT FOR FRESHNESS, ARTIFICIAL VANILLA FLAVOR), HIGH FRUCTOSE CORN SYRUP, MALT FLAVORING, POTASSIUM CHLORIDE, SALT, NATURAL AND ARTIFICIAL FLAVOR, VITAMIN A PALMITATE, BAKING SODA, ASCORBIC ACID (VITAMIN C), NIACINAMIDE, ZINC OXIDE, CALCIUM PANTOTHENATE, REDUCED IRON, VITAMIN B₆ (ALPHA TOCOPHEROL ACETATE [VITAMIN E], BHT [PRESERVATIVE], PYRIDOXINE HYDROCHLORIDE [VITAMIN B₆], RIBOFLAVIN [VITAMIN B₂], THIAMIN HYDROCHLORIDE [VITAMIN B₁], BETA CAROTENE [A SOURCE OF VITAMIN A], FOLIC ACID, VITAMIN B₁₂.

CONTAINS WHEAT AND SOY INGREDIENTS.

Exchange: 3 Carbohydrates
The dietary exchanges are based on the Exchange Lists for Meal Planning, ©2003 by The American Diabetes Association, Inc. and The American Dietetic Association.

Distributed by Kellogg Sales Co.
Battle Creek, MI 49016 USA
®, TM, © 2007 Kellogg NA Co.

†® American Heart Association

Visit Kelloggs.com for information on promotions, recipes, products, and FAQs.
To check your offer order status go to Kelloggs.com/orders
Phone us at 1-800-962-1413
Write to P.O. Box CAMB, Battle Creek, MI 49016-1986
Provide production code on package.

Pop-Tarts

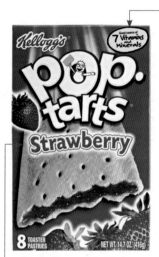

Yes, thankfully, there are actual strawberries in strawberry Pop Tarts. Problem is, it's the ninth ingredient in the list, six slots below high-fructose corn syrup.

■ The vitamin list? 10 percent of vitamin A, iron, niacin, thiamin, B₆, riboflavin, and folic acid. In accordance with USDA regulations, in order for a food product to claim that it is a "good source" of something, it must contain at least 10 percent of the recommended daily intake. The problem is that this system fails to consider the other junk that comes along with it, things like saturated fat and sugar. So Pop-Tarts can call itself a good source

of vitamins, and if your child eats 10 of these toaster pastries, she will have earned her daily intake of seven vitamins plus well over 2,000 calories. Sort of makes you wonder what a bad source of vitamins would be. So a 900-calorie pizza with 10 percent of the recommended daily intake of vitamin A can stamp "Good source of vitamin A!" on its box.

Unfortunately, two of the lowest numbers on the box also happen to be the most important, especially for something you might consider feeding to your kids for breakfast.

It's important to start the day with a bit of protein, as protein wakes up our metabolism and gets us burning calories early in the day.

Fiber is important because it helps control blood sugar levels, which makes it a potent defense mechanism against type 2 diabetes, a rising epidemic with kids in this country. And by slowing the rate at which food leaves the stomach, fiber is also a vital component of satiety, which means your child won't run out of fuel midmorning.

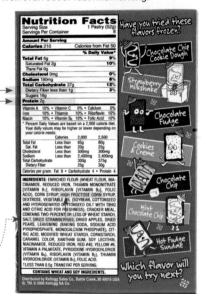

Dole Mandarins in Orange Gel

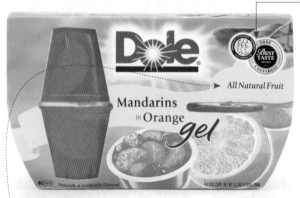

■ Chefs may know a thing or two about taste, but judging by the calorie bombs served up in most restaurants across the country, most care little of nutrition. They say so themselves on their Web site: "To receive a ChefsBest Certified Award, a product must meet the high quality standards set by the ChefsBest judges. Because of widely differing opinions, ChefsBest does not make a judgment on a product's stated nutritional or performance claims."

■ Unfortunately, "all natural" means very little when placed on a package, since the FDA doesn't have a definition for this claim. Although the fruit itself is real, it's gelled into a decidedly unnatural blend of additives and preservatives.

The ingredients include: sugar, natural and artificial flavors, sodium citrate, locust bean gum, malic acid, fumaric acid, potassium citrate, and FD&C yellow #6—a far cry from natural ingredients.

Dole puts this claim on a lot of their fruit cups, including those packaged with sugary syrup.

A medium mandarin, one of the naturally sweetest fruits on earth, contains 9 grams of sugar, so the remaining 13 grams are added sugars found in the gel.

That same medium tangerine has 47 calories and 2 grams of fiber, which means that with Dole's clever concoction here your kid gets twice the calories and half the fiber of the real thing.

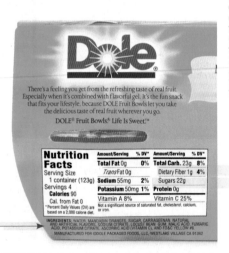

There's a feeling you get from the refreshing taste of real fruit. Especially when it's combined with flavorful gel. It's the fun snack that fits your lifestyle, because DOLE Fruit Bowls let you take the delicious taste of real fruit wherever you go.

DOLE® Fruit Bowls® Life Is Sweet.™

Nutrition Facts	Amount/Serving	% DV*	Amount/Serving	% DV*
Serving Size	**Total Fat** 0g	**0%**	**Total Carb.** 23g	**8%**
1 container (123g)	*Trans* Fat 0g		Dietary Fiber 1g	**4%**
Servings 4	**Sodium** 55mg	**2%**	Sugars 22g	
Calories 90	**Potassium** 50mg	**1%**	**Protein** 0g	
Cal. from Fat 0	Vitamin A 8%		Vitamin C 25%	
* Percent Daily Values (DV) are based on a 2,000 calorie diet.	Not a significant source of saturated fat, cholesterol, calcium, or iron.			

INGREDIENTS: WATER, MANDARIN ORANGES, SUGAR, CARRAGEENAN, NATURAL AND ARTIFICIAL FLAVORS, SODIUM CITRATE, LOCUST BEAN GUM, MALIC ACID, FUMARIC ACID, POTASSIUM CITRATE, ASCORBIC ACID (VITAMIN C), AND FD&C YELLOW #6.
MANUFACTURED FOR DDDLE PACKAGED FOODS, LLC, WESTLAKE VILLAGE CA 91362

Alternative Sweeteners

While there is a robust debate among scientists about the potential dangers of alternative sweeteners, research is still too new to make any final judgments. With little evidence to support cancer-causing claims made by those who oppose aspartame and its ilk, and a supermarket's worth of research clearly documenting the ill effects of sugar, we see no clear reason to cut out artificial sweeteners entirely, if it means decreasing sugar in your kid's diet. That being said, not all alternative sweeteners are created equal, and it's best to avoid excessively sweetened foods, artificial or not. When possible, shoot for natural ingredients and a short ingredients list.

ASPARTAME

What Is It? A low-calorie artificial sweetener made by joining two amino acids with an alcohol

How Sweet Is It? 180 times sweeter than sugar

Potential Dangers: Some researchers claim to have linked aspartame to brain tumors and lymphoma, but the FDA insists that the sweetener is safe for humans. A list of complaints submitted to the Department of Health and Human Services includes headaches, dizziness, diarrhea, memory loss, and mood changes. The Center for Science in the Public Interest states that children should avoid drinks sweetened with aspartame.

Found in: Nutra-Sweet, Equal, Diet Coke, Sugar Free Popsicle

Limit

ACESULFAME POTASSIUM

What Is It? A zero-calorie sweetener that often appears with sucralose or aspartame to create a flavor closer to sugar

How Sweet Is It? 200 times sweeter than sugar

Potential Dangers: In 2003, the FDA approved acesulfame-K for everything besides meat and poultry. Although the FDA does not recognize the sweetener as a carcinogen, some experts disagree. They point to flawed tests as the basis for the FDA's acceptance of the additive. Large doses have been shown to cause problems in the thyroid glands of rats, rabbits, and dogs.

Found in: Power-Ade Zero, Coke Zero, Breyers No Sugar Added Vanilla Ice Cream

Limit

SUCRALOSE

What Is It? A zero-calorie sugar derivative made by joining chlorine particles to sugar molecules

How Sweet Is It? 600 times sweeter than sugar

Potential Dangers: After reviewing more than 110 animal and human studies, the FDA decided in 1999 to approve sucralose for use in all foods. Sucralose opponents argue that the amount of human research is inadequate, but even groups like the Center for Science in the Public Interest have deemed it safe.

Found in: Splenda, Minute Maid Fruit Falls, Dannon Light & Fit

Safe

SUGAR ALCOHOLS

What Is It? A group of alcohols such as lactilol, sorbitol, and mannitol that provide roughly 25 percent fewer calories than sugar

How Sweet Is It? They vary from one alcohol to another, but generally they're slightly less sweet than sugar.

Potential Dangers: Sugar alcohols are applauded for not causing tooth decay and providing a smaller impact on blood sugar. Because they are not well digested, however, sugar alcohols may cause intestinal discomfort, gas, and diarrhea. Some people also report carb cravings after ingesting too much of these sweeteners.

Found in: Smuckers Sugar Free Breakfast Syrup, Wrigley's Gum, Jell-O Sugar Free cups

Limit

SACCHARIN

What Is It? A chemically complex zero-calorie sweetener

How Sweet Is It? 300 times sweeter than sugar

Potential Dangers: Between 1977 and 2000, the FDA mandated that saccharin-containing products carry a label warning consumers about the risk of cancer, due largely to the development of bladder tumors in saccharin-consuming rats. Saccharin still isn't in the clear. One recent study funded by Purdue and the National Institute of Health showed that rats with a saccharin-rich diet gained more weight than those with high-sugar diets.

Found in: Sweet'N Low

Avoid

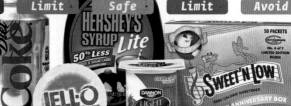

Cereal
Eat This

Kashi® 7 Whole Grain Honey Puffs (1 c)

120 calories
1 g fat (0 g saturated)
6 g sugars
2 g fiber

This cereal packs 22 grams of whole grains per serving.

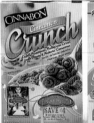

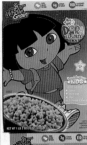

Dora the Explorer™ Cereal (¾ c/27 g)

100 calories
1.5 g fat
(0 g saturated)
6 g sugars
3 g fiber

Dora provides kids with a healthy mix of iron and B vitamins.

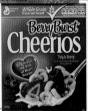

MultiGrain Cheerios® (1 c/29 g)

110 calories
1 g fat
(0 g saturated)
6 g sugars
3 g fiber

Of all the Cheerios-branded cereals, this one is second only to the original Cheerios.

Berry Burst Cheerios® (¾ c/27 g)

100 calories
1 g fat
(0 g saturated)
8 g sugars
2 g fiber

The "burst" comes in the form of real freeze-dried strawberries, raspberries, and blueberries.

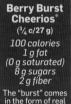

Kix® (1¼ c/30 g)

110 calories
1 g fat
(0 g saturated)
3 g sugars
3 g fiber

This low-cal cereal contains nearly half of your child's recommended daily intake of folic acid and iron.

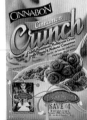

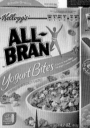

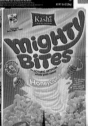

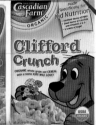

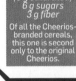

Cinnabon™ Cinnamon Crunch (1 c/40 g)

150 calories
1.5 g fat
(0 g saturated)
10 g sugars
3 g fiber

Much of the sugar comes from concentrated fruit juice and honey.

All-Bran® Yogurt Bites (1¼ c/56 g)

190 calories
3 g fat
(1.5 g saturated)
7 g sugars
10 g fiber

A single bowl has almost one-third of a child's daily fiber.

Kashi® Mighty Bites™ (1 c/33 g)

120 calories
1.5 g fat
(0 g saturated)
5 g sugars
3 g fiber

Kashi's cereals have a mix of healthy grains; this one contains 25% of the day's calcium and half of the day's iron.

Cascadian Farm® Clifford™ Crunch (1 c/30 g)

100 calories
1 g fat
(0 g saturated)
6 g sugars
5 g fiber

Whole grain oat and barley flours give this cereal a healthy boost of fiber.

Not That!

Cap'n Crunch®
(¾ c/27 g)

110 calories
1.5 g fat
(1 g saturated)
12 g sugars
1 g fiber

Yellow 5, used to color Cap'n Crunch, has been linked to hyperactivity and attention-deficit disorder.

Apple Cinnamon Cheerios®
(¾ c/30 g)

120 calories
1.5 g fat
(0 g saturated)
12 g sugars
1 g fiber

Grains are only good when they're not covered in sugar.

Corn Pops®
(1 c/31 g)

120 calories
0 g fat
14 g sugars
< 1 g fiber

The basic formula for this cereal is milled corn soaked in sugar and corn syrup.

Honey Smacks®
(¾ c/27 g)

100 calories
0.5 g fat (0 g saturated)
15 g sugars
1 g fiber

Calorie for calorie, this is the sweetest cereal in the supermarket.

Fruity Pebbles®
(¾ c/30 g)

110 calories
1 g fat
(1 g saturated)
11 g sugars
3 g fiber

Nature's Path EnviroKidz™ Organic Gorilla Munch® (¾ c/30 g)

120 calories
0 g fat
(0 g saturated)
8 g sugars
2 g fiber

The ratio of sugar to nutrients is concerningly high.

Golden Grahams®
(¾ c/31 g)

120 calories
1 g fat
(0 g saturated)
15 g sugars
1 g fiber

We're glad General Mills is commited to whole grains, but we can't get past all that sugar.

Yogurt Burst® Cheerios®
(¾ c/30 g)

120 calories
1.5 g fat
(0.5 g saturated)
9 g sugars
2 g fiber

It looks innocent, but almost one-third of this cereal's calories come from sugars.

French Toast Crunch®
(1 c/41 g)

173 calories
4 g fat
(0 g saturated)
15 g sugars
1 g fiber

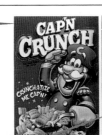

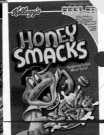
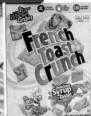

Cereal
Eat This

Quaker® Oatmeal Squares Brown Sugar (1 c)

210 calories
2.5 g fat
(0.5 g saturated)
10 g sugars
5 g fiber

All of the fiber of granola, without the sugar surge.

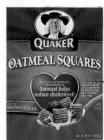

Frosted Mini-Wheats® Bite Size

(12 biscuits/30 g)

100 calories
0.5 g fat (0 g saturated)
6 g sugars
4 g fiber

Grape-Nuts® Flakes (¾ c/29 g)

110 calories
1 g fat
(0 g saturated)
4 g sugars
3 g fiber

A hint of sweetness, plus enough fiber to keep their bellies full until lunch.

Not only does it have 3 grams of protein, but it also has 45 percent of your child's daily iron and a whole host of B vitamins.

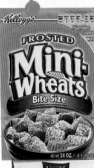

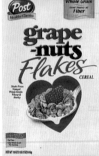

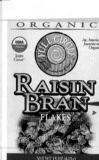

Kashi® GOLEAN® (1 c)

140 calories
1 g fat
(0 g saturated)
6 g sugars
10 g fiber

One of our favorite cereals, with enough sweetness for a kid to enjoy, plus major fiber to boot.

Full Circle® Raisin Bran (1 c)

190 calories
1 g fat
(0 g saturated)
13 g sugars
6 g fiber

Instead of being battered in sugar, Full Circle's raisins are coated in cane juice.

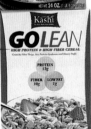

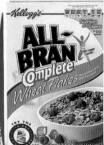

All-Bran® Complete® Wheat Flakes (1 c)

120 calories
1 g fat
(0 g saturated)
7 g sugars
7 g fiber

The same fiber hit for a fraction of the calories.

Cheerios® (1 c)

100 calories
2 g fat
(0 g saturated)
1 g sugars
3 g fiber

Classic for a reason: It's low-sugar, low-cal, and even contains a decent dose of fiber. It's screaming out for sliced banana.

Not That!

Quaker® Natural Granola Oats, Honey & Raisins
(1 c)
420 calories
6 g fat
(3.5 g saturated)
15 g sugars
3 g fiber

Frosted Flakes®
(¾ c/30 g)
110 calories
0 g fat
11 g sugars
1 g fiber

Where the Mini-Wheats use whole grain wheat, the Frosted Flakes use milled corn, a cheap and nutritionally empty filler food.

Smart Start® Original Antioxidants
(1 c)
190 calories
0.5 g fat
(0 g saturated)
14 g sugars
3 g fiber

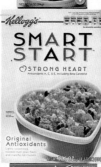

Raisin Nut Bran
(¾ c/49 g)
180 calories
3 g fat
(0.5 g saturated)
14 g sugars
5 g fiber

Sugar comes before raisins on the list of ingredients.

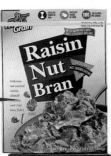

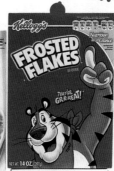

Kashi® GOLEAN® Crunch! Honey Almond Flax
(1 c/53 g)
200 calories
4.5 g fat
(0 g saturated)
12 g sugars
8 g fiber

Sugar and calories cancel out the fiber.

Rice Krispies®
(1¼ c/33 g)
120 calories
0 g fat
3 g sugars
0 g fiber

You can't afford to feed your kid a cereal with zero fiber.

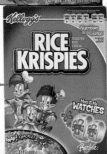

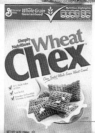

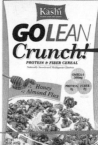

Wheat Chex®
(¾ c/47 g)
160 calories
1 g fat
(0 g saturated)
5 g sugars
5 g fiber

163

Hot Cereals

Eat This

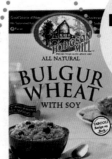

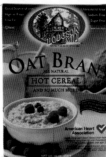

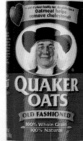

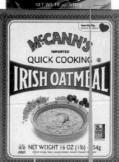

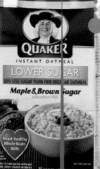

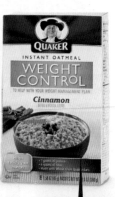

**Kashi®
GOLEAN®
Creamy Truly
Vanilla™
Instant Hot
Cereal**
(1 packet)

150 calories
2 g fat
(0 g saturated)
6 g sugars
7 g fiber

**Hodgson Mill®
Oat Bran Hot
Cereal** (¼ c dry)

120 calories
3 g fat
(1 g saturated)
0 g sugars
6 g fiber

Trading this for Malt-O-Meal for one week will add 35 grams of fiber to your child's diet.

**Old Fashioned
Quaker® Oats**
(½ c dry)

150 calories
3 g fat
(0.5 g saturated)
1 g sugars
4 g fiber

You can spare the 5 minutes it takes to cook Old Fashioned Oats—your kid's worth it.

**McCann's®
Quick & Easy
Steel-Cut Irish
Oatmeal**
(¼ c dry)

150 calories
2 g fat
(0 g saturated)
0 g sugars
4 g fiber

Steel-cut oats have a rich texture.

**Hodgson Mill®
Bulgur Wheat
with Soy Hot
Cereal** (¼ c dry)

115 calories
1 g fat
(0 g saturated)
0 g sugars
3 g fiber

Bulgur wheat has a gentle effect on blood sugar.

**Quaker®
Instant
Oatmeal
Weight Control
Cinnamon**
(1 packet)

160 calories
3 g fat
(0.5 g saturated)
1 g sugars
6 g fiber

Not That!

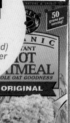

Quaker® Organic Instant Maple Brown Sugar
(1 packet)

150 calories
2 g fat (0 g saturated)
12 g sugars   3 g fiber

Forgo the heavily sweetened flavored varieties; the high sugar intake cancels out any benefit your kid might get from the fiber.

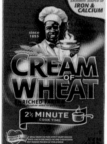

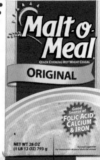

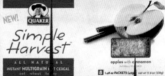

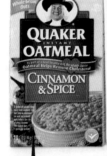

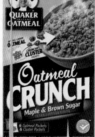

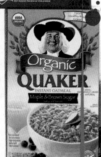

Quaker® Instant Oatmeal Cinnamon & Spice (1 packet)

170 calories
2 g fat
(0.5 g saturated)
15 g sugars
3 g fiber

Nature's Path® Organic Instant Original Hot Oatmeal (1 packet)

190 calories
4 g fat
(0 g saturated)
0 g sugars
4 g fiber

Quaker® Oatmeal Crunch Maple & Brown Sugar (1 packet)

190 calories
2.5 g fat
(0.5 g saturated)
14 g sugars
3 g fiber

Cream of Wheat Original Flavor (3 Tbsp dry)

120 calories
0 g fat
0 g sugars
1 g fiber

Oatmeal prevails in the battle of the classic hot cereals, packing more than double the fiber.

Malt-O-Meal® Original Hot Wheat Cereal (3 Tbsp dry)

130 calories
0.5 g fat
(0 g saturated)
0 g sugars
1 g fiber

No real nutrition makes Malt-O-Meal a breakfast worth passing on.

Quaker® Simple Harvest™ Apples with Cinnamon (1 packet)

150 calories
1.5 g fat
(0 g saturated)
12 g sugars
4 g fiber

165

Granola and Breakfast
Eat This

Quaker® Chewy® Peanut Butter Chocolate Chip Bar with 25% Less Sugar (1 bar)
100 calories
3 g fat
(1 g saturated)
5 g sugars
3 g fiber

Clif® Kid™ Organic Chocolate Brownie ZBar (1 bar)
120 calories
3 g fat
(1 g saturated)
12 g sugars
3 g fiber
More of all the things that matter most.

All-Bran® Apple Cinnamon Streusel Fiber Bar (1 bar)
130 calories
2.5 g fat
(1 g saturated)
10 g sugars
10 g fiber
One-third of a 10-year-old's fiber RDA.

If you need to reward a well-behaved kid, use a Rice Krispies Treat. It's the least dangerous of the sugary-snack bars.

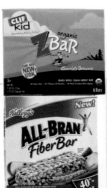

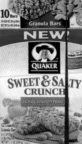

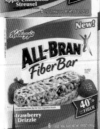

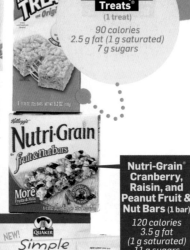

Rice Krispies Treats® (1 treat)
90 calories
2.5 g fat (1 g saturated)
7 g sugars

Nutri-Grain® Cranberry, Raisin, and Peanut Fruit & Nut Bars (1 bar)
120 calories
3.5 g fat
(1 g saturated)
11 g sugars
3 g fiber

All-Bran® Strawberry Drizzle Fiber Bar (1 bar)
120 calories
2.5 g fat
(1 g saturated)
9 g sugars
10 g fiber
Twice the protein and 10 times the fiber.

Quaker® Oats, Nuts & Honey Sweet & Salty Crunch (2 bars)
150 calories
6 g fat
(1 saturated)
8 g sugars
2 g fiber
Why not save 30 calories per serving?

Quaker® Chewy® 90 Calorie Peanut Butter Granola Bar (1 bar)
90 calories
2 g fat
(0 g saturated)
7 g sugars
1 g fiber
Light on the fiber, but also light on sugar.

Quaker® Simple Harvest™ Cinnamon Brown Sugar Bar (1 bar)
140 calories
3 g fat
(0 g saturated)
10 g sugars
2 g fiber

Kashi® GOLEAN® Crunchy! Chocolate Almond Protein & Fiber Bar (1 bar)
170 calories
5 g fat
(2.5 g saturated)
13 g sugars
5 g fiber

Bars

Not That!

Kudos® Peanut Butter Whole Grain Bars
(1 bar)
130 calories
6 g fat
(3 g saturated)
12 g sugars
1 g fiber

This bar would be more at home in the candy aisle.

Cascadian Farm® Organic Vanilla Chip Chewy Granola Bars
(1 bar)
140 calories
3 g fat (2 g saturated)
13 g sugars

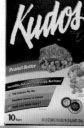

Nature Valley® Chewy Trail Mix Bars
(all flavors) (1 bar)
140 calories
4 g fat
(0.5 g saturated)
13 g sugars
1 g fiber

Crunchy Nut® Peanut Butter Sweet & Salty Granola Bars
(1 bar)
150 calories
8 g fat
(3 g saturated)
10 g sugars
2 g fiber

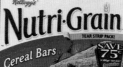
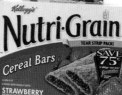

Quaker® Brown Sugar Cinnamon Oatmeal to Go
(1 bar)
220 calories
4 g fat
(1 g saturated)
19 g sugars
5 g fiber

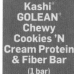

Kashi® GOLEAN® Chewy Cookies 'N Cream Protein & Fiber Bar
(1 bar)
290 calories
6 g fat
(4 g saturated)
35 g sugars
6 g fiber

Cinnamon Toast Crunch® Milk 'n Cereal Bars (1 bar)
180 calories
4 g fat
(2 g saturated)
15 g sugars
1 g fiber

75% of the sugar and less fiber than its parent cereal.

Health Valley® Peanut Crunch Chewy Granola Bars
(1 bar)
110 calories
2.5 g fat
(1 g saturated)
10 g sugars
<1 g fiber

40% of its calories are from sugar.

Nature Valley® Oats 'N Honey Granola Bars
(2 bars)
180 calories
6 g fat
(0.5 g saturated)
11 g sugars
2 g fiber

Nutri-Grain® Strawberry Cereal Bars
(1 bar)
140 calories
3 g fat
(0.5 saturated)
13 g sugars
<1 g fiber

Loaded with high-fructose corn syrup.

Just because it's organic doesn't mean it's good for you. This one has a load of sugar and very little protein or fiber.

Yogurt
Eat This

Oikos™ Greek Vanilla
(5.3 oz)

110 calories
0 g fat
11 g sugars

Dannon® All Natural Strawberry (4 oz)

110 calories
1 g fat
(0.5 g saturated)
19 g sugars

Dannon's All-Natural line is made with real fruit and no chemicals.

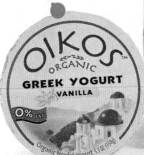

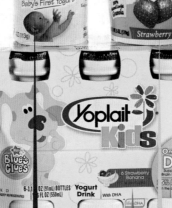

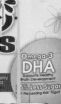

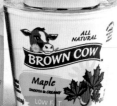

Greek-style yogurt involves straining the whey (the liquid part) from the yogurt, leaving a creamier cup with nearly twice the protein of regular American yogurt.

Stonyfield Farm® Organic YoBaby® Simply Plain
(1 c/4 oz)

90 calories
4.5 g fat
(1 g saturated)
6 g sugars

Unlike most children's squeezable and drinkable yogurts, this one's made with real fruit puree.

Yoplait® Kids™ Strawberry Banana Yogurt Drink (3.2 oz)

70 calories
1.5 g fat
(1 g saturated)
10 g sugars

Breyers® YoCrunch® Light Strawberry (6 oz)

120 calories
1 g fat
(0 g saturated)
11 g sugars

Take advantage of the creamy-crunchy blend to turn this yogurt-granola combo into a super healthy dessert.

Brown Cow Low Fat Maple (6 oz)

130 calories
2.5 g fat
(1.5 g saturated)
20 g sugars

This one contains almost one-quarter of your child's recommended daily calcium.

Not That!

Stonyfield Farm®
All Natural
O'Soy®
Strawberry
(6 oz)

170 calories
2.5 g fat
(0 g saturated)
27 g sugars

Some of the "healthier" brands tend to overdo it with the cane sugar.

Horizon®
Organic
Fat-Free Vanilla
(6 oz)

80 calories
0 g fat
24 g sugars

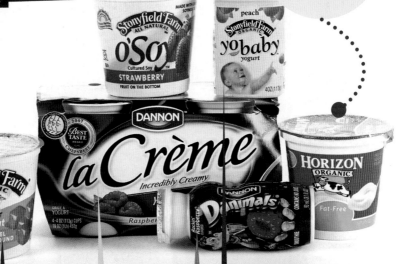

Stonyfield Farm®
Organic Lowfat
Caramel (6 oz)

180 calories
1.5 g fat
(1 g saturated)
35 g sugars

This cup of yogurt has 15 grams more sugar than a ½-cup serving of Stonyfield's After Dark Chocolate Ice Cream.

Dannon® la Crème
Raspberry (4 oz)

140 calories
5 g fat
(3 g saturated)
18 g sugars

If you want a creamy yogurt that tastes like dessert, try the Greek-style cups from Oikos.

Danimals®
Drinkables
Swingin'
Strawberry-
Banana™ (6 oz)

180 calories
3 g fat
(2 g saturated)
30 g sugars

Stonyfield Farm®
Organic YoBaby®
Peach (4 oz)

110 calories
4 g fat
(1 g saturated)
13 g sugars

This cup contains more than 3 grams of sugar per ounce of yogurt.

Who cares if the yogurt is organic if it still contains more sugar than a Häagen-Dazs ice cream bar?

169

Breakfast Breads and

Eat This

Still a sweet breakfast, but with 5 grams of protein and 4 grams of fiber.

Pastries

Not That!

Pepperidge Farm® Plain Bagels (1 bagel)

260 calories
1 g fat
(0 g saturated)
10 g sugars
3 g fiber

The refined flour found in white breads can cause blood sugar to soar. Studies found that the resulting metabolic changes from these foods caused obese boys to overeat.

Hostess® Blueberry Mini Muffins (1 pouch)

270 calories
15 g fat (2.5 g saturated)
19 g sugars
< 1 g fiber

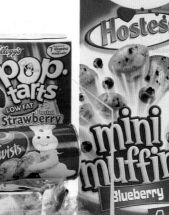

Remember this: Blueberries are good for you. Blueberry muffins are not.

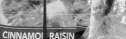

Hostess® Donettes® Frosted Mini Donuts (4 donuts)

240 calories
14 g fat (10 g saturated)
16 g sugars
<1 g fiber

There's nothing mini about the effects of frosted donuts. The main ingredient is sugar, and with zero fiber, your child will be hungry before first bell.

Thomas'® Cinnamon Raisin English Muffin (1 muffin)

140 calories
1 g fat
(0 g saturated)
9 g sugars
2 g fiber

Pillsbury® Flaky Cinnamon Twists with Glaze (2 twists)

180 calories
9 g fat (2.5 g saturated, 2.5 g trans)
10 g sugars
0 g fiber

If you're going to go through the effort of cooking, why waste the effort on something nutritionally empty?

Pop-Tarts® Low Fat Frosted Strawberry (1 pastry)

190 calories
3 g fat
(1 g saturated)
20 g sugars
< 1 g fiber

Low fat or not, this gooey tart packs unhealthy doses of high-fructose corn syrup.

Breakfast Condiments
Eat This

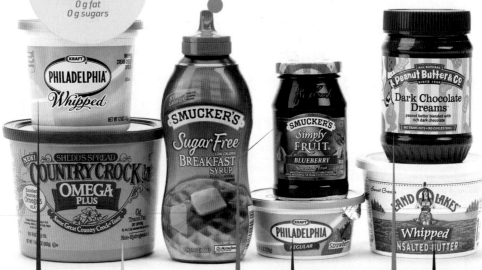

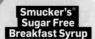

**Smucker's®
Sugar Free
Breakfast Syrup**
(¼ c)
*25 calories
0 g fat
0 g sugars*

**Kraft®
Philadelphia®
Whipped
Cream Cheese**
(2 Tbsp)

*60 calories
6 g fat
(3.5 g saturated)*

Easier to spread
and less caloric.
What more could
you want?

**Shedd's
Spread
Country
Crock® Omega
Plus**
(1 Tbsp)

*50 calories
5 g fat
(1 g saturated)*

Contains
310 milligrams of
omega-3 fats.

**Smucker's®
Simply Fruit®
Blueberry
Spreadable
Fruit** (2 Tbsp)

*80 calories
0 g fat
16 g sugars*

Perfect as a syrup
substitute. Most of
the sugars here
come from real fruit.

**Kraft®
Philadelphia®
Strawberry
Cream Cheese**
(2 Tbsp)

*90 calories
8 g fat
(4.5 g saturated)
4 g sugars*

Flavored with real
strawberry.

**Peanut Butter
& Co® Dark
Chocolate
Dreams®**
(2 Tbsp)

*170 calories
13 g fat
(2.5 g saturated)
7 g sugars*

**Land O Lakes®
Unsalted
Whipped
Butter** (1 Tbsp)

*50 calories
6 g fat
(3.5 g saturated)*

Whipping air into
the butter decreases
the caloric
density—plus it
makes for easier
spreading.

Not That!

Lite syrups are essentially just watered-down versions of regular syrups.

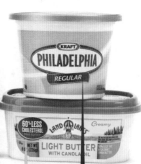

Mrs. Butterworth's® Lite Syrup
(¼ c)
100 calories
0 g fat
24 g sugars

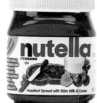

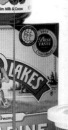

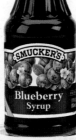

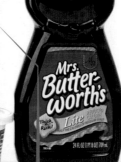

Land O' Lakes® Stick Margarine
(1 Tbsp)

100 calories
11 g fat
(2 g saturated, 2.5 g trans)

Stick margarine trades saturated fat for more-dangerous trans fats.

Nutella® (2 Tbsp)

200 calories
11 g fat
(2 g saturated)
20 g sugars

This chocolate-hazelnut spread may be a favorite in Europe, but it has no place on the breakfast table.

Horizon® Organic Cream Cheese (2 Tbsp)

110 calories
10 g fat
(6 g saturated)
0 g sugars

Smucker's® Blueberry Syrup (2 Tbsp)

200 calories
0 g fat
44 g sugars

Although it does have a small amount of blueberry puree, this syrup is still mostly corn syrup and high-fructose corn syrup.

Land O Lakes® Light Butter (1 Tbsp)

50 calories
6 g fat
(3.5 g saturated)

Not a bad choice, as far as butters go, but swap with the Crock and you'll trade saturated fat for healthy omega-3s.

Kraft® Philadelphia® Regular Cream Cheese (2 Tbsp)

90 calories
9 g fat
(5 g saturated)

Peanut Butter and Jell
Eat This

This is a great
alternative
to ultrasweet
grape jelly.

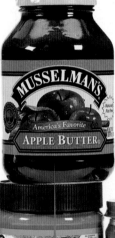

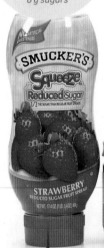

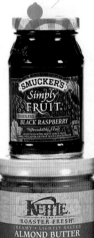

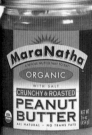

**Smucker's®
Reduced Sugar
Strawberry Fruit
Spread** (1 Tbsp)

*20 calories
0 g fat
5 g sugars*

Make the switch to
reduced sugar twice a
week and you'll save
your kid 4 cups of
added sugar by the end
of the year.

**Kettle™ Creamy
Almond Butter**
(1 oz)

*184 calories
16 g fat
(2 g saturated)*

The same smooth
sweetness of peanut
butter, almonds have
more heart-healthy
fats and antioxidants
than peanuts.

**Skippy® Natural
Creamy Peanut
Butter** (2 Tbsp)

*180 calories
16 g fat
(3.5 g saturated)*

Unlike most peanut
butters, Skippy Natural
doesn't contain
hydrogenated oils.

**Musselman's®
Apple Butter**
(3 Tbsp)

*90 calories
0 g fat
18 g sugars*

No actual butter in this
one, just apples cooked
down long and slow
until the fruit has a
creamy consistency.
Make this your kid's
favorite condiment.

**MaraNatha®
Crunchy &
Roasted Peanut
Butter** (2 Tbsp)

*190 calories
16 g fat
(2 g saturated)*

Just dry roasted
peanuts and sea salt.

Not That!

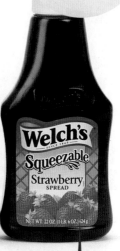

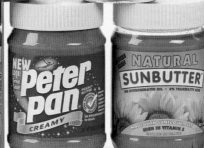

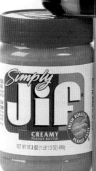

It might be organic, but the first ingredient is still sugar.

Smucker's® Organic Concord Grape Jelly
(1 Tbsp)
50 calories
0 g fat
12 g sugars

Simply Jif® Creamy Peanut Butter (2 Tbsp)
190 calories
16 g fat
(3 g saturated)
Contains fully hydrogenated vegetable oils.

Smucker's® Goober Grape® Peanut Butter and Grape Jelly Stripes (3 Tbsp)
240 calories
13 g fat
(2.5 g saturated)
21 g sugars
The Goober must be the mass of sugar holding this sludge together.

Peter Pan® Creamy Peanut Butter (2 Tbsp)
190 calories
17 g fat
(3.5 g saturated)

SunGold® Natural SunButter® (2 Tbsp)
200 calories
16 g fat
(2 g saturated)
This is a good alternative for kids with peanut allergies, but otherwise too high in calories for regular consumption.

Welch's® Squeezable Strawberry Spread (1 Tbsp)
50 calories
0 g fat
13 g sugars
Granted some of it is natural, but two tablespoons of this spread has nearly as much sugar as a Snickers bar.

Breads

Eat This

This is the best tortilla at your supermarket. It's a fiber-and-protein-rich rarity among wraps, and it contains only polyunsaturated and monounsaturated fats—both of which are good for you and your child.

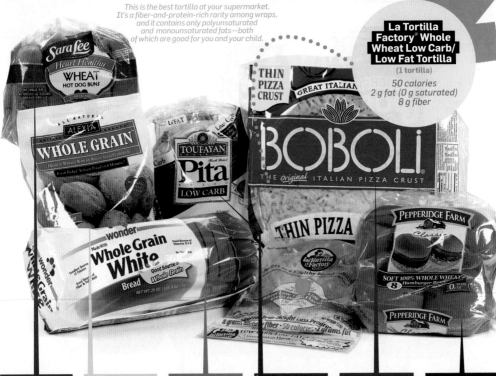

La Tortilla Factory® Whole Wheat Low Carb/Low Fat Tortilla
(1 tortilla)

50 calories
2 g fat (0 g saturated)
8 g fiber

Sara Lee® Heart Healthy Wheat Hot Dog Buns (1 bun)

110 calories
1 g fat
(0 g saturated)
2 g fiber

This small swap will still add a couple grams of fiber to your dog.

Alexia® Whole Grain Rolls
(bagged, frozen)
(1 roll)

90 calories
1 g fat
(0 g saturated)
3 g fiber

Frozen or not, this is as good as it gets for a dinner roll.

Wonder® Whole Grain White Bread (2 slices)

130 calories
2 g fat
(0.5 g saturated)
4 g fiber

If you must eat white bread, look for a white-wheat hybrid with at least 4 grams of fiber.

Toufayan® Low Carb Pita
(1 pita)

130 calories
2.5 g fat
(0 g saturated)
9 g fiber

Contains no sugar and an amazing 11 grams of protein.

Boboli® Thin Crust
(1 crust/12")

850 calories
17.5 g fat
(7.5 g saturated)
5 g fiber

Or try the new whole wheat thin crust, which has an impressive 25 grams of fiber per crust.

Pepperidge Farm® 100% Whole Wheat Buns (1 bun)

120 calories
2 g fat
(0 g saturated)
2 g fiber

The term "wheat" can be misleading. Make sure the label says "100% whole wheat."

Not That!

Mission® Garden Spinach Herb Wrap
(1 tortilla)
*210 calories
5 g fat (1.5 g saturated)
2 g fiber*

The "spinach" in this garden-herb wrap is actually spinach powder, which does not count as a serving of vegetables.

Pepperidge Farm® Farmhouse Sandwhich Rolls Country Wheat (1 roll)
*220 calories
4.5 g fat
(1 g saturated)
1 g fiber*

Boboli® Original Crust
(1 crust/12")
*1,120 calories
20 g fat
(8 g saturated)
8 g fiber*
Tack on 192 grams of carbs and more than 2,000 milligrams of sodium—and that's before toppings!

Toufayan® Wheat Flat Bread (1 piece)
*260 calories
9 g fat
(1.5 g saturated)
3 g fiber*
Just because it's thin doesn't mean it's light.

Wonder® Classic
(2 slices)
*120 calories
1 g fat
(0 g saturated)
0 g fiber*
Run-of-the-mill white breads have little to offer in the way of nutrition.

King's Hawaiian® 100% Whole Wheat Rolls
(1 roll)
*100 calories
3 g fat
(1 g saturated)
2 g fiber*
Whole wheat, sure, but loaded with sugar and margarine.

Sara Lee® Whole Grain White Hot Dog Buns (1 bun)
*120 calories
1.5 g fat
(0 g saturated)
1 g fiber*

Cheeses

Eat This

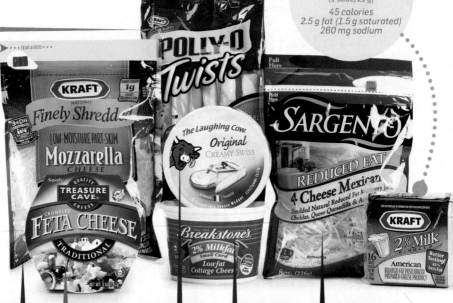

Not That!

Kraft® Deli Deluxe Sharp Cheddar
(2 slices/19 g)

110 calories
8 g fat (5 g saturated)
150 mg sodium

Kraft® Snackables® Cubes Natural Cheddar & Monterey Jack Cheeses
(5 pieces)

72 calories
7 g fat
(4.5 g saturated)
132 mg sodium

Why triple your kid's fat intake when a perfectly fine substitute is readily available?

Kraft® Natural Shredded Sharp Cheddar (¼ c)	**Horizon® Organic Cottage Cheese** (½ c)	**WisPride® Sharp Cheddar** (2 Tbsp/28 g)	**DiGiorno® Shredded Romano Cheese** (¼ c)	**Kraft® Finely Shredded Mild Cheddar** (¼ c)
110 calories *9 g fat* *(6 g saturated)* *180 mg sodium*	*120 calories* *5 g fat* *(3 g saturated)* *390 mg sodium*	*90 calories* *7 g fat* *(3.5 g saturated)* *170 mg sodium*	*110 calories* *8 g fat* *(5 g saturated)* *430 mg sodium*	*110 calories* *9 g fat* *(6 g saturated)* *180 mg sodium*
		There's nothing sharp about a cheese that's made with xantham gum.	The long aging process concentrates the fat and sodium levels in this cheese.	

Deli Meats
Eat This

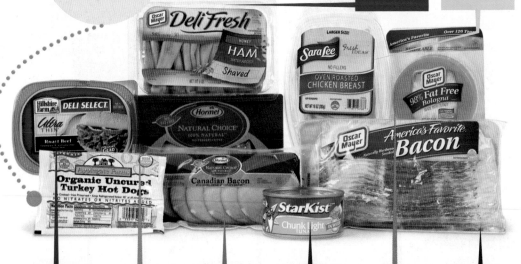

Applegate Farms® Organic Uncured Turkey Hot Dogs
(1 dog)

80 calories
6 g fat (2 g saturated)
350 mg sodium

You'd be hard pressed to find a better hot dog anywhere.

Oscar Mayer® Deli Fresh Honey Shaved Ham
(6 slices/51 g)

50 calories
1 g fat
(0 g saturated)
650 mg sodium

Sara Lee® Fresh Ideas Oven Roasted Chicken Breast
(6 slices/86 g)

68 calories
1 g fat
(0 g saturated)
645 mg sodium

Hillshire Farm® Deli Select® UltraThin™ Roast Beef
(2 oz)

60 calories
3 g fat
(1 g saturated)
450 mg sodium

Hormel® Natural Choice® 100% Natural Smoked Deli Turkey
(3 slices/56 g)

50 calories
1 g fat
(0 g saturated)
450 mg sodium

No added nitrates.

Hormel® Natural Choice® Canadian Style Bacon
(2 slices/56 g)

70 calories
2 g fat
(1 g saturated)
680 mg sodium

StarKist® Chunk Light Tuna in Water
(2 oz)

60 calories
0.5 g fat
(0 g saturated)
250 mg sodium

The water-packed tuna contains a fraction of the fat and calories.

Oscar Mayer® 98% Fat Free Bologna
(1 slice/28g)

25 calories
0.5 g fat
(0 g saturated)
240 mg sodium

Oscar Mayer® America's Favorite Bacon
(2 slices)

70 calories
6 g fat
(2 g saturated)
290 mg sodium

Whether in a BLT, or as a breakfast side, two slices of bacon is a relatively low-impact indulgence.

Not That!

Oscar Mayer Deli Fresh Grilled Chicken Breast Strips
(9 slices / 84 g)

110 calories
1.5 g fat
(1 g saturated)
690 mg sodium

Budding Baked Honey Ham Deli Cuts
(2 oz / 57 g)

80 calories
2.5 g fat
(1 g saturated)
650 mg sodium

Oscar Mayer Louis Rich ⅓ Less Fat Turkey Franks
(1 dog)

100 calories
8 g fat
(2.5 g saturated)
510 mg sodium

Oscar Mayer Turkey Bacon
(2 slices)

70 calories
6 g fat
(2 g saturated)
360 mg sodium

And here you were, thinking that you were doing yourself and your family a favor by using turkey bacon.

Oscar Mayer Turkey Bologna
(1 slice / 28 g)

50 calories
4 g fat
(1 g saturated)
270 mg sodium

StarKist Chunk Light Tuna in Vegetable Oil
(2 oz)

90 calories
4.5 g fat
(1 g saturated)
170 mg sodium

Tuna is a great source of protein; vegetable oil is not.

Hormel Turkey Pepperoni
(22 slices / 39 g)

90 calories
5 g fat
(2 g saturated)
830 mg sodium

Butterball Honey Roasted Turkey Breast
(7 slices / 56 g)

70 calories
1 g fat
(0.5 g saturated)
550 mg sodium

Hillshire Farm Deli Select Ultra Thin Hard Salami
(5 slices / 28 g)

110 calories
10 g fat
(4 g saturated)
500 mg sodium

This "thin" salami packs 125 milligrams of sodium per slice.

181

Trail Mix, Dried Fruit,
Eat This

Look for a brand with the fewest possible preservatives. And added sugars are absolutely unnecessary, since fruit has enough natural sweetness to satisfy a sweet tooth.

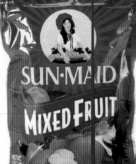

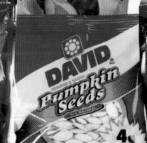

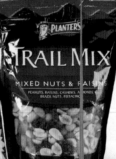

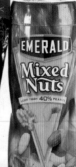

Sun-Maid® Mixed Fruit
(¼ c/40 g)

100 calories
0 g fat
17 g sugars

Sunsweet® Pitted Prunes
(5 prunes/40 g)

100 calories
0 g fat
12 g sugars
3 g fiber

Per gram, prunes provide fewer calories, more fiber, and less sugar than raisins.

DAVID® Roasted & Salted Pumpkin Seeds
(¼ c/30 g)

160 calories
12 g fat
(2.5 g saturated)
0 g sugars
940 mg sodium

Jacked full of manganese, magnesium, and iron.

Planters® Mixed Nuts and Raisins Trail Mix (1 oz)

150 calories
11 g fat
(1.5 g saturated)
6 g sugars

Ocean Spray® Craisins Orange Flavor
(¼ c/30 g)

98 calories
0 g fat
20 g sugars

When it comes to antioxidants, few fruits can match the concentration found in cranberries.

Emerald® Mixed Nuts (1 oz)

170 calories
16 g fat
(2.5 g saturated)
1 g sugars

Peanut-free, so your child gets more cashews, almonds, and walnuts, which have higher levels of healthy fats and antioxidants.

and Mixed Nuts
Not That!

Welch's® Mixed Fruit (¼ c/40 g)

130 calories
0 g fat
21 g sugars

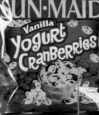

As if dried fruit weren't sweet enough already, Welch's adds extra sugar to the mix.

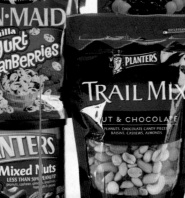

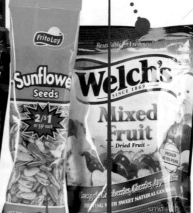

Planters® Mixed Nuts (1 oz)

170 calories
15 g fat (
2 g saturated)
1 g sugars

This mix lists peanuts as the main nut. Technically peanuts are legumes and are lower in healthy fats and antioxidants than more legitimate nuts.

Sun-Maid® Vanilla Yogurt Cranberries (¼ c/30 g)

120 calories
3.5 g fat
(3 g saturated)
20 g sugars

This is really more candy than fruit.

Planters® Nut & Chocolate Trail Mix (1 oz)

160 calories
10 g fat
(2.5 g saturated)
13 g sugars

The sugar doubles when chocolate pieces sneak into the mix.

Frito Lay® Sunflower Seeds (3 Tbsp hulled seeds/28 g)

200 calories
16 g fat
(2 g saturated)
150 mg sodium

Add in the shells and the sodium jumps to 1,230 milligrams.

Sun-Maid® Raisins (¼ c/40 g)

130 calories
0 g fat
29 g sugars
2 g fiber

Crackers

Eat This

With 3 grams of fiber and no added sugars, this is the best cracker for cheese, peanut butter, or just straight snacking.

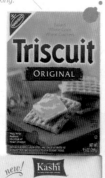

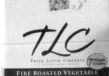

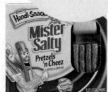

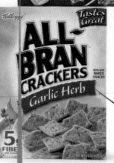

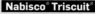

Nabisco® Triscuit®
(6 crackers/29 g)

120 calories
4.5 g fat (1 g saturated)
180 mg sodium

Kashi® TLC™ Fire Roasted Vegetable
(15 crackers/30 g)

130 calories
3.5 g fat
(0 g saturated)
210 mg sodium

Made with Kashi's signature 7 whole grains and real bell peppers, onions, and carrots.

Keebler® Club® Original Cracker
(4 crackers)

70 calories
3 g fat
(0.5 g saturated)
140 mg sodium

Nabisco® Premium® Toasted Onion Saltine Crackers
(10 crackers/30 g)

120 calories
3 g fat
(0 g saturated)
360 mg sodium

Nabisco® Triscuit® Roasted Garlic
(6 crackers/28 g)

120 calories
4.5 g fat
(0.5 g saturated)
140 mg sodium

This tasty twist on original Triscuits boasts 3 grams of fiber per serving.

Kraft® Handi-Snacks® Mister Salty® Pretzels 'n Cheez
(1 packet)

90 calories
3.5 g fat
(1 g saturated)
380 mg sodium

Pretzels make for safer dipping than breadsticks.

Kellogg's® All-Bran™ Garlic Herb Crackers
(18 crackers/30 g)

120 calories
6 g fat
(1 g saturated)
330 mg sodium

184

Not That!

Nabisco® Wheat Thins®
(16 crackers/31 g)

140 calories
6 g fat (1 g saturated)
260 mg sodium

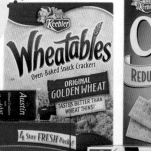

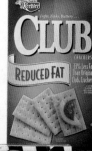

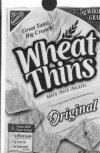

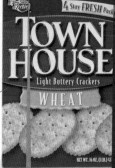

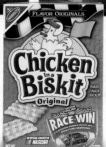

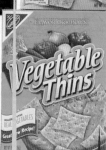

Keebler® Town House® Wheat
(10 crackers/32 g)

*160 calories
8 g fat
(2 g saturated)
280 mg sodium*

These wheat crackers have more partially hydrogenated oil than they do actual whole grain wheat.

Austin® Wheat Crackers with Cheddar Cheese (1 packet)

*200 calories
10 g fat
(2 g saturated,
4 g trans)
370 mg sodium*

Beware: more than a half-gram of trans fat per cracker!

Keebler® Wheatables®
(17 crackers/30 g)

*140 calories
6 g fat
(1.5 g saturated)
340 mg sodium*

These offer only 1 gram of fiber.

Nabisco® Chicken in a Biskit®
(12 crackers/31 g)

*160 calories
8 g fat
(1.5 g saturated)
300 mg sodium*

The liberal use of soybean and palm oils loads each of these crackers with nearly 1 gram of fat.

Keebler® Club® Reduced Fat Crackers
(5 crackers)

*70 calories
2 g fat
(0 g saturated)
180 mg sodium*

In exchange for one less gram of fat you get more sodium and double the sugar. Keep it original.

Nabisco® Vegetable Thins®
(21 crackers/30 g)

*150 calories
7 g fat
(2 g saturated)
320 mg sodium*

Thin in name only, these pack partially hydrogenated oils and high-fructose corn syrup.

185

Crunchy Snacks
Eat This

Pepperidge Farm® Cheddar Goldfish
(55 pieces/ 30 g)
140 calories
5 g fat
(1 g saturated)
250 mg sodium

Nabisco® Garden Harvest® Toasted Chips Apple Cinnamon
(16 chips/1 oz)
120 calories
3 g fat
(0 g saturated)
Half a serving of fruit in each bag.

Doritos® Spicy Nacho
(12 chips/1 oz)
140 calories
7 g fat (1 g saturated)
210 mg sodium

Not the quintessential healthful food option, but the lesser of two spicy evils in the full-flavor chip category.

Baked! Lay's® Original
(15 crisps/1 oz)
120 calories
2 g fat
(0 g saturated)
180 mg sodium
If you're going to have chips in your pantry, this is a good one to stock.

Smart Balance® Light Butter Microwave Popcorn
(4 c popped)
120 calories
4.5 g fat
(1.5 g saturated)
290 mg sodium

Garden of Eatin'® Nacho Cheese
(9 chips/1 oz)
140 calories
6 g fat
(0.5 g saturated)
140 mg sodium

Ritz® Snack Mix 100 Calorie Packs® (1 packet)
100 calories
3 g fat
(0.5 g saturated)
210 mg sodium
When it comes to self-contained snacks, you'd be hard-pressed to find a better one.

Baked! Lays® Barbecue Flavored
(14 chips/1 oz)
120 calories
3 g fat
(0.5 g saturated)
210 mg sodium

New York Style® Whole Wheat Pita Chips
(7 chips/1 oz)
110 calories
3.5 g fat
(1.5 g saturated)
350 mg sodium

Not That!

Seneca® Crispy Apple Chips
(12 chips/1 oz)
*140 calories
7 g fat
(1 g saturated)*

Nabisco® Cheez-It®
(27 crackers/30 g)
*160 calories
8 g fat
(2 g saturated)
250 mg sodium*

Pringles® Extreme® Blazin' Buffalo Wing
(15 chips/1 oz)
*150 calories
10 g fat (3 g saturated)
280 mg sodium*

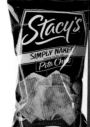
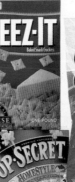
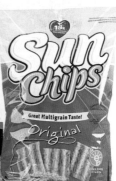

Stacy's® Simply Naked Pita Chips
(14 chips/1 oz)
*130 calories
5 g fat
(0.5 g saturated)
270 mg sodium*

Kettle™ Krinkle Cut™ Classic Barbeque
(1 oz)
*150 calories
9 g fat
(1 g saturated)
170 mg sodium*
Natural it may be, but light it is not.

Keebler® Toast & Peanut Butter Sandwich Crackers
(1 packet)
*200 calories
10 g fat
(1.5 g saturated)
410 mg sodium*

Tostitos® Multigrain
(8 chips/1 oz)
*150 calories
8 g fat
(1 g saturated)
135 mg sodium*
Opt for a thinner tortilla chip. It provides just as many salsa-dunks for a fraction of the calories.

Pop Secret® Homestyle Premium Popcorn
(4 c popped)
*180 calories
11 g fat
(1.5 g saturated,
5 g trans)
410 mg sodium*
The real secret is the amount of trans fat.

SunChips® Original
(16 chips/1 oz)
*140 calories
6 g fat
(1 g saturated)
120 mg sodium*
For all the good press they get, SunChips are only marginally better for you than real potato chips.

187

Dips

Eat This

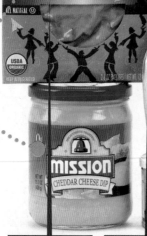
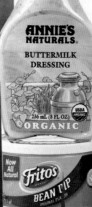
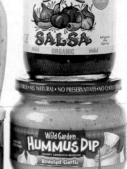

Mission® Cheddar Cheese Dip
(2 Tbsp)
45 calories
3 g fat (0.5 g saturated)
280 mg sodium

Drew's® All Natural Mild Salsa (2 Tbsp)
10 calories
0 g fat
100 mg sodium

There's no beating a pure, tomato-based salsa. Beyond being a low-calorie condiment, salsa also packs plenty of disease-fighting antioxidants.

Wholly Guacamole™
(2 Tbsp)
50 calories
4 g fat
(0.5 g saturated)
75 mg sodium

It might be a few more calories, but they come from real heart-healthy avocados—not oil and thickening agents.

Annie's Naturals® Organic Buttermilk Dressing
(2 Tbsp)
60 calories
6 g fat
(1 g saturated)
230 mg sodium

The exact flavors of the beloved ranch, with half the calories.

Fritos® Bean Dip Original Flavor
(2 Tbsp)
35 calories
1 g fat
(0 g saturated)
190 mg sodium

Pinto beans, like the ones used in this dip, are an excellent source of fiber.

Wild Garden® Roasted Garlic Hummus Dip
(2 Tbsp)
35 g calories
2 g fat
(0 g saturated)
70 mg sodium

Set up a plate of baby carrots, Triscuits, and hummus for a perfect after-school snack.

Not That!

Ruffles® Rich and Creamy Sour Cream & Chive
(2 Tbsp)

60 calories
5 g fat
(0.5 g saturated)
240 mg sodium

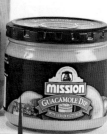

Pace® Mexican Four Cheese Salsa
(2 Tbsp)

90 calories
7 g fat (1.5 g saturated)
430 mg sodium

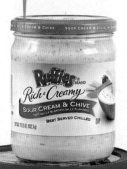
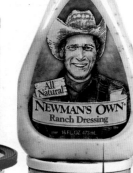
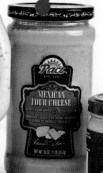

Taco Bell® Medium Salsa con Queso (2 Tbsp)

25 calories
2 g fat
(0 g saturated)
220 mg sodium

The first two ingredients are water and soybean oil.

Fritos® Mild Cheddar Dip (2 Tbsp)

50 calories
3.5 g fat
(5 g saturated)
330 mg sodium

This dip is easy to confuse with a bean dip, but its base is really milk, and it contains partially hydrogenated oils.

Newman's Own® Ranch Dressing (2 Tbsp)

140 calories
16 g fat
(2.5 g saturated)
310 mg sodium

What with the way kids are dipping these days, a bottle of this stuff in the fridge could be a major health hazard.

Mission® Guacamole Dip (2 Tbsp)

40 calories
3 g fat
(0 g saturated)
150 mg sodium

The first three ingredients are water, canola oil, and food starch. The only mention of avocado is the "avocado powder."

Cookies
Eat This

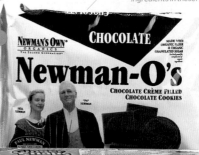

Unlike most cookies on the shelves, you'll actually recognize most of the ingredients in these.

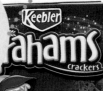

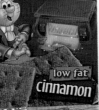

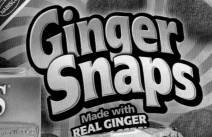

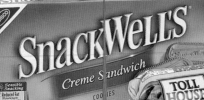

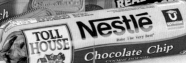

Newman's Own® Newman-O's® Chocolate Crème Filled Chocolate Cookies

(2 cookies/28 g)

130 calories
4.5 g fat (1.5 g saturated)
10 g sugars

Nabisco® Snack Well's® Creme Sandwich Cookies

(2 cookies/25 g)

110 calories
3 g fat (1 g saturated)
9 g sugars

Keebler® Low Fat Cinnamon Grahams

(1 sheet/28 g)

110 calories
1.5 g fat
(0 g saturated)
9 g sugars

As a rule, graham crackers crush cookies in the calorie and fat department. Up the satiety quotient by spreading the grahams with peanut butter.

Nestlé® Toll House® Chocolate Chip Cookie Dough (1 large cookie)

120 calories
6 g fat
(3 g saturated)
10 g sugars

Nearly identical as the Pillsbury version, but for one big difference: no trans fat.

Nabisco® Ginger Snaps®

(4 cookies/28 g)

120 calories
2.5 g fat
(0.5 g saturated)
11 g sugars

As far as classes of cookies go, ginger snaps are about as safe as it gets.

Not That!

They may look like friendly elves, but Keebler cookies are consistently some of the most caloric in the supermarket.

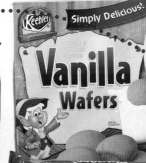

Keebler® E.L. Fudge® Original
(2 cookies/36 g)

180 calories
7 g fat (3 g saturated)
12 g sugars

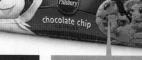

Keebler® Sandies® Simply Shortbread
(2 cookies/31 g)

170 calories
9 g fat (4 g saturated)
7 g sugars

We applaud Keebler for cutting back on the trans fats, but these cookies still contain partially hydrogenated oils—and 2 grams of saturated fat apiece.

Pillsbury® Ready to Bake Chocolate Chip Cookie Dough
(1 large cookie)

120 calories
6 g fat (2 g saturated, 2 g trans)
10 g sugars

The trans fat comes from the partially hydrogenated soybean and cottonseed oils in the recipe.

Keebler® Vanilla Wafers
(8 cookies/30 g)

140 calories
6 g fat (2 g saturated)
9 g sugars

Keebler® Vienna Fingers
(2 cookies/31 g)

150 calories
6 g fat (2 g saturated)
10 g sugars

Pudding
Eat This

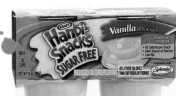

Kraft® Handi-Snacks® Sugar Free Vanilla Pudding

(1 c)

45 calories
1 g fat (.5 g saturated)
0 g sugars

You only gain 1 gram of fat and save 35 calories and 14 grams of sugar!

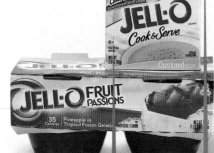

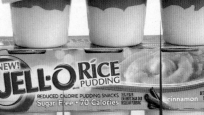

Jell-O® Fruit Passions® Pineapple in Tropical Fusion Gelatin (1 c)

35 calories
0 g fat
6 g sugars

Might as well use the Jell-O snack as an opportunity to slip in a serving of good fruit.

Jell-O® Cook & Serve Custard (¼ package)

80 calories
0 g fat
17 g sugars

Try instant custard over pudding. There's no point in eating saturated fat when what you're really craving is sugar.

Jell-O® Sugar Free/Fat Free Cook & Serve Chocolate Pudding (¼ package)

30 calories
0 g fat
0 g sugars

Jell-O® Sugar Free Cinnamon Rice Pudding (1 c)

70 calories
2 g fat (1.5 g saturated)
0 g sugars

Jell-O® Sugar Free Dulce De Leche Pudding (1 c)

60 calories
1 g fat (1 g saturated)
0 g sugars

Not That!

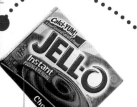

Food manufacturers love to remove fat only to replace it with a ton of sugar.

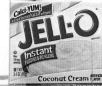

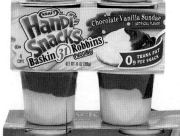

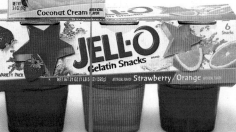

**Snack Pack®
Fat Free Tapioca
Pudding**
(1 c)

*80 calories
0 g fat
14 g sugars*

**Kraft® Handi-
Snacks® Baskin
Robbins
Chocolate
Vanilla Sundae**
(1 c)

*100 calories
1 g fat
(1 g saturated)
16 g sugars*

**Kozy Shack®
No Sugar Added
Rice Pudding**
(1 c)

*90 calories
3 g fat
(2 g saturated)
4 g sugars*

**Jell-O® Instant
Chocolate
Pudding** (1 c)

*100 calories
0 g fat
19 g sugars*

The first two
ingredients are sugar
and starch.

**Jell-O® Instant
Coconut Cream
Pudding & Pie
Filling** (¼ package)

*100 calories
2.5 g fat
(2.5 g saturated)
16 g sugars*

Don't let the "Calci-
YUM!" declaration on
the front of the box
fool you; there's no
calcium inside.

**Jell-O® Gelatin
Snacks
Strawberry/
Orange**
(1 c)

*70 calories
0 g fat
17 g sugars*

193

Juice

Eat This

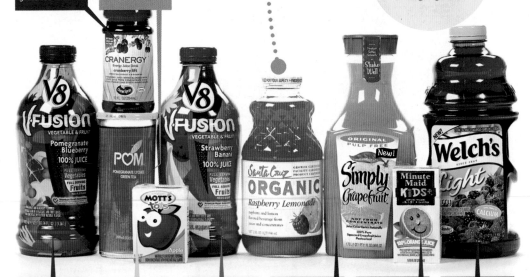

Ocean Spray® Cranergy® Cranberry Lift (12 oz)

50 calories
12 g sugars

This alternative to straight cranberry juice has an energizing mix of B vitamins and green tea extracts.

Pom® Pomegranate Lychee Green Tea (8 oz)

70 calories
16 g sugars

Part green tea and part pomegranate juice, this packs a walloping dose of antioxidants for the little ones.

Santa Cruz® Raspberry Lemonade (8 oz)

100 calories
22 g sugars

V8 V-Fusion® Pomegranate Blueberry 100% Juice (8 oz)

100 calories
0 g fat
23 g sugars

One serving of fruit *and* a serving of vegetables in every 8-ounce glass.

Mott's for Tots® Apple Juice (1 box/6.8 oz)

50 calories
13 g sugars

This is 100 percent apple juice diluted with purified water. The kids get the sweetness and the nutrition, but avoid the deluge of sugar.

V8 V-Fusion® Strawberry Banana Light (8 oz)

50 calories
0 g fat
10 g sugars

The Fusion line masks V8's vegetable blend with the sweetness of real fruit juice.

Simply Orange® Juice Company's Simply Grapefruit™ (8 oz)

90 calories
18 g sugars

This juice is entirely unadulterated.

Minute Maid® Kids+® 100% Orange Juice (1 box, 6.8 oz)

100 calories
20 g sugars

This orange juice is a step above most because it's fortified with a slew of good vitamins.

Welch's® Light Berry (8 oz)

70 calories
16 g sugars

Drink this and you'll lose nearly half the sugars without sacrificing the tasty and healthful allure of blueberries, blackberries, and raspberries.

194

Not That!

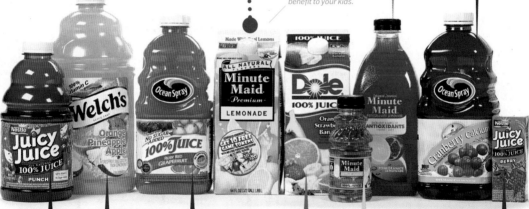

Minute Maid® Lemonade
(8 oz)

110 calories
29 g sugars

Minute Maid® Enhanced Pomegranate Lemonade
(8 oz)

110 calories
30 g sugars

The first two ingredients are water and high-fructose corn syrup.

Ocean Spray® Cranberry with Calcium
(8 oz)

150 calories
37 g sugars

This juice contains only 27 percent cranberry juice. The rest of the calories come from added sugars.

Lemonade is generally 10 percent lemon juice and 90 percent sugar water and provides little nutritional benefit to your kids.

Juicy Juice® 100% Juice Fruit Punch
(8 oz)

120 calories
26 g sugars

This diluted mix still holds 26 grams of sugar—equal to two servings of Edy's® Loaded Chocolate Peanut Butter Cup Ice Cream.

Welch's® Orange Pineapple Apple (8 oz)

140 calories
34 g sugars

One of the most sugar-laden "juices" in the supermarket.

Ocean Spray® Ruby Red Grapefruit 100% Juice
(8 oz)

130 calories
29 g sugars

The grapefruit juice is diluted with cheap, high-sugar fillers such as grape and apple juices.

Dole® Orange Strawberry Banana Juice
(8 oz)

120 calories
0 g fat
24 g sugars

Minute Maid® Apple Juice
(1 bottle/10 oz)

140 calories
32 g sugars

There's a simple reason why kids love apple juice so much: it's sweeter than most soft drinks. This bottle is no exception.

Nestlé® Juicy Juice® Berry All-Natural 100% Juice
(8 oz)

120 calories
0 g fat
27 g sugars

Children's Drinks
Eat This

Gatorade® G2®
(8 oz)
25 calories
7 g sugars
Gatorade's new light sports beverage provides all the electrolytes active kids will need without all the sugar or calories. Perfect for game day.

Minute Maid's line of water-based beverages for kids provides the hit of sweetness they crave, but without the heavy caloric cost. Plus each pouch packs a day's worth of vitamin C.

Minute Maid® Fruit Falls™ Tropical Water Beverage
(1 pouch)
5 calories
< 1 g sugars

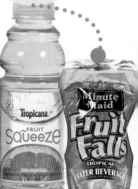

Nestlé® Nesquik® Chocolate No Sugar Added Powder
(2 Tbsp)
35 calories
1 g fat
(0.5 g saturated)
3 g sugars

Crystal Light® On The Go
(1 packet)
10 calories
0 g sugars
Check the serving size on the box, because they're almost always listed as ½ packet, while everyone will use the whole packet.

Crayons® All Natural Fruit Juice Drink
(1 can/8 oz)
90 calories
19 g sugars

Horizon® 2% Milk (1 container/ 8 oz) with 2 Tbsp Nesquik® Chocolate No Sugar Added Powder
155 calories
5.5 g fat
(3 g saturated)
15 g sugars

Tropicana® Light 'n Healthy (8 oz)
50 calories
10 g sugars

Tropicana® Fruit Squeeze™ Tropical Tangerine
(1 bottle)
35 calories
7 g sugars

196

Not That!

Capri Sun® Roarin' Waters® Tropical Fruit Water Beverage
(1 pouch)
35 calories
9 g sugars

Capri Sun® Sport™ Lightspeed Lemon Lime with Electrolytes
(1 pouch)
60 calories
16 g sugars

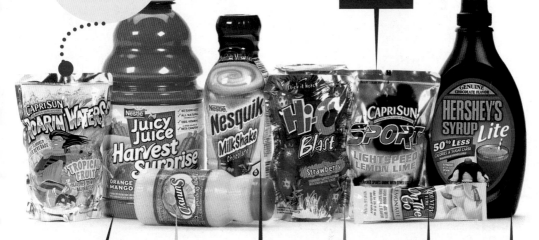

Nestlé® Juicy Juice® Harvest Surprise™ Orange Mango
(1 bottle, 8 oz)
130 calories
27 g sugars

Sunny D® Tangy Original
(1 bottle, 6.75 oz)
80 calories
16 g sugars
Basically diluted HFCS: All of the ingredients combined, aside from water and HFCS, make up less than 2 percent of the drink.

Nesquik® Chocolate Milkshake
(1 bottle/16 oz)
340 calories
10 g fat
(6 g saturated)
26 g sugars
Exercise portion control by making your own 8-ounce glass of chocolate milk.

Hi-C Blast® Strawberry
(1 pouch)
100 calories
26 g sugars

Country Time® Lemonade On The Go
(1 packet)
70 calories
18 g sugars
The first ingredient is sugar.

Hershey's® Lite Syrup
(2 Tbsp)
50 calories
0 g fat
10 g sugars
Even this is a step above regular Hershey's, which lists high-fructose corn syrup as its main ingredient.

197

Grains

Eat This

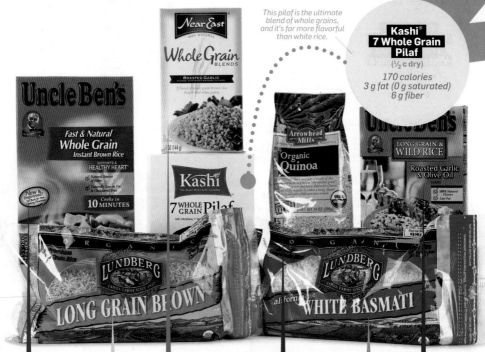

This pilaf is the ultimate blend of whole grains, and it's far more flavorful than white rice.

Kashi® 7 Whole Grain Pilaf
(½ c dry)
170 calories
3 g fat (0 g saturated)
6 g fiber

Uncle Ben's Fast and Natural™ Whole Grain Instant Brown Rice
(1 c prepared)
170 calories
1 g fat (0 g saturated)
2 g fiber

Lundberg Long Grain Brown (¼ c dry)
170 calories
1.5 g fat (0 saturated)
3 g fiber
Slightly higher in calories, but it's worth it to get the extra fiber.

Near East® Whole Grain Blends Roasted Garlic
(1 c, prepared with olive oil)
220 calories
5 g fat (0.5 g saturated)
5 g fiber

Arrowhead Mills® Quinoa
(⅓ c dry)
160 calories
2.5 g fat (0 g saturated)
3 g fiber
One of the world's most perfect foods, quinoa has a remarkable balance of protein, healthy fats, and fiber.

Lundberg® White Basmati Rice (¼ c dry)
170 calories
.5 g fat (0 g saturated)
1 g fiber
Basmati rice has a lower glycemic index than jasmine, so it better regulates blood sugar levels.

Uncle Ben's® Long Grain & Wild Rice, Roasted Garlic & Olive Oil
(1 c prepared)
180 calories
1 g fat (0 g saturated)
3 g fiber

Not That!

Minute® Premium White Rice
(½ c dry)
190 calories
0 g fat
0 g fiber

White rice is the black sheep of the grain family. It has high levels of carbohydrates and no fiber to slow digestion, which means that white rice will spike kids' insulin levels dangerously high.

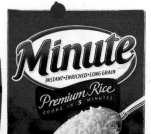
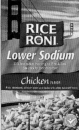
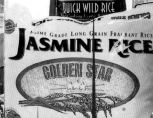
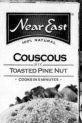
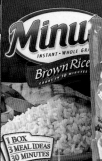
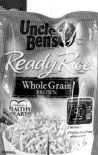

**Rice-A-Roni®
Lower Sodium
Chicken
Flavor Rice**
(1 c prepared)
270 calories
5 g fat
(1 g saturated)
2 g fiber

This side will cost one-third of the day's sodium.

**Golden Star®
Jasmine Rice**
(¼ c dry)
200 calories
.5 g fat
(0 g saturated)
0 g fiber

**Lundberg®
Quick Wild
Rice**
(¼ c dry)
150 calories
0.5 g fat
(0 g saturated)
2 g fiber

Wild beats white every time, but still can't compete with a superfood like quinoa.

**Near East®
Toasted Pine
Nut Couscous**
(1 c, prepared with olive oil)
230 calories
6 g fat
(1 g saturated)
2 g fiber

**Minute®
Brown Rice**
(¼ c dry)
150 calories
1.5 g fat
(0 g saturated)
2 g fiber

**Uncle Ben's®
Whole Grain
Brown Ready
Rice®**
(1 c prepared)
220 calories
4 g fat
(0 g saturated)
2 g fiber

Faster prep time means that the rice is more processed.

199

Noodles

Eat This

Ronzoni® Healthy Harvest® Whole Wheat Blend Thin Spaghetti (2 oz)

*180 calories
2 g fat
(0 g saturated)
6 g fiber*

Tons of fiber and protein.

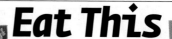

Kraft® Tangy Italian Spaghetti Classics®

(2 oz prepared)

*200 calories
1.5 g fat
(0.5 g saturated)
610 mg sodium*

For prepackaged pasta meals, Kraft Spaghetti Classics outshines Kraft Macaroni & Cheese by 3 grams of protein and 14 grams of fat.

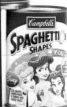

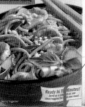

Ronzoni® Healthy Harvest® Whole Wheat Blend Extra-Wide Noodle Style Pasta (2 oz)

*180 calories
1 g fat
(0 g saturated)
15 mg sodium
6 g fiber*

Thai Kitchen® Bangkok Curry Instant Rice Noodle Soup

(1 package)

*190 calories
3.5 g fat
(0.5 g saturated)
870 mg sodium*

Low-calorie rice noodles are a decent alternative to ramen.

Simply Asia® Roasted Peanut Noodles (105 g)

*383 calories
14 g fat
(1 g saturated)
936 mg sodium*

Kids will love the simple, familiar flavors of this dish.

SpaghettiOs® Plus Calcium

(1 c)

*170 calories
1 g fat
(0.5 g saturated)
620 mg sodium*

Additional vitamin D and calcium come along with less fat.

Chef Boyardee® Cheesy Burger Macaroni (1 c)

*200 calories
5 g fat
(2.5 g saturated)
820 mg sodium*

It's better than Beefaroni, but still very high in sodium. Proceed with caution.

SpaghettiOs® Princess Fun Shapes (1 c)

*170 calories
1 g fat
(0.5 g saturated)
630 mg sodium*

Look for cans that say "plus calcium." Besides the calcium boost, they're lower in calories and sodium.

Not That!

Kraft® Macaroni & Cheese Dinner prepared with margarine and 2% milk
(1 c prepared)

410 calories
19 g fat (5 g saturated, 4 g trans)
710 mg sodium

Was there ever any doubt that "The Cheesiest" was not the healthiest?

Barilla® Angel Hair Pasta (2 oz)

200 calories
1 g fat
(0 g saturated)
2 g fiber

With less fiber than its whole wheat counterpart, white pasta moves through the stomach quickly and raises blood sugar levels.

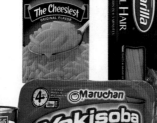
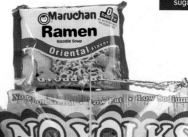
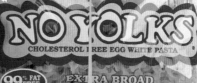

SpaghettiOs® A to Z's with Meatballs (1 c)

260 calories
9 g fat
(3.5 g saturated)
990 mg sodium

Small additions can tip the scale in a big way. The addition of meat means nine times the fat per serving.

Chef Boyardee® Beefaroni® (1 c)

260 calories
10 g fat
(4.5 g saturated)
990 mg sodium

SpaghettiOs® Raviolio's (1 c)

270 calories
8 g fat
(3.5 g saturated)
1,090 mg sodium

Canned pastas have dangerously high levels of sodium. A whole can contains more than half the RDA for sodium.

Maruchan® Yakisoba Teriyaki Flavor (1 bowl/113 g)

520 calories
20 g fat
(10 g saturated)
1,260 mg sodium

The teriyaki flavor brings with it more than half a day's worth of sodium.

Maruchan® Top Ramen Oriental Flavor (1 package)

380 calories
14 g fat
(7 g saturated)
1,760 mg sodium

This starving-student staple contains 77 percent of your kid's recommended daily sodium intake.

No Yolks® Cholesterol Free Egg White Pasta (2 oz)

210 calories
0.5 g fat
(0 g saturated)
3 g fiber

Don't fear the yolks—they're loaded with healthy fats and protein.

Sauces

Eat This

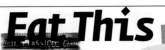

You don't have to bathe a wing in butter and fat to make it good. Stubb's is spicy and delicious without all the junk.

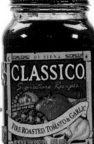

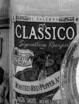

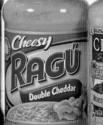

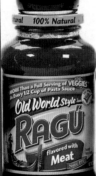

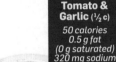

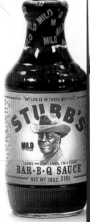

**Stubb's®
Mild Bar-B-Q Sauce**
(2 Tbsp)

15 calories
0 g fat
210 mg sodium

Classico® Fire Roasted Tomato & Garlic (½ c)

50 calories
0.5 g fat
(0 g saturated)
320 mg sodium

There's a reason Classico doesn't have a line of light sauces: It doesn't need one.

**Kikkoman®
Less Sodium
Soy Sauce**
(1 Tbsp)

10 calories
0 g fat
575 mg sodium

With half a day's sodium in a tablespoon of regular soy sauce, you can't afford not to make this simple swap.

**Ragú® Old
World Style®
Flavored with
Meat** (½ c)

70 calories
3 g fat
(0.5 g saturated)
570 mg sodium

You won't find a meat sauce with less calories or fat in the supermarket.

**Ragú® Double
Cheddar** (¼ c)

100 calories
9 g fat
(3 g saturated)
450 mg sodium

Break glass in case of emergency! Otherwise, leave all cheese-based sauces out of your pantry.

**Classico®
Roasted Red
Pepper
Alfredo** (½ c)

120 calories
10 g fat
(6 g saturated)
620 mg sodium

Far from a nutritional superstar, but this is the best of the Alfredo sauces.

**Cibo Naturals®
Artichoke
Lemon Pesto**
(¼ c)

210 calories
21 g fat
(2.5 g saturated)
260 mg sodium

An antioxidant-packed sauce that's perfect tossed with hot spaghetti.

202

Not That!

Kraft® Original Barbecue Sauce
(2 Tbsp)

50 calories
0 g fat
440 mg sodium

Beware of high levels of sodium in steak and BBQ sauces— even a drizzle or a dunk can carry a huge salt load.

Ragú® Light Tomato & Basil, No Added Sugar
(½ c)

60 calories
1.5 g fat
(0 g saturated)
330 mg sodium

Even Ragu's lightest effort still loses to Classico.

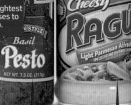
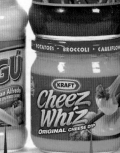
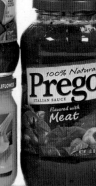
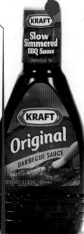

Melissa's® Italian Style Basil Pesto
(¼ c)

340 calories
34 g fat
(6 g saturated)
230 mg sodium

True, most of the fat comes from olive oil, but the calorie load is too great to justify.

Ragú® Light Parmesan Alfredo (½ c)

280 calories
20 g fat
(12 g saturated)
1,280 mg sodium

Despite being "light," this version has more calories and sodium.

Kraft® Cheez Whiz®
(¼ c)

180 calories
14 g fat
(3 g saturated)
880 mg sodium

Prego® Flavored with Meat Italian Sauce (½ c)

100 calories
4 g fat
(1 g saturated)
580 mg sodium

Prego almost always has more calories than the other popular brands.

La Choy® Soy Sauce
(1 Tbsp)

10 calories
0 g fat
1,160 mg sodium

La Choy has more sodium than any of the other major soy sauce brands.

Soups

Eat This

Each serving is lower in calories and loaded with protein and fiber.

Campbell's® Chunky™ Grilled Steak Chili with Beans
(1 c)
200 calories
3 g fat (1 g saturated)
870 mg sodium

Imagine® Organic Sweet Potato Soup
(1 c)
110 calories
1.5 g fat
(0 g saturated)
400 mg sodium
One-third of kids ages 12 to 19 are vitamin A deficient. This soup has 270 percent of the RDI.

Campbell's® Dora Fun Shapes
(½ c prepared)
70 calories
2 g fat
(0.5 g saturated)
580 mg sodium

Campbell's® Healthy Request® Select™ Mexican Style Chicken Tortilla (1 c)
130 calories
2.5 g fat
(1 g saturated)
480 mg sodium

Lipton® Soup Secrets® Noodle Soup with Real Chicken Broth
(1 c prepared)
62 calories
2 g fat
(0.5 g saturated)
720 mg sodium

Campbell's® Healthy Request® Homestyle Chicken Noodle Soup
(½ c prepared)
60 calories
2 g fat
(0.5 g saturated)
480 mg sodium

Campbell's® Chunky™ Grilled Sirloin Steak (1 c)
130 calories
2 g fat
(1 g saturated)
890 mg sodium
Contains 40 percent of your child's daily vitamin A requirement.

204

Not That!

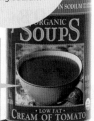

**Bush's Best®
Homestyle Chili**
(1 c)

*250 calories
17 g fat
(10 g saturated, 4 g trans)
810 mg sodium*

**Amy's® Organic
Low Fat Light
in Sodium
Cream of
Tomato Soup**
(1 c)

*100 calories
2 g fat
(1.5 g saturated)
690 mg sodium*

Amy's also adds in
11 grams of sugar.

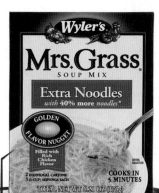

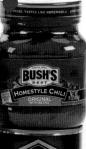

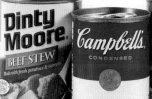

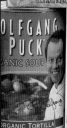

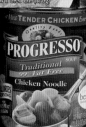

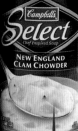

**Dinty Moore®
Beef Stew** (1 c)

*210 calories
10 g fat
(4 g saturated)
970 mg sodium*

After more than 70
years in American
pantries, this
ubiquitous stew has
been lapped by more
nutritionally minded
newcomers.

**Campbell's®
Chicken
Noodle Soup**
(1 c prepared)

*60 calories
2 g fat
(0.5 g saturated)
890 mg sodium*

This can may be
iconic, but it's also a
sodium bomb. Make
Healthy Request
your go-to soup.

**Wyler's® Mrs.
Grass® Soup
Mix Extra
Noodles**
(1 c prepared)

*110 calories
2 g fat
(0.5 g saturated)
700 mg sodium*

**Wolfgang
Puck® Organic
Tortilla Soup**
(1 c)

*160 calories
3.5 g fat
(1 g saturated)
980 mg sodium*

**Progresso®
Traditional
99% Fat Free
Chicken
Noodle** (1 c)

*100 calories
2 g fat
(0.5 g saturated)
950 mg sodium*

99% fat free, but
saltier than 99% of
soups out there.

**Campbell's®
Select™ New
England Clam
Chowder** (1 c)

*160 calories
8 g fat
(2 g saturated)
870 mg sodium*

Chowder is generally
a bad choice. This
one is mixed with
vegetable oil, butter,
and cream.

Canned & Frozen Produce
Eat This

Ore-Ida® Potatoes O'Brien with Onions and Peppers
(¾ c)

60 calories
0 g fat
20 mg sodium

More flavor, fewer calories. It's a simple swap that will save your family big on weeknights and weekend breakfasts.

Del Monte® Mandarin Oranges No Sugar Added
(½ c)

45 calories
0 g fat
6 g sugars

Great as a snack, or tossed with a simple dinner salad with almonds and vinaigrette.

Del Monte® Sliced Peaches in 100% Juice
(½ c)

60 calories
14 g sugars

Never buy a can of fruit with the word "syrup" on the label. 100 percent real fruit juice is always the way to go.

Del Monte® Sweet Peas No Salt Added (½ c)

60 calories
6 g sugars
10 mg sodium

Peas offer the same natural sweetness kids love about corn, but with a much better nutritional payoff, including big doses of B vitamins, fiber, and vitamin C.

Bush's® Dark Red Kidney Beans
(½ c)

105 calories
3 g sugar
260 mg sodium

Dark red kidney beans are high in fiber, folate, and a surprise powerhouse in the antioxidant department.

Birds Eye® Broccoli & Cauliflower
(1 c frozen)

25 calories
0 g fat
25 mg sodium

Because vegetables are picked and flash frozen immediately, they retain most of the same nutrients fresh vegetables offer.

Not That!

Roasted potatoes should never have trans fats. On second thought, no potatoes should.

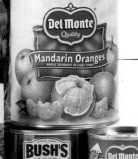

**Ore-Ida®
Roasted Potatoes**
(¾ c)

*130 calories
4.5 g fat (1 g saturated;
1.5g trans fat)
380 mg sodium*

**Del Monte®
Mandarin
Oranges in Light
Syrup** (½ c)

*80 calories
0 g fat
19 g sugars*

Few fruits are sweeter than mandarins, so why have them preserved in a sugary syrup?

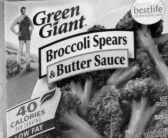

**Green Giant®
Broccoli Spears
& Butter Sauce**
(1 c frozen)

*40 calories
1.5 g fat
(1 g saturated)
330 mg sodium*

**Bush's® Original
Baked Beans**
(½ c)

*140 calories
12 g sugars
550 mg sodium*

With all the sugar, bacon, and salt cooked into baked beans, you're better off seasoning the beans yourself.

**Del Monte®
Whole Kernel
Corn No Salt
Added** (½ c)

*60 calories
7 g sugars
10 mg sodium*

**Del Monte®
Sliced Peaches
in Heavy Syrup**
(½ c)

*100 calories
23 g sugars*

Warning: Once your kids get hooked on sugar-spiked fruit, it'll be a challenge to get them to eat the real thing.

207

Frozen Breakfast Entr

Eat This

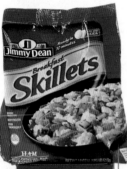

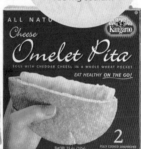

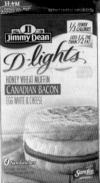

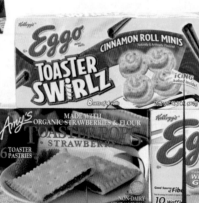

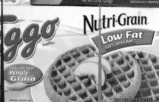

The 3 grams of fiber aren't as much as you'd get from a good bowl of cereal, but it's still a decent breakfast.

Eggo® Nutri-Grain® Low Fat Waffles
(2 waffles)
140 calories
2.5 g fat (0.5 g saturated)
410 mg sodium

Jimmy Dean® D-lights® Canadian Bacon, Egg White, & Cheese Sandwich
(1 sandwich)

230 calories
6 g fat
(3 g saturated)
790 mg sodium

Jimmy Dean® Ham Breakfast Skillets
(¼ package)

130 calories
4 g fat
(1 g saturated)
430 mg sodium

The simple swap of breakfast meat makes a difference of 11 grams of fat and 90 calories.

Amy's® Strawberry Toaster Pops
(1 toaster pop)

150 calories
3.5 g fat
(0 g saturated)
8 g sugars

Amy's filling is made from strawberry purée and strawberry juice concentrate.

Eggo® Toaster Swirlz™ Cinnamon Roll Minis
(4 mini rolls)

120 calories
3 g fat
(0.5 g saturated)
6 g sugars

One of the only cinnamon rolls you should feed a kid.

Quality Kangaroo® Cheese Omelet Pita (1 pita/106 g)

200 calories
7 g fat
(3 g saturated)
445 mg sodium

This pita a protein powerhouse with four times the fiber of the Toaster Scrambles pastry.

ées
Not That!

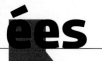

Eggo® Nutri-Grain® Whole Wheat Waffles
(2 waffles)

180 calories
6 g fat (1.5 g saturated)
420 mg sodium

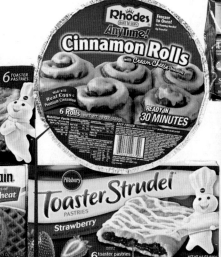

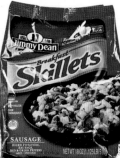

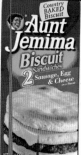

Pillsbury® Cheese, Egg, and Bacon Toaster Scrambles® (2 pastries/94 g)	Rhodes® Anytime Cinnamon Rolls (1 roll with icing/5 oz)	Pillsbury® Strawberry Toaster Strudel™ (1 pastry)	Jimmy Dean® Sausage Breakfast Skillets (¼ package)	Aunt Jemima® Sausage, Egg & Cheese Biscuit Sandwich (1 sandwich)
360 calories 24 g fat (7 g saturated, 2 g trans) 660 mg sodium	310 calories 9.5 g fat (2.5 g saturated) 21 g sugars High in fat and sugar, low in protein and fiber, this is the worst of breakfast formulas.	190 calories 9 g fat (3.5 g saturated, 1 g trans) 9 g sugars Be skeptical of toaster pastries—they're usually loaded with fat.	220 calories 15 g fat (5 g saturated) 590 mg sodium	340 calories 21 g fat (7 g saturated, 3 g trans) 830 g sodium Ban biscuits!

209

Frozen Snacks
Eat This

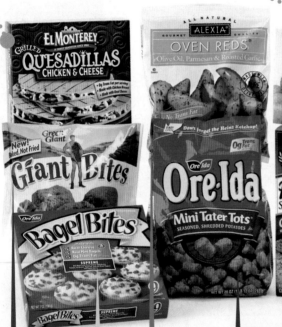

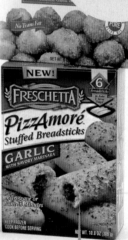

More protein and fewer calories.

El Monterey® Chicken and Cheese Grilled Quesadillas
(1 quesadilla/85 g)

190 calories
7 g fat (3 g saturated)
460 mg sodium

Green Giant® Broccoli and Cheese GiantBites™
(3 nuggets/85 g)

150 calories
7 g fat
(1 g saturated)
460 mg sodium

A sneaky way to get your kids to make friends with broccoli.

Bagel Bites® Supreme
(4 bites/88 g)

200 calories
6 g fat
(2.5 g saturated)
370 mg sodium

Not an ideal snack, but you could do a lot worse than four of these mini pizzas.

Alexia® Oven Reds
(12 pieces/85 g)

120 calories
3.5 g fat
(0.5 g saturated)
270 mg sodium

These fries are cut from red potatoes and cooked with olive oil.

Ore-Ida® Mini Tater Tots®
(19 pieces)

170 calories
9 g fat
(1.5 g saturated)
430 mg sodium

Not a substitute for fresh vegetables by any stretch of the imagination, but decent in a pinch.

Freschetta PizzAmoré Garlic with Savory Marinara Stuffed Breadsticks
(1 stick/51 g)

110 calories
3.5 fat
(1.5 g saturated)
330 mg sodium

Alexia® Breaded Mushrooms
(6 pieces/80 g)

110 calories
6 g fat
(0.5 g saturated)
280 mg sodium

The same rich, fried taste kids crave for half the calories and fat.

Not That!

Cedarlane™ Three Cheese Quesadillas
(1 quesadilla/85 g)

250 calories
11 g fat (6 g saturated)
420 mg sodium

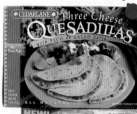

Microwave your own whole wheat quesadilla with low-fat cheese at home.

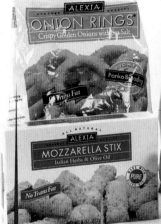

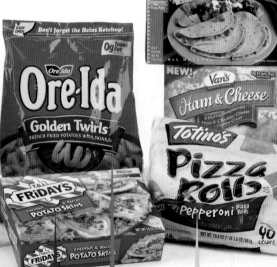

Alexia® Onion Rings *(6 rings/85 g)*	**Alexia® Mozzarella Stix** *(2 stix/37 g)*	**T.G.I. Fridays® Cheddar and Bacon Potato Skins** *(3 pieces)*	**Ore-Ida® Golden Twirls** *(1⅓ c/84 g)*	**Totino's® Pepperoni Pizza Rolls** *(6 rolls/85 g)*	**Van's® Ham & Cheese Stuffed Sandwiches** *(1 pocket/121 g)*
230 calories *12 g fat* *(1 g saturated)* *230 mg sodium*	*120 calories* *7 g fat* *(1 g saturated)* *220 mg sodium*	*210 calories* *12 g fat* *(4 g saturated)* *480 mg sodium*	*160 calories* *6 g fat* *(1 g saturated)* *400 mg sodium*	*220 calories* *10 g fat* *(3 g saturated)* *1.5 g trans)* *510 mg sodium*	*330 calories* *18 g fat* *(11 g saturated)* *470 mg sodium*
At 2 grams of fat per piece, these rings are best left frozen.		Better than the bombs they serve in the restaurant, but still pretty awful.	Choose a better potato cooked in a better oil, and you'll get a fry with half the fat.		Contains more than half a day's saturated fat.

Frozen Beef Dishes
Eat This

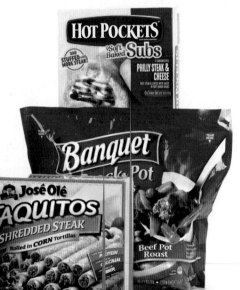

Stouffer's® Meatloaf
(1 package)

340 calories
18 g fat (8 g saturated)
780 mg sodium

Meatloaf trumps meatballs, with a fraction of the calories and saturated fat.

Michelina's Lean Gourmet® Salisbury Steak with Gravy and Mashed Potatoes
(1 package)

190 calories
6 g fat
(3 g saturated)
760 mg sodium

A lighter take on a normally heavy classic.

Smart Ones® Roast Beef in Portobello Vermouth Sauce with Broccoli and Cauliflower
(1 package)

190 calories
8 g fat
(2.5 g saturated)
680 mg sodium

José Olé® Shredded Steak Taquitos
(in corn tortillas)
(3 taquitos/113 g)

190 calories
7 g fat
(1.5 g saturated)
440 mg sodium

Serve with a scoop of salsa for a solid after-school snack.

Banquet® Crock-Pot Classics® Beef Pot Roast
(²⁄₃ c)

150 calories
3.5 g fat
(2 g saturated)
660 mg sodium

A safe bet for a quick meal, even if they come back for seconds.

Hot Pockets® Philly Steak & Cheese Soft Baked Subs
(1 sub)

270 calories
9 g fat
(2.5 g saturated)
870 mg sodium

Surprisingly, this is the safest selection in the Hot Pockets section.

Not That!

In the battle of the beefy comfort dishes, the mountain of pasta and cream-drowned meatballs loses everytime. All told, this entrée has more than half a kid's daily allotment of saturated fat.

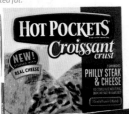

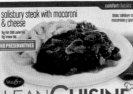

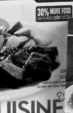

**Stouffer's®
Swedish Meatballs
(1 package)**

*560 calories
27 g fat (12 g saturated)
1,250 mg sodium*

**Hot Pockets®
Philly Steak and
Cheese Croissant
Crust (1 pocket)**

*340 calories
18 g fat
(9 g saturated)
550 mg sodium*

The combo of margarine and dense croissant adds up to nearly half a day's worth of saturated fat.

**Banquet® Crock-
Pot Classics®
Meatballs in
Stroganoff Sauce
(²⁄₃ c)**

*300 calories
14 g fat
(5 g saturated)
800 mg sodium*

The serving size is small, even for a kid, so count on higher calorie count.

**José Olé® Steak
& Cheese
Chimichanga
(1 chimichanga/142 g)**

*350 calories
15 g fat
(4.5 g saturated)
580 mg sodium*

The only thing worse for your kid than a burrito is a fried burrito.

**Lean Cuisine®
Steak Tips Dijon
(1 package)**

*280 calories
7 g fat
(2.5 g saturated)
650 mg sodium*

If you're going to feed the little ones something lean, you can do much better than this.

**Lean Cuisine®
Salisbury Steak
with Macaroni
& Cheese
(1 package)**

*280 calories
9 g fat
(4.5 g saturated)
610 mg sodium*

213

Frozen Poultry Dishes
Eat This

Corn tortillas are lower in calories and carbs and higher in fiber than flour tortillas.

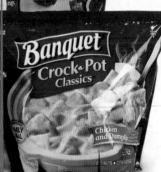

José Olé® Chicken Taquitos in Corn Tortillas
(3 taquitos/85 g)
190 calories
8 g fat (1 g saturated)
390 mg sodium

Kashi® Chicken Pasta Pomodoro
(1 package)
280 calories
6 g fat
(1.5 g saturated)
470 mg sodium
Multigrain penne pasta contributes to the 6 grams of fiber and 19 grams of protein in this skinny pasta.

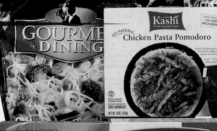

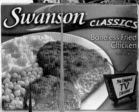

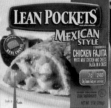

Swanson® Boneless Fried Chicken with Mashed Potatoes and Corn
(1 package)
230 calories
11 g fat
(2.5 g saturated)
790 mg sodium

Gourmet Dining Chicken Stir Fry
(8 oz)
200 calories
1.5 g fat
(0 g saturated)
870 mg sodium
Instead of white rice, this stir-fry uses lo mein noodles, which consist mostly of niacin-enriched durum semolina.

Lean Pocket® Mexican Style Chicken Fajita
(1 pocket)
240 calories
7 g fat
(3 g saturated)
660 mg sodium

Tyson® Any'tizers™ Buffalo Style Boneless Chicken Wyngs™
(3 pieces/84 g)
150 calories
7 g fat
(1.5 g saturated)
680 mg sodium

Banquet® Crock Pot® Classics Chicken and Dumplings (⅔ c)
200 calories
8 g fat
(2 g saturated)
940 mg sodium
Basically, this is just the guts of a potpie. There's a ton of trans fats living in the buttery-biscuit skin.

Not That!

The perfect example of how one word can nearly double the calorie, fat, and sodium counts.

José Olé® Chicken & Cheese Taquitos in Flour Tortillas

(2 taquitos/85 g)

240 calories
10 g fat (2.5 g saturated)
500 mg sodium

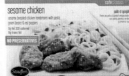

Lean Cuisine® Sesame Chicken

(1 package)

330 calories
9 g fat
(1.5 g saturated)
650 mg sodium

Many "lean" entrées replace fat with sugar. This one packs 14 grams of sugar, mostly found in the sauce.

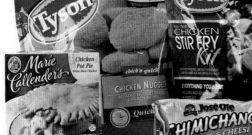

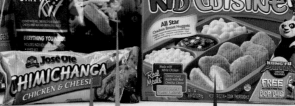

Marie Callender's® Chicken Pot Pie

(1 pie/10 oz)

670 calories
41 g fat
(14 g saturated,
2 g trans)
1,000 mg sodium

Potpies are consistently one of the worst foods you can feed to a kid.

Tyson® Chicken Nuggets

(5 nuggets/91 g)

280 calories
18 g fat
(4 g saturated)
480 mg sodium

Breaded with bleached wheat flour and fried in vegetable oil.

José Olé® Chicken & Cheese Chimichanga

(1 chimichanga/5 oz)

330 calories
12 g fat
(3 g saturated)
550 mg sodium

Tyson™ Chicken Stir Fry Meal Kit

(1.8 c frozen)

290 calories
4 g fat
(1 g saturated)
1,130 mg sodium

A majority of American's sodium intake comes from packaged foods; this is one of the worst offenders.

Kid Cuisine® All Star Chicken Breast Nuggets with Corn, Mac & Cheese, and Chocolate Pudding (1 package)

430 calories
17 g fat
(4 g saturated)
640 mg sodium

Frozen Fish Dishes
Eat This

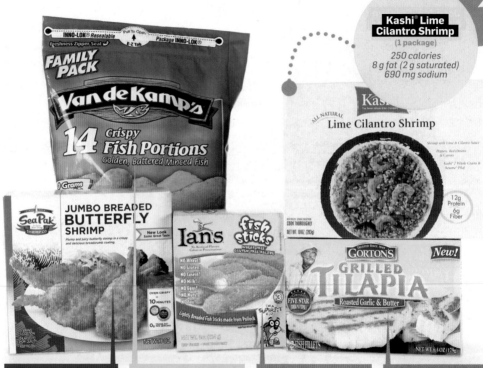

Kashi® Lime Cilantro Shrimp
(1 package)

250 calories
8 g fat (2 g saturated)
690 mg sodium

FAMILY PACK

Van de Kamp's

14 Crispy **Fish Portions**
Golden, Battered Minced Fish

JUMBO BREADED **BUTTERFLY SHRIMP**

Ian's fish sticks

Lime Cilantro Shrimp

GORTON'S New!
GRILLED **TILAPIA**
Roasted Garlic & Butter

Sea Pak® Jumbo Breaded Butterfly Shrimp (4 shrimp/84 g)

210 calories
10 g fat
(1.5 g saturated)
480 mg sodium

While it's best to get your kid used to non-fried seafood, these numbers are super reasonable.

Van de Kamp's® Crispy Fish Portions
(1 portion)

140 calories
7 g fat
(2.5 g saturated)
440 mg sodium

Microwave a potato and serve it with the fish for a complete meal.

Ian's® Fish Sticks
(4 sticks/93 g)

190 calories
6 g fat
(1 g saturated)
310 mg sodium

When it comes to the normally perilous fish sticks, these are as good as it gets.

Gorton's® Roasted Garlic and Butter Grilled Tilapia
(1 fillet)

80 calories
2.5 g fat
(0.5 g saturated)
150 mg sodium

Grilled means good in the world of frozen foods.

Not That!

Bertolli® Shrimp Scampi & Linguine
(½ package)

560 calories
25 g fat (11 g saturated)
670 mg sodium

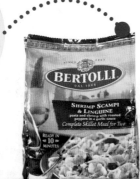

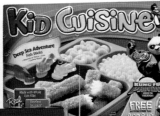

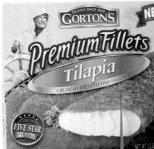

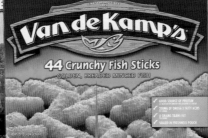

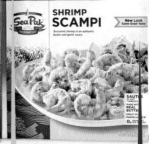

Gorton's® Crunchy Breaded Tilapia (1 fillet)

250 calories
12 g fat
(3.5 g saturated)
480 mg sodium

That thin layer of breading might seem innocent, but it effectively triples the calories and quadruples the fat found in this fish fillet.

Van de Kamp's® Crunchy Fish Sticks (6 sticks/114 g)

230 calories
11 g fat
(4 g saturated)
370 mg sodium

Tartar sauce will tack on another 200 calories to the total. Dunk in cocktail sauce or ketchup, instead.

Kid Cuisine® Deep Sea Adventure Fish Sticks (1 meal)

390 calories
12 g fat
(2.5 g saturated)
500 mg sodium

The abysmal sides included in Kid Cuisine meals (see: mac and cheese and gummi bears) make them consistently dubious picks.

Sea Pak® American Shrimp Scampi (6 shrimp/4 oz)

330 calories
29 g fat
(10 g saturated)
460 mg sodium

The shrimp itself is innocent, but scampi is Italian for a heavy dose of oil and butter.

Frozen Vegetarian
Eat This

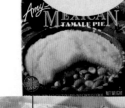
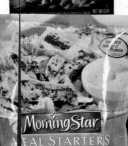
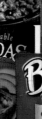
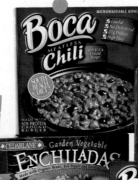
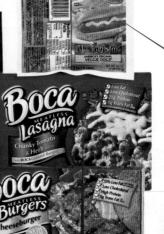

Boca® Meatless Chili
(1 package)

*150 calories
1 g fat (0 g saturated)
650 mg sodium*

Super-packed with fiber and protein.

Amy's® Mexican Tamale Pie
(1 pie)

*150 calories
3 g fat
(0 g saturated)
590 mg sodium*

Beneath the cornmeal crust lies a rich deposit of fiber-packed vegetables.

MorningStar Farms® Meal Starters™ Chik'n Strips
(12 strips/85 g)

*140 calories
3.5 g fat
(0.5 g saturated)
510 mg sodium*

Great low-cal treat with a massive dose of soy protein.

Cedarlane™ Garden Vegetable Enchiladas
(2 enchiladas)

*280 calories
6 g fat
(3 g saturated)
620 mg sodium*

Boca® Meatless Cheeseburger
(1 patty)

*100 calories
4.5 g fat
(1.5 g saturated)
320 mg sodium*

Boca® Chunky Tomato and Herb Meatless Lasagna
(1 package)

*290 calories
5 g fat
(2 g saturated)
880 mg sodium*

MorningStar Farms® Original Veggie Dogs™
(1 hot dog)

*80 calories
0.5 g fat
(0 g saturated)
580 mg sodium*

Not That!

**Amy's®
Chili & Cornbread
Whole Meal**
(1 package)

*340 calories
6 g fat (2.5 g saturated)
680 mg sodium*

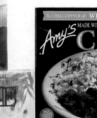

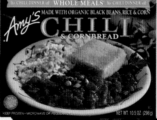

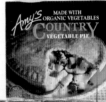

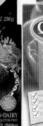

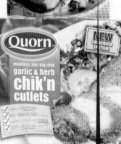

**MorningStar
Farms® Veggie
Corn Dogs**
(1 corn dog)

*150 calories
4 g fat
(0.5 g saturated)
500 mg sodium*

**Amy's®
Cheese
Lasagna**
(1 package)

*380 calories
14 g fat
(8 g saturated)
680 mg sodium*

**MorningStar
Farms®
Grillers Prime®**
(1 patty)

*170 calories
9 g fat
(1 g saturated)
360 mg sodium*

**Amy's®
Black Bean
Vegetable
Enchilada**
(2 enchiladas)

*360 calories
12 g fat
(1 g saturated)
780 mg sodium*

**Quorn™
Meatless and
Soy-Free
Garlic & Herb
Chik'n Cutlets**
(1 cutlet/100 g)

*200 calories
9 g fat
(1 g saturated)
570 mg sodium*

**Amy's®
Country
Vegetable Pie**
(1 pie)

*370 calories
16 g fat
(9 g saturated)
580 mg sodium*

We've yet to find a
healthy potpie
anywhere in
America.

219

Frozen Pasta
Eat This

Mama Rosie's® Cheese Lasagna
(1 package)

290 calories
7 g fat
(3 g saturated)
680 mg sodium

Trade alfredo for marinara and meatballs and ditch the bread and you'll cut the calories and sodium in half.

Stouffer's® Spaghetti with Meatballs
(1 package)

350 calories
12 g fat (4 g saturated)
660 mg sodium

Kashi® Pesto Pasta Primavera
(1 package)

290 calories
11 g fat
(2 g saturated)
750 mg sodium

Michelina's® Authenitico™ Macaroni & Cheese
(1 package)

230 calories
3.5 g fat
(2 g saturated)
540 mg sodium

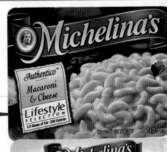

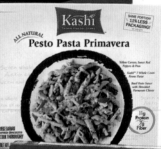

Michelina's® Lean Gourmet Spaghetti & Meat Sauce
(1 package)

300 calories
6 g fat
(2 g saturated)
540 mg sodium

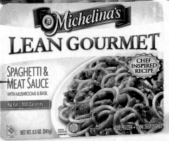

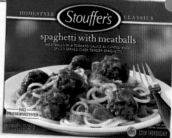

Not That!

Marie Callender's® Fettuccini Alfredo & Garlic Bread
(1 package)
770 calories
46 g fat (16 g saturated, 1 g trans)
1,300 mg sodium

Alfredo sauce means a rich, buttery, artery-clogging cream sauce, and this garlic bread adds an extra dose of high-fructose corn syrup and partially hydrogenated oils.

Stouffer's® Five Cheese Lasagna
(1 c/237 g)
330 calories
14 g fat
(8 g saturated)
870 mg sodium

Amy's® Pesto Tortellini Bowl
(1 package)
430 calories
19 g fat
(8 g saturated)
640 mg sodium

Banquet® Macaroni and Cheese Meal
(1 package)
390 calories
11 g fat
(6 g saturated)
1,100 mg sodium

Kid Cuisine® Twist & Twirl Spaghetti with Mini Meatballs and Brownie
(1 package)
420 calories
12 g fat (4 g saturated)
690 mg sodium

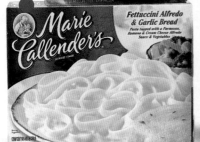
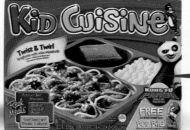

221

Frozen Pizza
Eat This

Hot Pockets can be a great way to exercise portion control, as long as you avoid the oily crust used for their regular line of products. Lean Pockets replace the oil with 20 grams of whole grains.

Lean Pockets® Whole Grain Supreme Pizza
(1 pizza)

220 calories
7 g fat (2.5 g saturated)
490 mg sodium

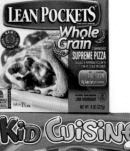

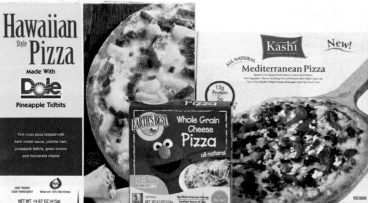

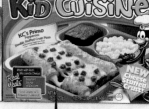

Dole® Hawaiian Style Pizza (⅓ pizza)

290 calories
13 g fat
(7 g saturated)
800 mg sodium

Ham proves the perfect lean meat topping for a pizza, trouncing pepperoni and sausage in the fat and calorie categories.

Earth's Best® Sesame Street Frozen Whole Grain Cheese Pizza (1 pizza)

190 calories
6 g fat
(3 g saturated)
380 mg sodium

This is one of the few TV-backed products worth buying.

Kashi® Mediterranean Pizza (⅓ pizza)

290 calories
9 g fat
(4 g saturated)
640 mg sodium

Instead of vegetable oil, Kashi uses olive oil, which makes much of the fat here the heart-friendly kind.

Kid Cuisine® KC's Primo Pepperoni Pizza with Corn & Brownie (1 package)

480 calories
15 g fat
(5 g saturated)
710 mg sodium

Not That!

Red Baron may call this a pizza for one, but it contains a full day of saturated fat and nearly a full day of sodium.

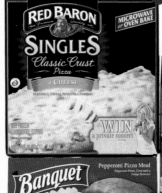

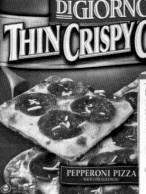

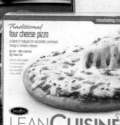

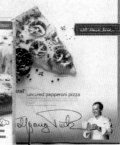

Banquet® Pepperoni Pizza Meal with Corn and Brownie
(1 package)

550 calories
29 g fat
(5 g saturated,
0.5 g trans)
890 mg sodium

DiGiorno® Thin Crispy Crust Pepperoni Pizza
(⅙ pizza)

320 calories
15 g fat
(7 g saturated)
790 mg sodium

The thin crust keeps the carbs down, but the fatty meats jack the calories and sodium up.

Lean Cuisine® Four Cheese Pizza (1 pizza)

360 calories
8 g fat
(3.5 g saturated)
690 mg sodium

Four cheeses and lean are mutually exclusive terms.

Wolfgang Puck's® All-Natural Uncured Pepperoni Pizza (⅓ pizza)

360 calories
19 g fat
(7 g saturated)
870 g sodium

Ice Cream

Eat This

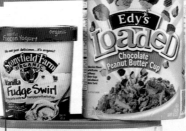

*"Double Churn"
is Breyer's code word
for low-fat, which is
good news for you and
the unsuspecting
family.*

Breyer's®
Double Churn Extra
Creamy Vanilla
Bean Ice Cream
(1/2 c)

100 calories
3 g fat (2 g saturated)
13 g sugars

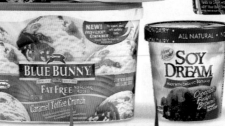

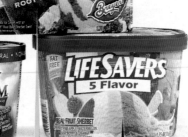

**Stonyfield
Farm® Nonfat
Vanilla Fudge
Swirl Frozen
Yogurt** (½ c)

120 calories
0 g fat
22 g sugars

**Blue Bunny®
No Sugar
Added Fat Free
Caramel
Toffee Crunch**
(½ c)

90 calories
0 g fat
4 g sugars

You won't find an
ice cream with less
sugar than this one.

**Soy Dream®
Non-Dairy
Chocolate
Fudge
Brownie** (½ c)

130 calories
7 g fat
(1.5 g saturated)
12 g sugars

A great sweet
option for lactose-
intolerant little ones.

**Breyers®
A&W™ Root
Beer Float**
(½ c)

130 calories
4.5 g fat
(3 g saturated)
16 g sugars

Not a bad scoop,
considering a real
Root Beer float has
about 400 calories.

**Life Savers®
5 Flavor Real
Fruit Sherbert**
(½ c)

110 calories
0 g fat
21 g sugars

Generally speaking,
fruity sherberts
make for a
relatively safe
fat-free scoop.

Not That!

Häagen-Dazs® Extra Rich Light Vanilla Bean Ice Cream
(1/2 c)

200 calories
7 g fat (4 g saturated)
25 g sugars

While we applaud Häagen-Dazs for the simplicity of their ice cream—only seven ingredients in this scoop—their "light" ice creams are worse than most brands' regular lines.

Ben & Jerry's® All Natural Peanut Butter Cup™ (1/2 c)

360 calories
26 g fat
(13 g saturated)
23 g sugars

One of Ben & Jerry's most dubious flavors, with nearly a full day of saturated fat per serving.

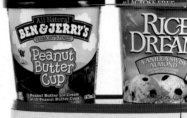

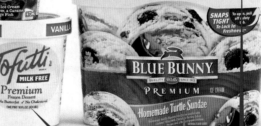

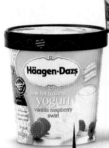

Häagen-Dazs® Vanilla Raspberry Swirl Low-Fat Frozen Yogurt (1/2 c)

160 calories
1.5 g fat
(0.5 g saturated)
25 g sugars

Ben & Jerry's® All Natural Phish Food® Light (1/2 c)

210 calories
6 g fat
(4.5 g saturated)
23 g sugars

Made with skim milk, but liquid sugar and corn syrup are still the second and third ingredients.

Tofutti® Vanilla Milk Free Premium Frozen Dessert (1/2 c)

180 calories
11 g fat
(2 g saturated)
8 g sugars

Blue Bunny® Homemade Turtle Sundae (1/2 c)

180 calories
9 g fat
(5 g saturated)
19 g sugars
Take advantage of Blue Bunny's slimmer line of ice creams.

Rice Dream® Vanilla Swiss Almond (1/2 c)

190 calories
10 g fat
(2.5 g saturated)
18 g sugars

225

Frozen Treats
Eat This

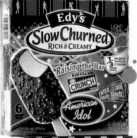

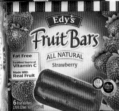

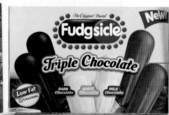

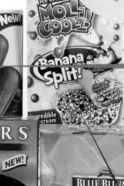

Edy's/Dreyer's® Slow Churned® Vanilla with Nestlé Crunch® Bar
(1 bar)
150 calories
8 g fat (6 g saturated)
10 g sugars

Fudgesicle® Triple Chocolate
(1 fudgesicle)
60 calories
1.5 g fat (1 g saturated)
9 g sugars

A good rule of thumb: Stuff with "sicle" in the name makes for a safe indulgence.

Edy's/ Dreyer's® Strawberry Fruit Bars
(1 bar)
80 calories
0 g fat
20 g sugars

Popsicle® Orange, Cherry and Grape Ice Pops
(1 popsicle)
45 calories
0 g fat
8 g sugars

Classic, and still one of the best frozen treats you can use to reward your kids.

The Skinny Cow® Low Fat Chocolate Peanut Butter Ice Cream Sandwich
(1 sandwich)
150 calories
2 g fat (1 g saturated)
15 g sugars

Breyers® Oreo Ice Cream Sandwiches
(1 sandwich)
160 calories
6 g fat (2 g saturated)
13 g sugars

Your kid's better off eating this than three regular Oreos.

Blue Bunny® Orange Dream Bar
(1 pop)
80 calories
1.5 g fat
14 g sugars

Blue Bunny has some of the best and some of the worst products in the freezer. Be sure to read the label.

MolliCoolz™ Incredible Banana Split Ice Cream Beads (1 c/71 g)
129 calories
10 g fat (7 g saturated)
5 g sugars

The smartest choice in the bite-size dessert category.

Not That!

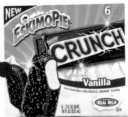

Eskimo Pie® Vanilla Ice Cream Bar with Nestlé Crunch® Coating

(1 bar)

210 calories
14 g fat (10 g saturated)
12 g sugars

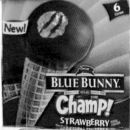

Rice Dream® Vanilla Bar

(1 bar)

230 calories
14 g fat
(9 g saturated)
16 g sugars

They may be lactose-free, but they still contain half a day's worth of saturated fat.

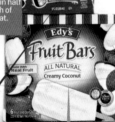

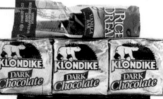

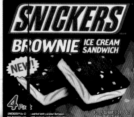

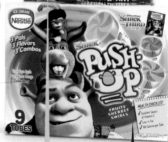

Edy's/Dreyer's® Strawberry Dibs®

(26 pieces/105 g)

370 calories
26 g fat
(16 g saturated)
22 g sugars

The "chocolate" coating is made with coconut and palm oil.

Edy's™ Fruit Bars All Natural Creamy Coconut (1 bar)

120 calories
3 g fat
(2.5 g saturated)
15 g sugars

Keep your kid's popsicles under 100 calories.

Klondike® Dark Chocolate Bar

(1 bar)

250 calories
17 g fat
(12 g saturated)
17 g sugars

The "dark chocolate" is actually a "chocolate flavored coating," which lists vegetable oils as its first ingredient.

Snickers® Brownie Ice Cream Sandwich

(1 sandwich)

210 calories
9 g fat
(4.5 g saturated)
18 g sugars

Nestlé Push Ups® "Shrek"

(1 push up)

80 calories
1 g fat
(0.5 g saturated)
13 g sugars

Not a terrible choice, but still has nearly double the calories of a Popsicle.

Blue Bunny® The Champ!® Strawberry Cone (1 cone)

220 calories
12 g fat
(9 g saturated)
21 g sugars

227

5

Conquering the
Cafeteria

AT SCHOOL

EAT
THIS
NOT
THAT!

FOR
KIDS!

Conquering the Cafeteria

There are few places on earth as terrifying as the school lunchroom.

First, there's the social intrigue over who's sitting with whom, who's not sitting with whom, and who gets picked on if they sit with the wrong whom. It's sort of like *Lord of the Flies* with spaghetti sauce, with tribes and cliques huddled together in a tremulous social pecking order. Add in grumpy, graying lunch ladies, stringent hall monitors, and the stress of trying to eat your lunch while dodging flying chicken fingers, and lunch can be a serious hazard to a kid's social standing.

School lunches shouldn't be hazardous to your child's health. Yet the lunchroom is, in most of America's school districts, a nutritional minefield.

Sure, the National School Lunch Program (NSLP), instituted in 1946, has made some positive strides toward improving the nutritional quality of school lunches. Under the program's guidelines, a proper school lunch must derive on average 30 percent or less of its calories from fat and must serve two or more fruit and vegetable items each day. So if your child sticks with the prescribed school lunch—mushy green beans and all—he or she will supposedly get a meal that at least hews to some modicum of nutritional responsibility, lacking though it might be in palate appeal. And the program does seem to be making a difference in some quarters: According to one study, students who report eating NSLP meals consume greater amounts of all nutrients except vitamin C, compared with students who eat meals from other sources.

But sending your child to school with a couple of dollars for lunch certainly doesn't guarantee that he's going to come home with a belly full of goodness. Despite the NSLP guidelines, many school districts are having a heck of a time measuring up to its standards. In a recent study by the National Institutes of Health, the average lunch got 35.9 percent of its

calories from total fat and 12.6 percent from saturated fat, exceeding the guidelines of 30 and 10 percent, respectively. The problem? Funding. A recent analysis found that federal reimbursements cover only about half of the real cost of providing healthy meals for our children, and almost 85 percent of school food service programs receive no financial support from their school districts.

And in addition to the breakdown in the school lunch program, there are other hazards lurking in the school cafeteria.

SCREWY LUNCH SCHEDULES

First, the school day usually revolves around coordinating a fleet of buses, an army of students, and a complex schedule of academics—a schedule made ever more complicated by the increasing federal regulation of school course loads. Trying to fit time for lunch into that complex web can be difficult. Indeed, a survey conducted by Penn State University found that, of 228 high schools, one in four schools scheduled lunch periods before 10:30 A.M. Who wants to eat lunch at a time when most parents are still finishing their coffee? And researchers found that an earlier

lunch start predicted that a larger number of students would be buying their food not from the school lunch program, but from . . .

THE SNACK BAR

About 90 percent of public schools now offer à la carte items, or as your kids might know them, "snack bar" foods. A study in the *Journal of the American Dietetic Association* found that middle-school students with access to snack bar foods consume significantly fewer fruit and vegetable servings than students who eat only NSLP meals. And a study at the University of Minnesota found that when students had access to snack bars at school, their consumption of both fat and saturated fat ballooned. Why do schools offer these less-healthy, à la carte foods? One word: money. To compensate for a lack of adequate funding, schools need to finance the feeding of our children in other ways, and à la carte foods offer an easy solution. The Penn State study found that the average school in Pennsylvania earned almost $700 a day—or nearly $14,000 a month—from à la carte food sales. And beyond the snack bars, there's another hazard lurking in your local school.

THE VENDING MACHINES

In addition to snack bar offerings, contracts from soft-drink manufacturers and vending-machine companies (and incentives from soft-drink bottlers based on sales) are another significant way that schools have found to finance their activities. Consider these eye-opening statistics:

✖ The average secondary school in America now has 12 vending machines on its property. Research shows that the greater the number of vending machines on the property, the fewer the fruits and vegetables students ate, and the fewer the students who took advantage of the school lunch program.

✖ During the past 2 decades, soft drink consumption among adolescents ages 11 to 17 has increased 100 percent. No wonder: In a survey of 228 high school food service directors in Pennsylvania, two-thirds reported having soft-drink advertisements in their school.

✖ A study of 2,000 middle school students in Texas found that 72 percent of the sweetened beverages, 80 percent of the soft drinks, and 39 percent of the candy they consumed came from vending machines.

Sadly, all of this could be avoided if schools were willing to intervene. In a 2008 study at the Center for Obesity Research and Education at Temple University, five Philadelphia-area elementary schools replaced high-sugar, high-fat vending machine snacks with juice, water, low-fat milk, and healthy snacks; provided nutritional education to the students; and gave away raffle tickets for wise food choices. The result: Over a 2-year period, the obesity rate in those five schools fell to half of what it was in similar elementary schools.

But until healthy eating becomes a priority, it's up to you, the parent, to make the smart choices. To help your child navigate the nutritional no-man's-land of the school cafeteria, arm him or her with this easy-to-follow guide. It may take a little coaxing—putting a kid with a little cash in his pocket next to a vending machine is like putting a local politician next to an empty podium—but by explaining that he'll not only look and feel better, but also become better at sports, at school, at play, and at all the things he enjoys doing, you'll inspire him to make the right choices.

How Our Schools Are Failing Our Kids

Established in 1946, the National School Lunch Program (NSLP) was supposed to guarantee that all public school children in America received a proper school lunch that averaged 30 percent or less of its calories from fat and 10 percent or less from saturated fat and offered two or more fruit and vegetable items each day. But as governments at every level have been draining funds away from our schools, one essential element of our children's lives—nutrition—has gotten the short end of the breadstick. Under the NSLP, the federal government reimburses school districts just $2.47 per day for every meal for children who qualify for free lunches, $2.07 per day for students who qualify for reduced-price fare, and a whopping $0.23 for students who pay full price. Ann Cooper, director of nutrition services for the Berkeley Unified School System, estimates that schools spend about $1.68 per meal on payroll and overhead. For actual food costs, that leaves cafeteria managers with all of 72 cents for each meal. Here is just a small sample of numbers underscoring the need for reform in our school lunch programs:

- In February 2008, 37 million pounds of meat were recalled from school lunches.

- In a recent study by the Center for Science in the Public Interest, 46 percent of states received an F on their School Food Report Card.

- In a study on school lunches in Harwich, Massachusetts, 50 percent of lunches were found to come from leftovers.

- In a study of 22 of the largest 100 elementary school districts in the United States, the Physicians Committee for Responsible Medicine rated the lunches students received based on how well those programs helped protect against obesity and chronic disease, promoted healthy nutrition, and taught children about healthy eating. Sadly, less than half of school programs rated an A or B. Nearly one in four received an F, including school districts in Missouri, Utah, Texas, West Virginia, and Alaska.

Breakfast

Eat This

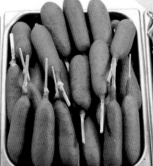

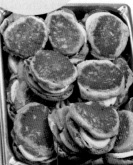

Scrambled eggs and bacon
250 calories
10 g fat (4 g saturated)
550 mg sodium

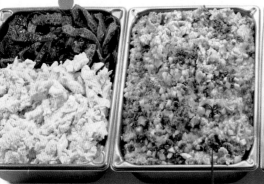

A study from St. Louis University found that people starting their day with eggs consumed 264 fewer calories than people eating bagels for breakfast. The reason? Protein and good fat are important elements of satiety, working diligently to keep your kid's belly full and prevent those midmorning cravings that lead to empty calorie consumption.

Apple-cinnamon oatmeal
280 calories
3 g fat
(0 g saturated)
5 g carbohydrates

True, the calories from oatmeal come mostly from carbohydrates, but with each bowl comes a dose of soluble fiber, which helps slow the absorption of the carbs, keeping kids' blood sugar levels—and thus their energy and concentration levels—more stable.

Pancake on a stick
220 calories
13 g fat (4 g saturated)
350 mg sodium

The same concept as a sausage biscuit: carbs wrapped around a fatty piece of meat for a portable breakfast. Neither are paradigms of nutrition, but pancakes pack a fraction of the calories and fat found in the dreaded biscuit. Warning: If your kid has a penchant for syrup-dipping, the calories here can jump quickly.

Ham and egg on an English muffin
240 calories
8 g fat
(3 g saturated)
610 mg sodium

Not even the most malicious cafeteria cook could mess this one up: low-calorie bread, an egg, and a few slices of lean ham. Protein and healthy fat are two great ways to wake up; the only thing that's missing is fiber, and that can be corrected easily enough by using a whole grain English muffin.

Not That!

Blueberry muffin
*360 calories
14 g fat (2 g saturated)
32 g sugars
2 g fiber*

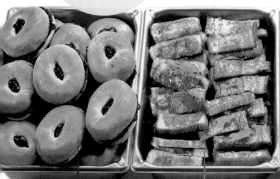

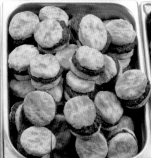

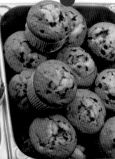

Bagel with jelly
*390 calories
12 g fat (1 g saturated)
385 mg sodium*

Bagels may look harmless, but behind each bite is a mouthful of refined carbohydrates. When a flood of quick-burning carbs enters the bloodstream, blood sugars rise rapidly and your body panics and begins to store fat. Jelly only makes matters worse, since most jellies found in school cafeterias have more sugar in them than fruit.

French toast with syrup and margarine
*450 calories
18 g fat
(5 g saturated)
67 g carbohydrates*

The only thing vaguely nutritious about French toast is the egg in which the bread is battered, but even that is drowned out by a flood of melted margarine and sugary syrup.

Sausage biscuit
*400 calories
22 g fat
(12 g saturated,
3 g trans)
1,100 mg sodium*

Here's the standard biscuit recipe: flour, lard, buttermilk. So it's not hard to imagine how this greasy, sausage-stuffed breakfast sandwich packs such a wallop. The fact that biscuits are one of the biggest transporters of trans fats only makes the need to avoid this breakfast bomb all the more vital.

Is blueberry pie healthy just because it packs a serving of fruit? Same problem here. Don't be fooled by the fruit façade: Muffins consist primarily of highly refined flour and sugar—hardly the breakfast of champions the masquerading muffin purports itself to be.

Lunch

Eat This

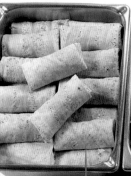
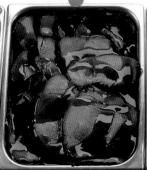
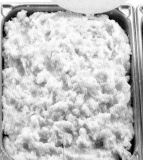
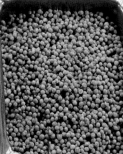

Roast beef and gravy

*240 calories
11 g fat
(4 g saturated)
625 mg sodium*

Bean burrito

*300 calories
12 g fat
(3 g saturated)
650 mg sodium*

The tortilla is a less-than-ideal vehicle for anything, but in this case, the benefit of the beans trumps the troubles of the tortilla. The ½ cup of beans inside this burrito pack massive amounts of fiber, protein, and—as one of nature's best sources of antioxidants—plenty of disease-fighting phytochemicals.

Made from a lean cut of beef, a few slices of roast beef prove to be a relatively low-fat, low-calorie source of protein. And since cafeteria gravies are invariably of the "instant" variety, the only minor threat they pose is of adding a bit of extra sodium to the meal.

Mashed potatoes

*170 calories
8 g fat (3 g saturated)
300 mg sodium*

Chances are this pile of potatoes comes from a box of instant mashed potatoes, which are made from potato flakes.

Green peas

*75 calories
0 g fat
120 mg sodium*

Peas are a great source of vitamin K, an important bone strengthener, which makes them a perfect segue to the type of playground high jinks that normally follow school lunch. They're also packed with thiamin, niacin, and riboflavin, all vital for energy production, which means kids might actually be able to keep their eyes open once recess is over.

Not That!

Turkey wrap
375 calories
14 g fat
(5 g saturated)
575 mg sodium

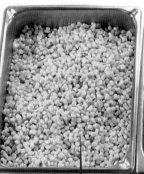

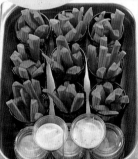

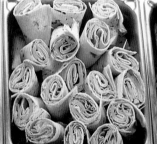

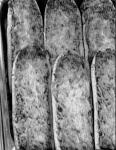

Corn niblets

100 calories
0 g fat
135 mg sodium

Not exactly a nutritional nightmare—in fact, corn does provide some meaningful nutrients like B vitamins and fiber. But corn is also one of nature's sweetest vegetables, which is why most of our packaged foods are sweetened with various forms of this processed staple crop. Save it for the summer barbecue.

Carrots with ranch

230 calories
16 g fat
(5 g saturated)
400 mg sodium

If it takes ranch dressing to get your kids to eat their vegetables, it's just not worth it. Two ounces of the stuff has more calories than an entire scoop of mashed potatoes.

Wraps start with the dreaded tortilla, to which the lunch ladies add fatty dressing (usually ranch or Italian), cheese (usually processed), and produce (usually token shreds of lettuce). What your kid is left with is something healthy in name only.

French bread cheese pizza

440 calories
19 g fat
(8 g saturated)
930 mg sodium

The thick, doughy crust used by most school cafeterias packs on a heavy carb and sodium load, plus it provides the structural integrity for a haphazard application of cheese, which doubles down on the calorie count.

237

Lunch

Eat This

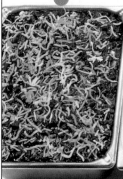

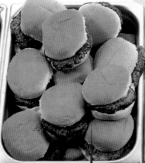

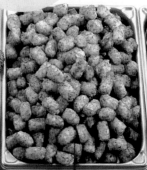

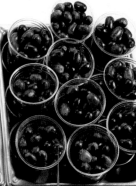

Chili with shredded cheese
300 calories
12 g fat
(4 g saturated)
570 mg sodium

This cheesy, gooey mess is actually good for your kid? Hard to believe, but beyond being packed with enough protein to keep her full and focused the rest of the school day, a bean-laced bowl of red gives your kid plenty of fiber and disease-fighting antioxidants. Tastes great, more filling, fights against cancer. What more could you want?

Hamburger

350 calories
15 g fat
(5 g saturated)
650 mg sodium

Topped with ketchup, mustard, and hopefully a few pieces of produce (lettuce, onions, tomatoes, pickles), the humble hamburger proves to be a relatively reasonable choice, especially when compared to some of the hidden dangers lurking in the cafeteria.

Tater Tots

150 calories
7 g fat (1 g saturated)
200 mg sodium

Cafeteria tots are invariably of the frozen variety. The upside is that they usually avoid the harsh fry treatment in favor of a simple bake, which keeps the calorie count down.

Red grapes (1 c)

104 calories
0 g fat
23 g sugars

Perhaps the most dependable fruit in the cafeteria. With tight budgets, cafeterias are often forced to buy fruit—apples, peaches, and pears, especially—in cans, which means they come with a thick coating of sugar syrup. Grapes, on the other hand, are dependably fresh and loaded with the same healthy antioxidants mom and dad enjoy in a glass of red wine.

Not That!

Grilled cheese

*350 calories
16 g fat
(7 g saturated)
650 mg sodium*

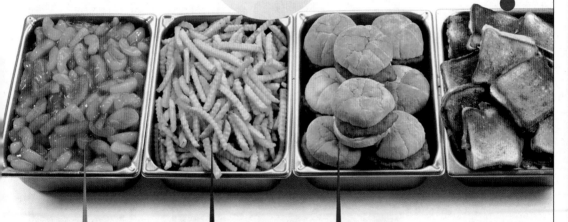

Cinnamon apples

*200 calories
6 g fat (2 g saturated)
30 g sugars*

Cinnamon apples are
the perfect example of taking
a perfectly good thing
like an apple and messing
it up with a load of unnecessary
sugar and often butter
or margarine.
In the words of Pink Floyd
(sorta): Hey, teachers,
leave our fruit alone!

French fries

*310 calories
18 g fat
(7 g saturated)
400 mg sodium*

French fries probably
won't be lucky enough to
avoid the boiling oil,
which is where they soak up
most of their saturated fat.
They might be America's
favorite side dish, but
more often than not,
they contain as many calories,
or more, than the entrée
sharing the plate with them.

**Crispy chicken
sandwich**

*400 calories
19 g fat
(7 g saturated)
735 mg sodium*

If they're going to take
an innocent chicken breast,
bread it, deep-fry it,
and cover it in mayo,
your kid may as well opt for
the hamburger.
When it comes to chicken
sandwiches, if it ain't grilled,
then it ain't worth eating.

*Bread and cheese
fried in butter?
Kinda hard to imagine how this
would be good for anyone.
At least at home you can pair it
with a cup of tomato soup
and make sure your kid gets
something nutritious out
of the meal.*

239

Candy

Eat This

High in sugar, yes, but much of that sugar comes from actual fruit. All told, chewy snacks contain 100 percent of the recommended daily intake of vitamin C.

C2

C3

Good & Plenty®
(1 box)

170 calories
0 g fat
27 g sugars

Seems like licorice fell out of favor with the little ones a while back, which is too bad, since as far as candy goes, it's a pretty good go-to.

Nutter Butter Bites (1 package)

170 calories
7 g fat
(2 g saturated)
10 g sugars

Guaranteed to become instant friends with peanut-butter fans young and old—which isn't such a bad thing, if your regular fix is of the Reese's variety.

York® Peppermint Pattie (1 pattie)

140 calories
2.5 g fat
(1.5 g saturated)
25 g sugars

The most reasonable of all the mainstream candies, with half the calories of a Snickers® bar.

Kit Kat® Bar
(1 package)

220 calories
11 g fat
(7 g saturated)
22 g sugars

In the wide world of crunchy, sweet choco-late bars, Kit Kat is as low-cal as they come. Plus, breakable pieces means you can save some for later.

Nestlé® Crunch® Bar (43.9 g)

220 calories
11 g fat
(7 g saturated)
24 g sugars

Give up two grams of saturated fat and get a load of crunch in return. Who wouldn't want to make that swap?

Not That!

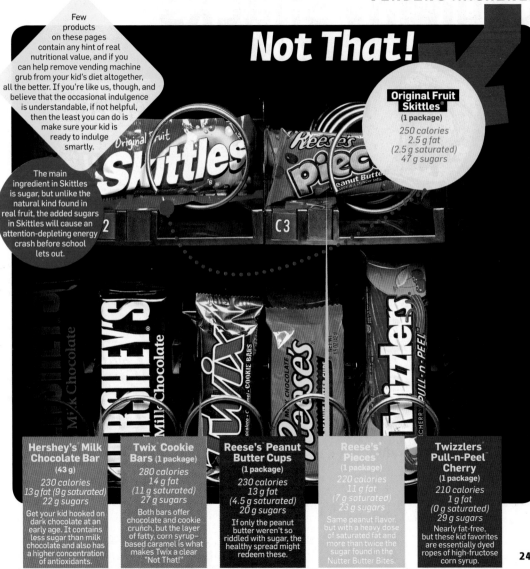

Few products on these pages contain any hint of real nutritional value, and if you can help remove vending machine grub from your kid's diet altogether, all the better. If you're like us, though, and believe that the occasional indulgence is understandable, if not helpful, then the least you can do is make sure your kid is ready to indulge smartly.

The main ingredient in Skittles is sugar, but unlike the natural kind found in real fruit, the added sugars in Skittles will cause an attention-depleting energy crash before school lets out.

Original Fruit Skittles (1 package)

250 calories
2.5 g fat
(2.5 g saturated)
47 g sugars

Hershey's Milk Chocolate Bar (43 g)

230 calories
13 g fat (9 g saturated)
22 g sugars

Get your kid hooked on dark chocolate at an early age. It contains less sugar than milk chocolate and also has a higher concentration of antioxidants.

Twix Cookie Bars (1 package)

280 calories
14 g fat (11 g saturated)
27 g sugars

Both bars offer chocolate and cookie crunch, but the layer of fatty, corn syrup–based caramel is what makes Twix a clear "Not That!"

Reese's Peanut Butter Cups (1 package)

230 calories
13 g fat (4.5 g saturated)
20 g sugars

If only the peanut butter weren't so riddled with sugar, the healthy spread might redeem these.

Reese's Pieces (1 package)

220 calories
11 g fat (7 g saturated)
23 g sugars

Same peanut flavor, but with a heavy dose of saturated fat and more than twice the sugar found in the Nutter Butter Bites.

Twizzlers Pull-n-Peel Cherry (1 package)

210 calories
1 g fat (0 g saturated)
29 g sugars

Nearly fat-free, but these kid favorites are essentially dyed ropes of high-fructose corn syrup.

241

Crunchy Snacks

Eat This

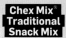

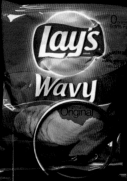

Chex Mix® Traditional Snack Mix

(1 oz)

130 calories
4 g fat
(0.5 g saturated)
380 mg sodium

This mix of Chex cereal, pretzels, and rye chips has 60 percent less fat than regular potato chips, but beware of the high sodium counts and the misleading serving sizes on the packages. Keep consumption down to one ounce at a time.

B 3

B 4

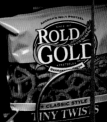

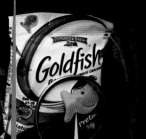

Baked! Lay's® Potato Chips (1 oz)	**Rold Gold® Tiny Twists Pretzels** (1 oz)	**Nacho Cheese Doritos®** (1 oz)	**Lays® Wavy Potato Chips** (1 oz)	**Goldfish® Pretzel Baked Snack Crackers** (1.3 oz)
110 calories *1.5 g fat* *(0 g saturated)* *150 mg sodium*	*110 calories* *1 g fat* *(0 g saturated)* *580 mg sodium*	*150 calories* *8 g fat* *(1.5 g saturated)* *180 mg sodium*	*150 calories* *10 g fat* *(1 g saturated)* *180 mg sodium*	*140 calories* *1.5 g fat* *(0 g saturated)* *530 mg sodium*
Baked Lays chips offer all of the crunch without any of the saturated fat. This is as guilt-free as chip munching gets.	Pretzels are low in calories, but because of the high sodium count, keep your kid's intake to an ounce at a time.	Made from whole corn instead of corn meal. Shed another 20 calories switching over to Baked! Doritos.	When it comes to snacking, portion control is key. An ounce of chips is more than enough for an afternoon snack.	Yes, high in sodium, but the fat and calorie advantage makes up for the saltiness.

242

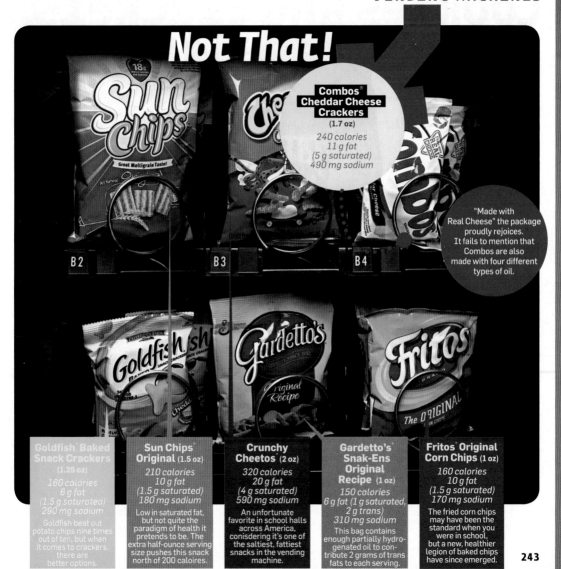

Not That!

Combos® Cheddar Cheese Crackers (1.7 oz)

240 calories
11 g fat
(5 g saturated)
490 mg sodium

B 2   B 3   B 4

"Made with Real Cheese" the package proudly rejoices. It fails to mention that Combos are also made with four different types of oil.

Goldfish® Baked Snack Crackers (1.25 oz)

160 calories
6 g fat
(1.5 g saturated)
290 mg sodium

Goldfish beat out potato chips nine times out of ten, but when it comes to crackers, there are better options.

Sun Chips® Original (1.5 oz)

210 calories
10 g fat
(1.5 g saturated)
180 mg sodium

Low in saturated fat, but not quite the paradigm of health it pretends to be. The extra half-ounce serving size pushes this snack north of 200 caloires.

Crunchy Cheetos® (2 oz)

320 calories
20 g fat
(4 g saturated)
590 mg sodium

An unfortunate favorite in school halls across America, considering it's one of the saltiest, fattiest snacks in the vending machine.

Gardetto's® Snak-Ens Original Recipe (1 oz)

150 calories
6 g fat (1 g saturated, 2 g trans)
310 mg sodium

This bag contains enough partially hydrogenated oil to contribute 2 grams of trans fats to each serving.

Fritos® Original Corn Chips (1 oz)

160 calories
10 g fat
(1.5 g saturated)
170 mg sodium

The fried corn chips may have been the standard when you were in school, but a new, healthier legion of baked chips have since emerged.

243

Cookies and Crackers
Eat This

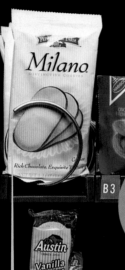

Make Ritz the peanut butter cracker of choice. The Ritz taste better and have 15 percent fewer calories than the Austin variety—and no trans fats!

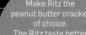

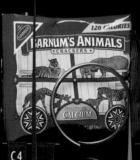

Ritz Bits® Peanut Butter Sandwiches
(1 package)
170 calories
10 g fat (2 g saturated)
280 mg sodium

B2   B3   B4   B

C3   C4

Pepperidge Farm® Milano® Cookies (1 package)

180 calories
10 g fat
(5 g saturated)
11 g sugars

The thin chocolate cookies are the best in the Pepperidge Farm line.

Austin® Vanilla Cremes (1 package)

170 calories
7 g fat
(2.5 g saturated)
11 g sugars

This is one of the safer packages of Austin crackers. It's trans fats–free and has 30 fewer calories than almost every other variety.

Rice Krispies Treats® Bar (1)

150 calories
3.5 g fat
(1 g saturated)
12 g sugars

Rice Krispies Treats are deceptively decent, mostly because the bulk of the bar is made from a fairly innocuous cereal.

Kraft® Cinnamon Bagel-fuls (1)

200 calories
4 g fat
(2.5 g saturated)
8 g sugars
190 mg sodium

Not one of Kraft's bagel-and-cream-cheese fusions has more that 200 calories or 6 grams of fat. Sweet!

Nabisco® Barnum's Animals® Crackers (1 package)

120 calories
3.5 g fat
(1 g saturated)
7 g sugars

As far as cookies are concerned, Barnum's Animals are a tame bunch.

Not That!

Far too many of Austin's prepackaged crackers contain trans fats. This small package contains 2 grams, which is why you should never fail to look over the label before passing a snack down to your child.

Austin® Cheese Crackers with Peanut Butter
(1 package, 39 g)
200 calories
10 g fat (1.5 g saturated;
2 g trans)
400 mg sodium

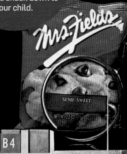

B 2   B 3   B 4   B 5

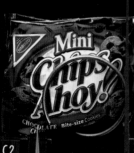

C2   C3   C4

Mini Chips Ahoy! Chocolate Chip
(1 package)
170 calories
8 g fat
(2.5 g saturated)
10 g sugars
The cookies might be smaller, but their caloric load is just as big.

Pop-Tarts Brown Sugar Cinnamon
(2 pastries)
420 calories
14 g fat
(4.5 g saturated)
31 g sugars
The caloric equivalent of two doughnuts, loaded with HFCS and partially hydrogenated vegetable oil.

Little Debbie Double Decker Oatmeal Creme Pie (1)
470 calories
18 g fat
(5 g saturated,)
39 g sugars
As densely caloric as anything your kid will encounter in the vending machine.

Keebler Vanilla Sugar Wafers
(1 package)
400 calories
21 g fat
(4 g saturated,
8 g trans)
34 g sugars
The trans fattiest vending machine snack we've seen. A single serving has three times a safe daily intake.

Mrs. Fields Semi-Sweet Chocolate Chip Cookie (1)
330 calories
16 g fat
(10 g saturated)
28 g sugars
The cookie queen has a thing for saturated fat—this cook has more than half a day's worth.

Beverages

Drink This

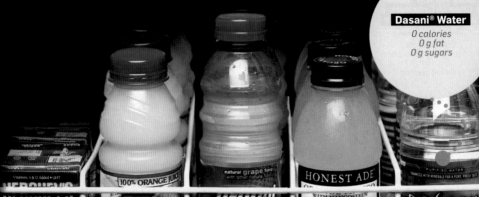

Dasani® Water

0 calories
0 g fat
0 g sugars

If you're really concerned about your kid's nutrient intake, give her a children's multivitamin—she can wash it down with a cold glass of H₂0.

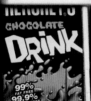

Hershey's Chocolate Drink
(8 oz)

130 calories
1 g fat
(0 g saturated)
26 g sugars

This chocolate drink has two advantages over Yoo-Hoo: Milk is higher up on the ingredient list, and the portion size is smaller.

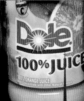

Dole® 100% Orange Juice
(15.2 oz)

210 calories
0 g fat
42 g sugars

100% fruit juice will never lose a nutritional contest to psuedo juice. Still, OJ intake should be limited in favor of eating the actual fruit.

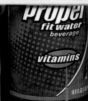

Propel® Fitness Water, Grape
(16.9 oz)

25 calories
0 g fat
4 g sugars

If your family is going to drink "fitness" waters or "functional beverages," make sure they have less than 50 calories and 10 grams of sugar per bottle.

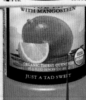

Honest Ade® Orange Mango
(16.9 oz)

100 calories
0 g fat
25 g sugars

Learn to love the Honest line of drinks in your household: They offer a kid-pleasing sweetness with a lower concentration of sugar than most major brands.

246

Not That!

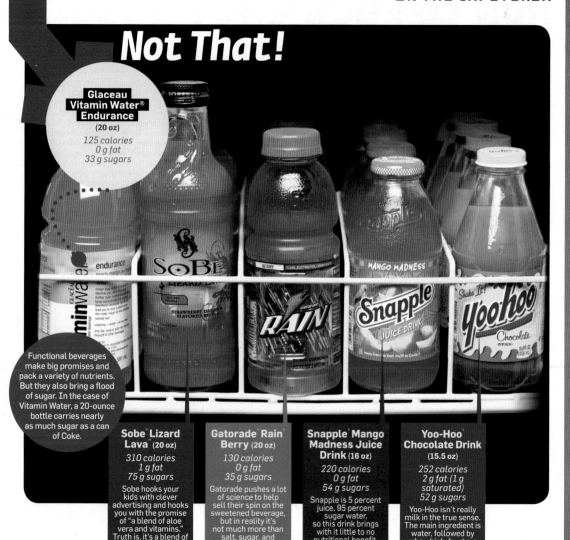

Glaceau Vitamin Water® Endurance (20 oz)

125 calories
0 g fat
33 g sugars

Functional beverages make big promises and pack a variety of nutrients. But they also bring a flood of sugar. In the case of Vitamin Water, a 20-ounce bottle carries nearly as much sugar as a can of Coke.

Sobe® Lizard Lava™ (20 oz)

310 calories
1 g fat
75 g sugars

Sobe hooks your kids with clever advertising and hooks you with the promise of "a blend of aloe vera and vitamins." Truth is, it's a blend of water and high-fructose corn syrup.

Gatorade® Rain® Berry (20 oz)

130 calories
0 g fat
35 g sugars

Gatorade pushes a lot of science to help sell their spin on the sweetened beverage, but in reality it's not much more than salt, sugar, and potassium blended into water.

Snapple® Mango Madness Juice Drink (16 oz)

220 calories
0 g fat
54 g sugars

Snapple is 5 percent juice, 95 percent sugar water, so this drink brings with it little to no nutritional benefit.

Yoo-Hoo® Chocolate Drink (15.5 oz)

252 calories
2 g fat (1 g saturated)
52 g sugars

Yoo-Hoo isn't really milk in the true sense. The main ingredient is water, followed by whey, high-fructose corn syrup, and sugar. Then comes milk.

247

How to Pack the Perfect

Concerned that the sludge they're slopping at the cafeteria is ruining your kid's appetite, and maybe even his waistline? Then it's time to take control of the midday meal by packing a heroic lunch for your loved ones each morning. Not only will you ensure optimum nutrition, you'll also be able to cater to his likes and dislikes, which means there's a darn good shot he'll actually eat this lunch, rather than leaving it behind in the rush to get to the playground.

A good lunch is a balanced one, formed around a dependable main course and punctuated with a solid supporting cast of nutrient-packed sides, a low- or no-calorie drink, and even a little treat. Mix and match like you would when ordering Chinese takeout—though, unlike General Tso's chicken and sweet-and-sour goop, this stuff is actually good for your kid. Master the mix and your kid will be the envy of every mystery meat-eating student in the second grade. Here are the four elements to a perfectly packed lunch.

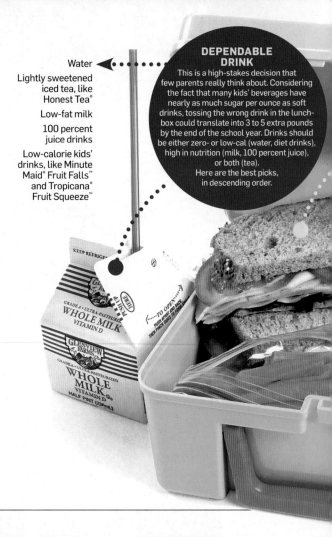

Water

Lightly sweetened iced tea, like Honest Tea®

Low-fat milk

100 percent juice drinks

Low-calorie kids' drinks, like Minute Maid® Fruit Falls™ and Tropicana® Fruit Squeeze™

DEPENDABLE DRINK

This is a high-stakes decision that few parents really think about. Considering the fact that many kids' beverages have nearly as much sugar per ounce as soft drinks, tossing the wrong drink in the lunch-box could translate into 3 to 5 extra pounds by the end of the school year. Drinks should be either zero- or low-cal (water, diet drinks), high in nutrition (milk, 100 percent juice), or both (tea). Here are the best picks, in descending order.

School Lunch

STURDY ANCHOR
Avoid a lunch built on refined carbohydrates, as the intake of quick-burning carbs will leave your kid with an energy and attention deficit for the rest of the day. Focus instead on protein, fiber, and healthy fats that will help keep your kid satisfied, keep his metabolism running high, and provide some meaningful nutrition along the way.

FOR SANDWICHES
Meats should be lean (no salami or bologna), breads should be whole wheat, and condiments should be used sparingly.

Turkey or roast beef and Swiss sandwich on wheat bread (sans mayo, but loaded with produce, if you can get away with it)

Sliced ham, cheese, and Triscuits®

PB&J (made on whole wheat bread with a pure-fruit jelly like Smucker's® Simply Fruit®)

Thermos of hot soup

Grilled chicken breast

Hard-boiled eggs

Tuna or cubed chicken tossed with light mayo, mustard, celery, and carrot

SIDES WITH SUBSTANCE
Only one in four kids consumes the recommended five servings of fruits and vegetables daily, so pack a lunch sans produce and you're missing a golden opportunity to slip some much-needed nutrients back into their diets. As long as you have at least one piece of fruit or a serving of vegetables, adding a second crunchy snack is fine.

Carrot sticks

Celery sticks

Apple slices with peanut butter

Fruit salad

Banana, pear, peach, or any other whole fruit

Grapes

Olives

Almonds and raisins (mixed 50-50)

Triscuits®

Small bag of pretzel sticks or Goldfish® pretzels

Baked! Lay's®

LOW-IMPACT TREAT
You've gotta give them something they can brag to their friends about, right? Some general rules of the lunchtime reward: A treat should have no trace of trans fats (many cookies and pastries do), less than 12 grams of sugar, and no more than 100 calories. If you can eke some extra nutrition out of it, all the better.

Fruit leather

Squeezable yogurt

Low-fat, low-sugar chocolate pudding

Sugar-free Jell-O®

Rice Krispies Treats®

A square of chocolate (the darker the better)

6

AT HOME

251

You, in Charge!

In the sanctity of your own kitchen is where you have the most control over your children's nutritional well-being. But while in your mind you may envision lazy Sundays spent lovingly cooking up a kitchen full of homemade chicken soup, the reality of our lives is often less Martha Stewart, more Speed Racer: Weekends are about charging through chores, plowing through paperwork, and chauffeuring the kids from soccer practice to sleepovers. That's American family life in the 21st century, and there's no evidence that things are going to slow down anytime soon.

Indeed, the notion of the home-cooked meal is beginning to fall by the wayside. Between 1977 and 1998, the percentage of our food calories consumed at home dropped precipitously—from 82 percent to less than 65 percent. Meanwhile, among children ages 2 to 18, intake of salty snacks and pizza has increased 132 percent. And a lack of home cooking and set mealtimes means that our children have become habitual snackers: In 1977, the average child had one snack a day, but by 1996 that number had doubled. Twice the snacks? Twice the calories.

So knowing what to prepare at home—and finding recipes that are both satisfying and nutritious—can be a challenge. The following food choices will help you cook up foods that make sense for your family—and keep your family out of the grasp of fast-food marketers.

♦ Saucing your noodles with a meaty marinara instead of creamy Alfredo will cut 200 calories from the dish—72 of which come from saturated fat.

♦ Upgrading from an Idaho to a baked sweet potato will save more than just a few calories: The swap will double the amount of fiber and save your kid from a vitamin A deficiency.

♦ Whipping up a pot of chili instead of a pot of mac 'n cheese will skim 110 calories and 9 grams of fat from your child's dinner.

Sneaky Parent! These Tricks Are for Kids!

How puppies, ice cream, and monkey runs can help you save your children (and yourself!) from obesity.

● **BREAK THE FAMILY FAST.** University of Massachusetts researchers found that skipping breakfast makes you 4.5 times more likely to be obese. And waiting longer than 90 minutes after waking to break your fast can increase your chances of obesity by nearly 50 percent. "To keep your family's metabolisms stoked all day, serve them whole grain waffles drizzled with melted peanut butter and a sliced banana in place of syrup," says Cynthia Sass, RD, CSSD, and former spokesperson for the American Dietetic Association. That will ratchet up the fiber, cut down on sugar, and keep them coming back for more.

● **JOIN IN THE TEAM PRACTICE.** When you take the kids to a sports practice, bring along your gym shoes and jog the track while they're playing, says Jen Mueller, MEd, CPT, the in-house personal trainer for sparkpeople.com. When there's a game, "follow the action on the field by walking up and down the sidelines," says Mueller. You'll not only keep yourself fit, but you'll also set an example for the kids to follow into their own adulthood.

● **BUY SMALLER PLATES.** A recent study found that when presented with large portions, people consume 30 percent more food—and calories. Another study revealed that children don't regulate their food based on how much they've eaten during the day, which means that portion size is critical to how many calories they consume. Use smaller plates, and make sure that your kids eat the same foods that you eat.

● **SIT UP STRAIGHT.** Teaching your kids good posture will encourage a sense of assurance—and protect them against back pain later in life. When sitting at the dinner table, have everyone imagine that there's a string tied from a shirt button at heart level to their belt buckle. See who can sit for the longest without collapsing the string. Do this for 5 minutes a few times each day, and you'll straighten up slumping shoulders.

● **BE STRICT ABOUT BEDTIME.** A University of Chicago study found that people who don't get enough sleep have lower levels of the hormones that control appetite, putting them at risk for obesity. A follow-up study of 9,588 Americans found that those who slept for 4 hours or less per night were 234 percent more likely to be obese. The National Sleep Foundation recommends that children ages 5 to 12 get 10 to 11 hours of sleep each night and that adolescents get $8^1/_2$ to $9^1/_2$.

● **SPRING FOR A PUPPY.** Kids won't exercise with you? Make your child walk the dog every morning. A recent study from Northwestern Medical School, in Chicago, found that people who walked their dogs for 20 minutes a day, 5 days a week, lost an average of 14 pounds during the course of a year.

● **INSTITUTE A 15-MINUTE RULE.** Make it a family rule that there will be 15 minutes of roughhousing between the time Mom and Dad get home from work and the kids go off to bed. Researchers from the University of Bristol measured the activity of 5,500 12-year-olds and found that just 15 minutes a day spent doing moderate physical activity (equivalent to a brisk walk) reduces the chances of being obese by up to 50 percent. Keep playing for another 15 minutes, and you'll burn 240 calories—about the same amount you would burn on a moderate bike ride, according to a study in the *Journal of Sports Medicine and Physical Fitness.*

● **PUSH SMALL PEOPLE AROUND.** Researchers at Texas A&M University found that running with a jogging stroller can push your heart rate up 10 beats per minute higher than when you run solo. Try the Baby Jogger Switchback Quick-Fold Trailer/Jogger, $600. rei.com

● **REWARD THEM WITH ICE CREAM.** British researchers conducted MRI scans and found that a single spoonful of ice cream triggers the pleasure centers in the brain. Plus, 1/2 cup of vanilla ice cream gives you 17 milligrams of choline, which recent USDA research showed lowered blood levels of

homocysteine by 9 percent. That translates into protection from cancer, heart attack, stroke, and dementia. Best pick: Dreyer's® Slow Churned® Rich and Creamy Light. One serving has only 2 grams of saturated fat.

● **PUT THEIR STOMACHS IN SUMMER SCHOOL.** A new study in the *American Journal of Public Health* surveyed 5,380 kindergartners and first graders and found that they were gaining weight at twice the rate over the summer months that they do during the school year. Researchers speculate that increased calorie consumption is to blame. A moderately active child should consume about 1,400 calories a day. In summer, continue to structure their meals just like a school day: breakfast by 9, lunch at noon, and a snack at 3.

● **KICK THE CAN.** Soda is the single largest source of calories

in the American diet, according to a 2005 study conducted by the Center for Science in the Public Interest. And popular energy drinks like Red Bull® are so packed with sugar that they completely inhibit your ability to burn fat, negating any metabolism-boosting effect the caffeine might have had. Swap water for sugary beverages and your kid will consume 150 fewer calories a day and drop an average of 15 pounds a year.

● **ENTER THE FAMILY OLYMPICS.** If you're serious about getting your kids moving, here are some parent-kid exercises put together by Michael Mejia, MS, CSCS, advisor to the Center for Sports Parenting.

6- TO 8-YEAR-OLDS:
Monkey runs.
Shuffle sideways for 10 yards and back. Turn around and repeat, leading with the other foot.

9- TO 11-YEAR-OLDS:
Driveway shuttles. Place six objects—tennis balls on red plastic cups, for instance—at the end of the driveway. Take turns sprinting to retrieve the objects.

12- TO 16-YEAR-OLDS:
Timed suicides. Sprint as fast as you can for 5 yards, then turn and sprint back to the starting line. Turn around and sprint for 10 yards, and then back. Continue sprinting, increasing the distance by 5 yards each time. Cover as much ground as you can in 30 seconds.

A Week of Perfect Eating

First of all, if you're cooking at home, congratulations. You've just made one of the most important decisions you can make with regard to your family's health and well-being. Besides the ineffable joy that is (or should be) the family meal, by cooking and eating as a unit, you ensure ultimate control over every last piece of food that hits the plate. A study from the *Journal of the American Dietetic Association* found that the more family meals a kid consumes, the higher his or her intake of fruits, vegetables, grains, and nutrients will be. The fewer packages you use, the more control you have.

Still, some of the most explosive calorie landmines may be lurking in your dusty old recipe books. A study from New York University found that classic recipes in the *Joy of Cooking* have grown in serving size significantly over the years. And though it's easy enough to figure out what tastes good to your family, it's never quite as simple to know what's good for them. When the difference between potpie and pot roast could mean more than 400 calories, it's clear parents could use a hand on the home front. That's what this chapter is all about, helping you decide which of your weeknight standbys should be stood by, and which deserve to be deserted.

All of the numbers in this section are for kid-size portions—4 to 6 ounces of the entrée and ½ cup for side dishes, unless otherwise noted. If some of these numbers on the Not That! side are cause for concern, just consider that mom- and dad-size portions will have about 50 percent more calories, fat, sodium—everything. Stick to 5 or 6 days of "Eat This"–worthy meals throughout the week, and you'll earn the right to a night of indulging outside of the kitchen.

*Find more tips, tricks, and savvy strategies for feeding your family well at **eatthis.com***

Sunday

Eat This

Meat Loaf Dinner

with baked sweet potato and roasted asparagus

540 calories
13 g fat
(3 g saturated)
850 mg sodium

The ketchup-covered loaf proves to be a fairly innocent weeknight standby. If the cook uses ground beef with anything more than 10 percent fat content, though, the fat and calorie counts begin to grow substantially.

The numbers in this section do not include desserts. While we wanted to give you dessert options for each night, it's not necessary (or advised) to end every meal with a bowl of ice cream or a slice of pie. Sometimes, a piece of fruit or nothing at all should be enough.

Baked Sweet Potato
(1 medium)

160 calories
0 g fat
100 mg sodium

Lower in calories and carbs and higher in fiber than an Idaho potato, sweet potatoes have a gentler effect on kids' blood sugar. Plus, they're loaded with vision-protecting beta-carotene.

Meat Loaf

280 calories
10 g fat
(3 g saturated)
600 mg sodium

Roasted Asparagus

100 calories, 3 g fat
(0 g saturated), 150 mg sodium

Make asparagus kid-friendly by dusting them with fresh grated parmesan cheese before roasting in the oven.

Jell-O (½ c)

80 calories
0 g fat
19 g sugars

In the world of sugar-clotted desserts, Jell-O proves to be a reasonable indulgence. But if you're the type of parent to let the kids get trigger happy with the whipped cream canister, then double the calories and add 10 grams of fat.

Not That!

Chicken Casserole Dinner

with baked potato and roasted asparagus

660 calories
20 g fat
(6 g saturated)
1,220 mg sodium

This everything-but-the-kitchen-sink approach to dinner has been a perennial favorite of busy moms for decades. Problem is, casseroles include starchy pasta, salty broth, and plenty of cream or butter or both. Kill the dairy and the pasta, increase the veggies, and use low-sodium broth, and you'll have a casserole worth concocting.

Italian Ice

130 calories
0 g fat
30 g sugars

Ice might sound innocent, but not when it's packed with more sugar than most candy bars. If your kid wants something cold and icy, try a classic Popsicle®, which has about 50 calories and 15 grams of sugar.

Roasted Asparagus

100 calories, 3 g fat
(0 g saturated), 150 mg
sodium

Chicken Casserole

380 calories
17 g fat
(6 g saturated)
1,020 mg sodium

Baked Potato (1 medium)

180 calories
0 g fat
50 mg sodium

Still not a bad option for your family, assuming that you can keep them from stuffing the potato full of cheese, sour cream, and bacon bits. The best topping of all? Salsa: It adds just 10 calories, plus a host of nutrients.

257

Monday
Eat This

Chili Dinner

with buttered dinner roll and sautéed broccoli with almonds

530 calories
21 g fat
(7 g saturated)
925 mg sodium

Make a batch from lean ground beef, onions, tomatoes, and plenty of beans, and you'll be doing your family a favor, packing their bellies full of fiber, protein, and antioxidants.

Buttered Dinner Roll (1)

130 calories
5 g fat (2 g saturated)
210 mg sodium

A small pat of butter actually helps lower the glycemic impact of high-carb foods like rolls and baked potatoes, which means they produce less of a spike in your kid's blood sugar.

Chili

300 calories
10 g fat (4 g saturated)
625 mg sodium

Sautéed Broccoli
with almonds

100 calories
6 g fat (1 g saturated)
90 mg sodium

Broccoli is packed full of fat-soluble vitamins, which means they're better absorbed through your body when paired with a bit of fat. Skip the steaming and sauté the vegetable in a bit of olive oil.

Peach Cobbler

240 calories
10 g fat (4 g saturated)
22 g sugars

This Southern favorite has one major virtue: It's made primarily from fresh peaches, which bring the antioxidant beta-carotene to table. Use crushed almonds and rolled oats for the topping instead of flour and butter and you'll cut another 80 calories.

Not That!

Macaroni and Cheese Dinner

with biscuit and sautéed broccoli with almonds

730 calories
36 g fat
(10.5 g saturated)
1,220 mg sodium

Pasta with milk, butter, and a small mountain of cheese: How could it possibly be healthy? Either adapt the recipe on page 268, or save more decadent versions of mac and cheese for a reward or a special occasion, rather than letting it to become a staple in your child's diet.

Banana Pudding

with wafers and whipped cream

350 calories
15 g fat (6 g saturated)
42 g sugars

This common comfort dessert is fruit-based in name only. Most of the sugar is added sugar, not naturally occuring sugar from the banana.

Sautéed Broccoli

with almonds

100 calories
6 g fat (1 g saturated)
90 mg sodium

Mac 'n Cheese

410 calories
19 g fat
(5.5 g saturated)
710 mg sodium

Biscuit (1)

220 calories
11 g fat (4 g saturated;
3 g trans fats)
420 mg sodium

Between the refined flour, the lard, and the copious amounts of salt, there's nothing in a biscuit that belongs on your dinner table.

259

Tuesday
Eat This

Pot Roast Dinner
with creamed corn and tomato soup

520 calories
22 g fat
(7 g saturated)
885 mg sodium

This classic wintertime one-pot wonder brings big, hearty flavor to the table with little empty nutrition cluttering up the plate. Plus, what better way to get your kids to eat their carrots and onions than to cook them low and slow, until they no longer taste like something grown in the ground?

Pot Roast

320 calories
12 g fat
(4 g saturated)
410 mg sodium

Tomato Soup (1 c)

80 calories
3 g fat (1 g saturated)
300 mg sodium

A study from Penn State found that people who ate soup before a meal consumed 135 fewer calories than those who went straight into the meal. If you're using canned soup, just be sure to score the reduced sodium version.

Creamed Corn

120 calories
7 g fat (2 g saturated)
175 mg sodium

Most of the creaminess in creamed corn doesn't come from the fatty dairy product, but from the corn itself, which releases its starch to thicken the dish and give it a rich taste and texture.

Scoop of Vanilla Ice Cream
with chocolate sauce

200 calories
10 g fat (6 g saturated)
26 g sugars

As far as desserts go, this is a pretty safe indulgence, especially if you use Breyer's Creamery Style Vanilla to make it.

875 calories
44 g fat
(17 g saturated)
1,320 mg sodium

Not That!

Beef Stroganoff Dinner

with creamed spinach and iceberg salad

This is a clear case of the good (mushrooms, onions, lean beef), the bad (cream, sour cream, buttered noodles), and the ugly (most renditions look like a car crash on a plate).

Slice of Chocolate Cake (4" slice)

400 calories
20 g fat (12 g saturated)
38 g sugars

Decadence defined. Too bad part of that definition includes more than half a day's worth of saturated fat and a small bucket of sugar.

Creamed Spinach

200 calories
10 g fat (4 g saturated)
240 mg sodium

Yes, spinach is nutritionally superior to corn, but each serving comes with up to a quarter cup of heavy cream. Cut the calories dramatically by using milk-and-flour-based bechamel sauce instead.

Iceberg Salad with carrots, tomatoes, and blue cheese dressing

200 calories
14 g fat (6 g saturated)
330 mg sodium

It's tempting to use any means necessary to get your kids to eat vegetables, but blue cheese dressing cancels out any possible benefits gleaned from the carrots and tomatoes.

Beef Stroganoff

475 calories
20 g fat (7 g saturated)
750 mg sodiumv

Wednesday

Eat This

Spaghetti Dinner

with mixed green salad and Pillsbury breadstick

550 calories
19.5 g fat
(6.5 g saturated)
1,005 mg sodium

Learn to adjust the pasta-to-sauce ratio in your house to skew heavily toward sauce. It might not be traditional, but it will cut calories and carbs dramatically.

Mixed Green Salad
with light balsamic vinaigrette

100 calories
6 g fat (1 g saturated)
270 mg sodium

Made of a variety of baby lettuces, prewashed mixed greens make the perfect staple for quick weeknight salads. Pick up a bag in the refrigerator section of the produce aisle.

Spaghetti and Meatballs

380 calories
12 g fat
(5 g saturated)
550 mg sodium

Pillsbury® Breadstick
(1)

70 calories
1.5 g fat (0.5 saturated)
185 mg sodium

One of the only times that one of those twist-and-pop cans yields something nutritionally reasonable.

Sliced Strawberries
with whipped cream

120 calories
6 g fat (2 g saturated)
16 g sugars

The simplest dessert on the planet is also one of the healthiest and most adored. Whip the cream fresh at home, adding just a touch of sugar for a bit of sweetness.

Not That!

Fettuccine Alfredo Dinner

with Caesar salad and garlic bread

1,040 calories
52 g fat
(25 g saturated)
1,625 mg sodium

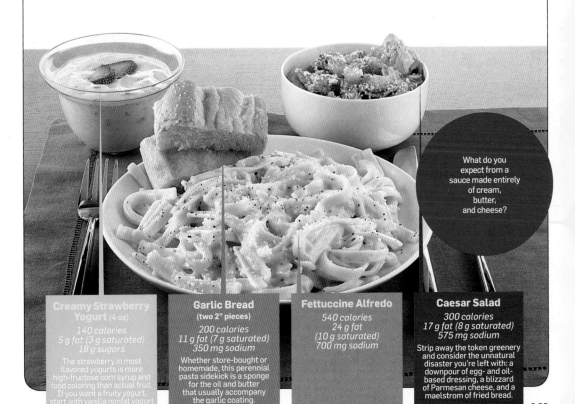

What do you expect from a sauce made entirely of cream, butter, and cheese?

Creamy Strawberry Yogurt (4 oz)

140 calories
5 g fat (3 g saturated)
18 g sugars

The strawberry in most flavored yogurts is more high-fructose corn syrup and food coloring than actual fruit. If you want a fruity yogurt, start with vanilla nonfat yogurt and add fresh fruit at home.

Garlic Bread
(two 2" pieces)

200 calories
11 g fat (7 g saturated)
350 mg sodium

Whether store-bought or homemade, this perennial pasta sidekick is a sponge for the oil and butter that usually accompany the garlic coating.

Fettuccine Alfredo

540 calories
24 g fat
(10 g saturated)
700 mg sodium

Caesar Salad

300 calories
17 g fat (8 g saturated)
575 mg sodium

Strip away the token greenery and consider the unnatural disaster you're left with: a downpour of egg- and oil-based dressing, a blizzard of Parmesan cheese, and a maelstrom of fried bread.

263

Thursday
Eat This

Roast Chicken Dinner

with Stove Top Stuffing and peas and pearl onions

412 calories
13 g fat
(4 g saturated)
874 mg sodium

You can cut extra calories here by removing the chicken skin, but what many fat-fearing nutritionists won't tell you is that animal fat, like the kind found in chicken skin, actually contains many of the same heart-healthy fats found in olive oil and avocados.

Roast Chicken
225 calories
10 g fat
(4 g saturated)
350 mg sodium

Stove Top® Stuffing, Chicken Flavor
(½ c prepared)
107 calories
1 g fat (0 g saturated)
429 mg sodium

Not exactly an ideal side, especially because of the high sodium levels, but it's good in a pinch and vastly superior to Rice-A-Roni.

Peas and Pearl Onions
80 calories
2 g fat (0 g saturated)
95 mg sodium

A great freezer staple. The fiber in the peas and the chromium in the onions both help to regulate blood sugar levels.

Chocolate Pudding
120 calories
3.5 g fat (2 g saturated)
16 g sugars

Made primarily from milk and chocolate, you could do worse than serve the occasional post-dinner scoop of pudding. It doesn't hurt that a serving of pudding also offers your kids a nice dose of bone-strengthening vitamin D.

Not That!

Chicken and Dumplings Dinner

with Rice a Roni and peas and pearl onions

670 calories
24.5 g fat
(7 g saturated)
1,465 mg sodium

Soul-soothing though it may be, the creamy, buttery base for this dish offers little comfort for the waistline. Making matters worse, those bloated dumplings, being just flour, salt, and water, offer nothing more than a heaping helping of quick-burning carbs.

Chocolate Chip Cookie

200 calories
14 g fat (4 g saturated)
15 g sugars

Every kid deserves a warm, homemade chocolate chip cookie on occasion, but it's just too high in calories—a function of the butter, sugar and refined flour used to make these treats—to make for a reliable weeknight dessert.

Peas and Pearl Onions

80 calories
2 g fat (0 g saturated)
95 mg sodium

Rice-A-Roni® Rice Pilaf (½ c prepared)

155 calories
4.5 g fat (1g saturated)
600 mg sodium

This is no treat, not even for San Franciscans. The stratospheric sodium count is bad enough, but the 1.5 grams of trans fats (trans fats in rice? why?!) just adds insult to injury.

Chicken and Dumplings

435 calories
18 g fat
(6 g saturated)
770 mg sodium

Friday
Eat This

Blackened Catfish Dinner
with black beans and glazed carrots

370 calories
8 g fat
(1 g saturated)
615 mg sodium

Catfish is a lean, omega-3–rich fish with few contaminants and a very mild taste—pretty much the best fish imaginable to serve a kid. The blackening seasoning serves two important functions: It boosts the mild flavor (and makes fish-phobic kids forget what they're eating) and because most spices contain active compounds, it adds an armory of antioxidants.

Blackened Catfish
180 calories
6 g fat (1 g saturated)
470 mg sodium

Glazed Carrots
80 calories
1 g fat (0 g saturated)
140 mg sodium

Make your carrots extra appealing by cooking them slowly in a bit of chicken stock and honey until they're tender, but still firm. Your kids will crave them!

Black Beans
110 calories
1 g fat (0 g saturated)
5 mg sodium

No, this isn't a mistake. Wild rice might have fewer calories than black beans, but it also offers considerably less nutrition. A cup of cooked black beans provides 15 grams of fiber, 15 grams of protein, and a huge dose of antioxidants.

Applesauce (1 c)
90 calories
0 g fat
18 g sugars

Make sure you stock your pantry with a good brand free of added sugars. How can you tell? Just read the back label. It should have apples, maybe cinnamon, maybe citric acid to help prevent spoiling. But no added sugar!

Not That!

Crab Cake Dinner

with wild rice and glazed carrots

565 calories
22 g fat
(5 g saturated)
845 mg sodium

The crab isn't the problem with these cakes—it's the binding of mayo, bread crumbs, and eggs, followed by face time with an oily frying pan, that does them in. Add tartar sauce to the equation, and you're looking at an extra 200 calories and 10 grams of fat. Want to have your crab cake and eat it, too? Cut the mayo, add an extra egg white to the mix, and bake the cakes in a 400°F oven for 20 minutes.

Fruit Cocktail (1 c)

160 calories
0 g fat
40 g sugars

"Cocktail" is the food industry's euphemism for "soaking in a viscous sugary syrup."

Wild Rice

85 calories
1 g fat (0 g saturated)
5 mg sodium

Wild rice ain't all that it's cracked up to be. While it's better than plain white rice, it still only offers 3 grams of fiber per cup and little other nutritional value. Make the switch to quinoa, which is rich in fiber and healthy fats and contains all vital amino acids.

Glazed Carrots

80 calories
1 g fat (0 g saturated)
140 mg sodium

Crab Cakes

400 calories
20 g fat
(5 g saturated)
700 mg sodium

267

10 Kid Favorites Made Healthy

Good food and good nutrition don't have to be mutually exclusive. Grab a little sous chef and redefine the fatty foods they love.

From cheese-covered mountains of mac and cheese to hulking helpings of sloppy joes, it just so happens that kids' favorite foods to eat are also some of the worst things they could be putting in their bodies. Coincidence? Not likely. So what's a parent to do, ban them from eating these foods? You'll make enemies faster than a Yankees fan at Fenway. Allow them to eat with impunity? No way.

To help you out, we've recast 10 of the most troublesome kid favorites in a healthier light. All scream out for a young sous chef's help, so enlist your kid to bread the chicken fingers or melt the cheese for the mac. Getting them involved will only further solidify these recipes as staples in your household.

MAC 'N CHEESE

- ½ Tbsp butter
- 2 Tbsp all-purpose flour
- 1 c 1% low-fat milk
- 1 ½ c reduced-fat extra sharp Cheddar cheese
- ¼ c fresh grated Parmesan cheese
- 4 c cooked whole wheat macaroni or penne
- ¼ c bread crumbs (preferably panko)

Preheat the oven to 400°F. Melt the butter in a large saucepan over medium heat and add the flour, cooking and stirring until it's fully incorporated and lightly golden. Add the milk slowly, whisking constantly to work out any lumps that may form. Cook for 3 to 5 minutes, until the mixture thickens slightly. Stir in the Cheddar and Parmesan, and cook until fully melted. Toss the sauce with the pasta, place in a large baking dish, and top with the bread crumbs. Bake for 30 minutes, until the bread crumbs are toasted and a crust has formed on top. Makes 4 servings.

Per serving: 340 calories, 9 g fat, 412 mg sodium

FETTUCCINE ALFREDO

- 1 Tbsp butter
- ¼ c minced onion
- 1 Tbsp all-purpose flour
- 1¼ c skim milk
- 1 c freshly grated Parmesan cheese
- 2 Tbsp reduced-fat cream cheese
- Pinch of nutmeg
- Salt and pepper
- 4 cups cooked whole wheat fettuccine

In a large saucepan over medium heat, heat the butter. Add the onion and cook for 2 minutes. Add the flour and cook for another 2 minutes, stirring constantly, until the flour gives off a nutty aroma. Add the milk gradually, whisking as you do to prevent the flour from clumping. Simmer for 5 to 10 minutes, until the sauce has thickened, then add the Parmesan, cream cheese, nutmeg, and salt and pepper to taste. (Remember, Parmesan is already really salty.) Toss the sauce with the cooked fettuccine and serve right away.

265 calories, 5 g fat, 128 mg sodium

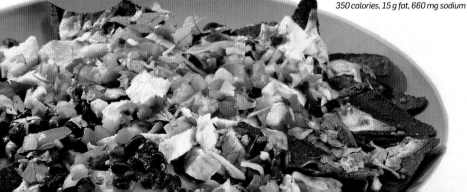

NACHO AVERAGE NACHOS
Mozzarella stands in for fatty cheddar, and black bean chips boost fiber and slice calories. Add a big scoop of black beans and salsa for a blast of antioxidants.

PEPPERONI PIZZA

1   c tomato sauce
4   whole wheat English muffins, split open to make 8 halves
1   tsp dried basil
½   tsp onion powder
1   c low-moisture mozzarella cheese
8   slices of turkey pepperoni

Preheat the oven to 400°F. Spread the tomato sauce evenly on the English muffin halves. Top with the basil, onion powder, cheese, and pepperoni, in that order. Bake for 15 to 20 minutes, until the cheese is fully melted and lightly browned. Makes 4 servings.

260 calories, 9 g fat, 750 mg sodium

NACHOS

1   bag black bean chips
1   can black beans, drained
1 ½ c shredded, low-moisture mozzarella cheese
1   c cooked shredded or chopped chicken
1   c favorite tomato salsa
½   c chopped fresh cilantro

Preheat the oven to 400°F. Arrange the chips in a single layer on a large nonstick baking sheet. Cover evenly with the beans, then the cheese. Cook for 15 minutes, until the cheese is slightly melted. Remove from the oven, spread the chicken evenly over the nachos, and return the nachos to the oven. Cook for another 10 minutes, or long enough to warm up the chicken and brown the cheese. Remove and top with your family's favorite salsa and the cilantro. Makes 6 servings.

350 calories, 15 g fat, 660 mg sodium

SLOPPY JOES

- 1 tsp olive oil
- 1 lb lean ground turkey
- 1 medium onion, diced
- 1 carrot, peeled and diced
- 1 medium green bell pepper, diced
- 2 cloves garlic, minced
- ½ c ketchup
- 1 Tbsp chili powder
- 2 tsp Worcestershire sauce
- Salt and pepper, to taste
- 4 whole wheat hamburger buns, warmed

Heat a large nonstick skillet over medium heat. Add the olive oil, turkey, onion, carrot, pepper, and garlic. Sauté, stirring occasionally, until the turkey is cooked and the onions are translucent, 7 to 10 minutes. Add the ketchup, chili powder, and Worcestershire. Reduce the heat to low and simmer for at least 15 minutes. Serve with the buns. Makes 4 servings.

300 calories, 4.5 g fat, 720 mg sodium

CHEESE FRIES

- 1½ lbs russet potatoes (about 2 medium), washed, dried, and cut into ½-inch wedges
- 1 Tbsp olive oil
- Salt and pepper
- 1 c shredded low-fat Cheddar cheese
- ½ bunch green onions, thinly sliced

Preheat the oven to 450°F. Toss the potatoes with the oil and a few pinches of salt and pepper. Arrange the potatoes in a single layer on a baking sheet. Bake for 25 minutes, until lightly browned. Remove the sheet from the oven, stir, then sprinkle the potatoes evenly with the cheese and return to the oven. Bake until the cheese is fully melted, another 10 to 15 minutes. Top with the green onions and serve. Makes 4 servings.

217 calories, 6 g fat, 220 mg sodium

APPLE CINNAMON PANCAKES

- ½ c all-purpose flour
- ½ c whole wheat flour
- 1 Tbsp sugar
- 1 tsp baking powder
- ½ tsp baking soda
- ½ tsp salt
- ½ tsp ground cinnamon
- 1 c low-fat buttermilk
- ½ Tbsp vegetable oil
- 1 large egg
- ½ c crushed walnuts
- 1 Granny Smith apple, peeled and diced
- Cooking spray

Combine both flours, sugar, baking powder, baking soda, salt, and cinnamon in a large bowl. In a separate bowl, combine the buttermilk, oil, and egg. Combine the wet and dry mixtures and add in the walnuts, stirring until blended but still slightly lumpy.

Coat a griddle or nonstick skillet with cooking spray and place over medium heat. When it's hot, spoon about ¼ cup of the batter per pancake onto the griddle. Place small chunks of apple on the raw pancake batter. Turn the pancakes over when the tops are covered with bubbles and the edges look cooked. Serve with syrup and butter. Makes 4 servings.

246 calories, 9 g fat, 344 mg sodium

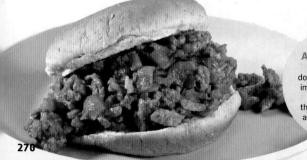

NOT YOUR AVERAGE JOE
Lean turkey downsizes the caloric impact, while a slew of vegetables ups the nutrition without arousing suspicion.

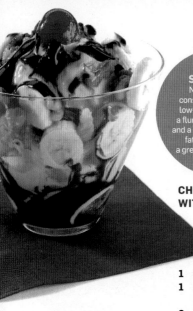

CHICKEN STRIPS WITH HONEY MUSTARD

½ tsp salt
½ tsp pepper
½ tsp chili powder (optional)
1 c panko bread crumbs
1 lb boneless, skinless chicken breast tenders
2 eggs, lightly beaten
¼ c of your family's favorite mustard
2 Tbsp honey

Preheat the oven to 375°F. Combine the salt, pepper, and chili powder with the bread crumbs, and mix. Dip the chicken in the egg, then in the spiced bread crumbs. Place on a nonstick baking sheet and bake for 12 to 15 minutes, turning once, until the chicken is firm and the bread crumbs are browned. While the chicken cooks, mix together the mustard and honey. Makes 4 servings.

238 calories, 4 g fat, 583 mg sodium

ICE CREAM SUNDAES

2 c vanilla ice cream
2 c sliced banana
¼ c chopped walnuts
¼ c hot fudge sauce
4 maraschino cherries

Place one large (½ cup) scoop of ice cream in each of four bowls. Divide the bananas and walnuts among the bowls, drizzle a tablespoon of hot chocolate sauce on each, and top with a maraschino cherry. Makes 4 servings.

268 calories, 9 g fat, 31 g sugars

FRENCH TOAST STICKS WITH HOT BANANA DIP

2 very ripe bananas
1 tsp brown sugar
¼ cup orange juice
2 tsp vanilla extract
4 egg whites
¼ cup skim milk
½ tsp ground cinnamon
Pinch ground nutmeg
8 slices whole wheat bread
Powdered sugar

Combine the bananas, brown sugar, orange juice, and half of the vanilla in a small sauce pan and cook over medium-low heat for 3 to 5 minutes. Mash the banana with the back of a fork until the sauce is mostly smooth and set aside.

Combine the egg whites, milk, remaining vanilla, cinnamon, and nutmeg in a large, shallow dish. Whisk. Warm up a nonstick pan or skillet covered with nonstick spray over medium heat. Lay individual slices of wheat bread in the mixture, then transfer to the pan or skillet. Cook for 2 to 3 minutes a side until brown and crispy. Remove the toast and slice into ½" thick sticks. Dust with powdered sugar and serve with the hot banana dip for dunking. Skip the syrup!

260 calories, 2.5 g fat, 16 g sugars

Thanksgiving

Eat This

White Meat Turkey Dinner

with homemade cranberry sauce, mashed potatoes and gravy, green bean casserole, and dinner roll

575 calories
22 g fat
(4.5 g saturated)
1,010 mg sodium

Americans consume more calories on Thanksgiving than on any other day of the year, but that's no reason to abandon all sense of proportion. Match 4 ounces of white meat with a few ½-cup servings of vegetables and you can keep the calorie count well under 1,000, an appropriate threshold for this yearly gorgefest.

Pumpkin Pie
(1 medium slice/
⅛ pie)with low-fat
whipped cream

335 calories
15 g fat
(6.5 g saturated)
42 g carbohydrates

A relatively safe play when it comes to pies.

**Green Bean
Casserole** (½ c)

100 calories
6 g fat
(1 g saturated)
200 mg sodium

Higher in fat and calories than corn, but also higher in nutrients. Can the Cream of Mushroom and fried onions and make it with fresh green beans and sautéed onions.

Turkey Breast
(4 oz) with homemade
cranberry sauce
(2 Tbsp)

225 calories
4 g fat (0 g saturated)
250 mg sodium

You won't find leaner meat than turkey breast. And homemade cranberry sauce allows you to control the sugar content.

Mashed Potatoes
(½ c) with
turkey gravy (¼ c)

140 calories
7 g fat (2 g saturated)
340 mg sodium

Homemade mashed potatoes aren't nearly as bad as most people think, especially if the cook uses 2% milk and has a light hand with the butter.

Dinner Roll (1)

110 calories
5 g fat
(1.5 g saturated)
220 calories

While it would be ideal to cut bread out of the meal entirely, this special occasion might require a sturdy vessel for sopping up gravy.

Not That!

Dark Meat Turkey Dinner

with jellied cranberry sauce, candied sweet potatoes, corn, and stuffing

780 calories
31 g fat
(15 g saturated)
1,285 mg sodium

This is no different from millions of plates that will come together on Turkey Day this year, but unfortunately, this seemingly average spread nearly satisfies an 8-year-old's requirements for calories, fat, and sodium for an entire day.

Stuffing (½ c)

175 calories
14 g fat (6 g saturated)
420 mg sodium

Flecked with butter and doused in salty broth, stuffing might be essential to your feast, but make sure to serve tiny portions. Cooking it inside the bird only makes matters worse.

Candied Sweet Potatoes with Marshmallow Topping (½ c)

225 calories
8 g fat (5 g saturated)
270 mg sodium

This dish suffers from an unnecessary tidal wave of sugar. Sweet potatoes are sweet enough; drop the marshmallows and brown sugar.

Dark Turkey Meat (4 oz) with jellied cranberry sauce (½" slice)

310 calories
8 g fat (4 g saturated)
320 mg sodium

Leg meat will always be fattier than breast meat. And a slice of canned cranberry sauce adds 22 grams of sugar.

Corn (½ c)

70 calories
1 g fat (0 g saturated)
275 mg sodium

In November, corn usually comes in the canned variety, which can be long on sodium and short on nutrition.

Pecan Pie (1 small slice/⅛ pie)

450 calories
21 g fat
(4 g saturated)
65 g carbohydrates

Much of the fat in this pie is of the heart-healthy variety found in pecans and other nuts. But the rest of the calories come from the thick slick of corn syrup.

273

Christmas

Eat This

Beef Tenderloin Dinner

with roasted new potatoes, green beans
with almonds, and dinner roll

535 calories
24 g fat
(7 g saturated)
800 mg sodium

Beef makes a
surprisingly lean centerpiece
for this holiday extravaganza.
Just make sure it's tenderloin or
sirloin and not fatty ribeye
or strip steak. Beef in any form
packs plenty of iron and zinc,
two nutrients many kids,
especially girls,
don't get enough of.

**Roasted New
Potatoes** (½ c)

*100 calories
5 g fat (1 g saturated)
170 mg sodium*

One of the healthiest
ways to prepare any
vegetable.

Beef Tenderloin
(4 oz)

*210 calories
10 g fat
(4 g saturated)
300 mg sodium*

**Green Beans with
Almonds** (½ c)

*95 calories
4 g fat (0 g saturated)
120 mg sodium*

Add crunch and a dose
of heart-healthy fats to
plain vegetables.

Dinner Roll
with butter

*130 calories
5 g fat
(2 g saturated)
210 mg sodium*

**Chocolate
Fondue**
(1 oz) with fruit (½ c)

*200 calories
8 g fat
(4 g saturated)
18 g sugars*

Not That!

Honey Baked Ham Dinner

with mashed potatoes with gravy, salad, and cornbread

760 calories
38 g fat
(14 g saturated)
2,190 mg sodium

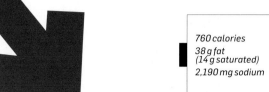

Don't make this the saltiest holiday ever! From the sodium-soaked ham to the Italian dressing and cornbread, this meal collectively has more salt than six large orders of McDonald's French fries.

Cheesecake
(1 slice/ 1/8 cake)

370 calories
19 g fat
(9 g saturated)
28 g sugars

Cornbread
with butter

190 calories
9 g fat (4 g saturated)
360 mg sodium

Simultaneously sweeter and saltier than a normal dinner roll.

Salad
with croutons and Italian dressing

240 calories
12 g fat
(4 g saturated)
390 mg sodium

Glazed Honey-Baked Ham (4 oz)

190 calories
10 g fat
(4 g saturated)
1,100 mg sodium

Fairly lean, but way too high in sodium.

Mashed Potatoes
with gravy (1/2 c)

140 calories
7 g fat (2 g saturated)
340 mg sodium

It beats other potato treatments, but can't contend with roasting.

275

Fourth Of July

Eat This

Hot Dog Meal

with beans, cole slaw, and fruit salad

615 calories
21.5 g fat
(4 g saturated)
1,095 mg sodium

Want to cut this calorie count in half without arousing any suspicions in a discerning kid's palate? Swap out the normal beef or pork frank for an Applegate Farms' All Natural Turkey Dog.

Fruit Salad (½ c)
55 calories
0 g fat
5 mg sodium

Baked Beans (½ c)
150 calories
1.5 g fat (0 g saturated)
250 mg sodium

Cole Slaw (½ c)
170 calories
10 g fat (2 g saturated)
210 mg sodium

Hotdog
with ketchup,
mustard and relish
240 calories
10 g fat
(2 g saturated)
630 mg sodium

Not That!

Cheeseburger Meal

with corn on the cob, potato salad, and iceberg salad

1,025 calories
54 g fat
(18 g saturated)
1,670 mg sodium

For a truly healthy burger, start with 95% lean ground beef. Use skim-milk mozzarella for cheese and pack as much produce as you can possibly fit in between a toasted whole wheat bun.

Cheeseburger
500 calories
25 g fat (9 g saturated)
850 mg sodium

Potato Salad (½ c)
190 calories
12 g fat (3 g saturated)
430 mg sodium

Corn on the Cob
with butter
160 calories
6 g fat (4 g saturated)
150 mg sodium

Iceberg Salad
with honey mustard dressing
175 calories
11 g fat (2 g saturated)
240 mg sodium

Birthday Party

Eat This

Beef Taco Meal

(2) with chips and salsa and a virgin daiquiri

610 calories
24 g fat
(8 g saturated)
1,140 mg sodium

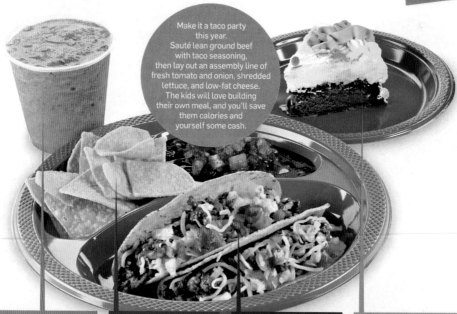

Make it a taco party this year. Sauté lean ground beef with taco seasoning, then lay out an assembly line of fresh tomato and onion, shredded lettuce, and low-fat cheese. The kids will love building their own meal, and you'll save them calories and yourself some cash.

Virgin Daiquiri (8 oz)

80 calories
0 g fat
16 g sugars

Blend together a can of pineapple chunks and their juices, a bag of frozen strawberries, the juice of two limes, 1 tablespoon of sugar, and a few cups of ice. This is enough to keep six kids from the soda.

Tortilla Chips
(1 oz) with salsa (⅛ c)

130 calories
5 g fat (1 g saturated)
390 mg sodium

Get your kids hooked on salsa at an early age. It's the ultimate condiment—loaded with disease-fighting lycopene, just 10 calories a serving, and 100% fat-free.

2 Beef Tacos
with cheese, lettuce, and tomato

400 calories
19 g fat
(7 g saturated)
750 mg sodium

Ice Cream Cake (⅛ cake)

330 calories
18 g fat (8 g saturated)
30 g sugars

Why give kids a huge serving of cake and a separate scoop of ice cream, when you can combine the two? They'll be so excited they won't notice that they're getting a smaller serving of each.

278

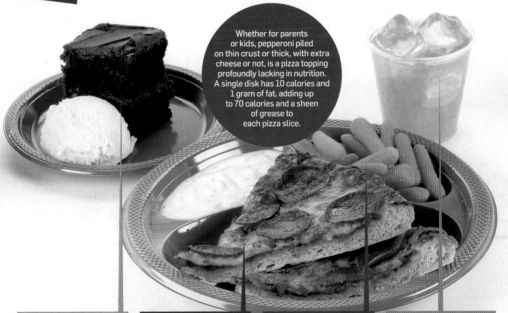

Not That!

Pepperoni Pizza Meal

with baby carrots and pink lemonade

860 calories
45 g fat
(18 g saturated)
1,740 mg sodium

Whether for parents or kids, pepperoni piled on thin crust or thick, with extra cheese or not, is a pizza topping profoundly lacking in nutrition. A single disk has 10 calories and 1 gram of fat, adding up to 70 calories and a sheen of grease to each pizza slice.

Chocolate Cake with Ice Cream

420 calories
24 g fat (10 g saturated)
39 g sugars

The standard birthday closer is a certifiable trainwreck of calories, fat, and sugar. If they must have their cake and eat it too, cut the slices small.

Pepperoni Pizza
(2 slices of 14" pie)

600 calories
30 g fat
(14 g saturated)
1,450 mg sodium

Baby Carrots (1/2 c) with ranch dip (2 Tbsp)

160 calories
15 g fat (4 g saturated)
290 mg sodium

Don't let a perfectly healthy snack become a mere utensil used to bring fatty ranch from plate to mouth. Carrots are fine on their own.

Pink Lemonade (8 oz)

100 calories
0 g fat
28 g sugars

No, this is not juice. Most lemonades consist of 10% lemon juice and 90% sugar water. If not for the bit of vitamin C from the lemon, your kid might as well drink a soda.

279

The Holiday Candy Scorecard

Not all candy was created equal.
It's your job to steer kids to the lesser of all evils.

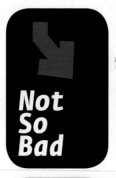

Not So Bad

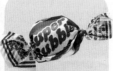

**FARLEY'S®
SUPER BUBBLE
BUBBLE GUM**
(3 pieces, 15 g)
*45 calories, 0 g fat,
9 g sugars*

WONKA NERDS
(1 small box, 13 g)
*50 calories, 0 g fat,
6 g sugars*

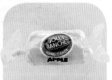

**JOLLY RANCHER®
HARD CANDY**
(3 pieces, 14 g)
*50 calories,
0 g fat,
7 g sugars*

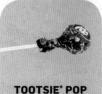

TOOTSIE® POP
(1 pop, 17 g)
*60 calories, 0 g fat,
10 g sugars*

**NECCO®
SWEETHEARTS**
(½ box, 14 g)
*55 calories, 0 g fat,
13.5 g sugar*

**CHARM'S®
BLOW POP®**
(1 pop, 18 g)
*60 calories,
0 g fat,
13 g sugars*

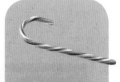

**BOB'S® CANDY
CANES**
(1 piece, 14 g)
*60 calories, 0 g fat,
14 g sugars*

Americans consume nearly 8 billion pounds of candy a year, and much of that can be attributed to the collective appetite of sugar-happy kids. From Halloween handouts to convenience store chocolate bars, the difference between a smart choice and a perilous one could mean pounds to your kid's waistline. Just to be extra clear: Nothing you see on these four pages has even a trace of redeeming nutritional value. Even the lowest-calorie options here will pack on major pounds if consumed recklessly. But knowing the relative winners and losers should help your kids save thousands of calories over the course of a year.

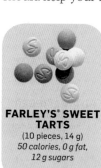

FARLEY'S® SWEET TARTS
(10 pieces, 14 g)
*50 calories, 0 g fat,
12 g sugars*

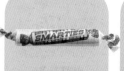

SMARTIES®
(2 rolls, 14 g)
*50 calories, 0 g fat,
12.5 g sugars*

SPANGLER® DUM DUM POPS®
(2 pops, 13 g)
*51 calories, 0 g fat,
10 g sugars*

NOW AND LATER®
(4 pieces, 18 g)
*54 calories, 0.5 g fat
(0 g saturated),
11 g sugars*

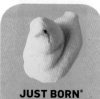

JUST BORN® MARSHMALLOW PEEPS®
(2 chicks, 17 g)
*64 calories, 0 g fat,
14.5 g sugars*

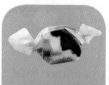

SWEET'S SALT WATER TAFFY
(3 pieces, 18 g)
*69 calories, 1 g fat
(0.5 g saturated),
10 g sugars*

3 MUSKETEERS®
(1 "fun" size bar, 15 g)
*63 calories, 2 g fat
(1.5 g saturated),
10 g sugars*

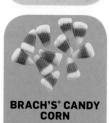

BRACH'S® CANDY CORN
(13 pieces, 20 g)
*70 calories, 0 g fat,
14 g sugars*

SEE'S® ASSORTED VALENTINE'S CHOCOLATES
(1 piece, 14 g)
70 calories, 4 g fat
(2 g saturated),
7 g sugars

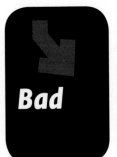

Bad

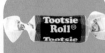

TOOTSIE ROLL®
(3 pieces)
70 calories, 1.5 g fat
(0.5 g saturated),
9.5 g sugars

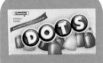

DOTS® CANDY
(1 box, 21 g)
70 calories, 0 g fat,
11 g sugars

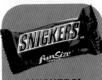

SNICKERS®
(1 "fun" size bar, 17 g)
80 calories, 4 g fat
(1.5 g saturated),
8.5 g sugars

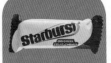

STARBURSTS®
(4 pieces, 20 g)
80 calories, 2 g fat
(1.5 g saturated),
11.5 g sugars

SKITTLES®
(1 "fun" size pack, 20 g)
80 calories, 1 g fat
(1 g saturated),
15 g sugars

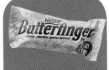

BUTTERFINGER® BAR
(1 "fun" size bar, 19 g)
85 calories, 3.5 g fat
(2 g saturated),
8.5 g sugars

REESE'S PEANUT BUTTER CUPS® MINIATURES
(2 pieces, 16 g)
84 calories, 4.5 g fat
(1.5 g saturated),
7.5 g sugars

HERSHEY'S® MINIATURES
(milk chocolate, Special Dark®, Krackel®, and Mr. Goodbar®)
(2 pieces, 17 g)
84 calories, 5.5 g fat
(2.5 g saturated), 8.5 g sugars

CADBURY® MILK CHOCOLATE MINI EGGS
(6 eggs, 20 g)
90 calories, 5 g fat
(3 g saturated),
12 g sugars

M&MS®
(1 "fun" size bag)
100 calories, 4.5 g fat
(2.5 g saturated),
13 g sugars

JELLY BELLY® 40 FLAVORS JELLY BEANS
(20 beans, 23 g)
70 calories, 0 g fat, 14 g sugars

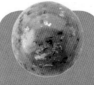

JAWBREAKERS
(3 pieces, 17 g)
70 calories, 0 g fat, 16 g sugars

FERRERO ROCHER® FINE HAZELNUT CHOCOLATES
(1 piece, 13.5 g)
73 calories, 5 g fat (1.5 g saturated), 4.5 g sugars

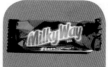

MILKY WAY®
(1 "fun" size bar, 17 g)
75 calories, 3 g fat (2 g saturated), 10 g sugars

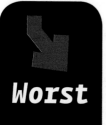

Worst

BRACH'S® MILK MAID® CARAMELS
(2 pieces, 19 g)
80 calories, 2.5 g fat (2 g saturated), 18 g sugars

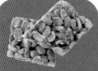

PEANUT BRITTLE
(1" chunk, 20 g)
90 calories, 3 g fat (1.5 g saturated), 7 g sugars

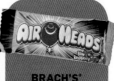

BRACH'S® AIRHEADS®
(2 pieces)
90 calories , 1 g fat (0 g saturated), 12 g sugars

HERSHEY®'S MILK CHOCOLATE KISSES®
(4 kisses, 18 g)
101.5 calories, 5.5 g fat (3.5 g saturated), 9 g sugars

RUSSELL STOVER® CHOCOLATE BUNNY
(½ bunny, 21.5 g)
115 calories, 7 g fat (4 g saturated), 11.5 g sugars

HOMEMADE FUDGE
(one 2" cube)
119 calories, 1.5 g fat 1.5 g saturated), 23.5 g sugars

CADBURY® CREME EGG
(1 egg, 34 g)
150 calories, 5 g fat (3 g saturated), 22 g sugars

The Ultimate Smoothie

Hopefully one of the major nutritional shortcomings of the average American kid's diet has become apparent in these pages: Kids don't consume enough fruits and vegetables. Parents need to find as many strategies as possible for boosting the presence of produce in their loved ones' diets. Luckily, the fruit failing is an easy fix: Toss it in a blender—or better yet, let them load it up with their favorite fresh and frozen fruits—add ice and juice and blast away. Each of the following liquid concoctions has between 200 and 300 calories (perfect for breakfast or a snack), can be made with fresh or frozen fruit, and takes about 60 seconds to make.

THE BRAIN BOOSTER

Try this one before a big test. Blueberries and raspberries are both loaded with antioxidants that help protect the brain from free-radical damage, which can improve cognitive processing. The berries here aren't just super food for your brain; they also offer an important cancer-fighting bonus.

½ c fresh or frozen blueberries
½ c fresh or frozen raspberries
¾ c pineapple orange juice
½ c low-fat vanilla yogurt
1 c ice (about 6 cubes)

270 calories, 2 g fat (0 g saturated), 57 g carbohydrates

THE METABOLISM CHARGER

Kids already have an edge over adults in the metabolism department, but that doesn't mean you shouldn't get their bodies into full calorie-burning mode early on. This smoothie employs the help of protein-packed yogurt and green tea, which contains antioxidants called catechins that are known to boost metabolism.

½ c brewed green tea, cooled to room temperature
½ c nonfat vanilla yogurt
1 c mango
½ Tbsp honey
1 c ice (about 6 cubes)

260 calories, 0 g fat, 61 g carbohydrates

Selector

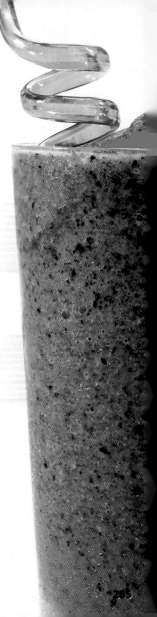

THE IMMUNIZER

Beyond the vision-protecting capacity of beta-carotene, found abundantly in orange fruits and vegetables, researchers also believe the powerful carotenoid is vital for fortifying the immune system, which means this beta blast could be the first line of defense against sickness.

1   c ice (about 6 cubes)
1   apricot, sliced and pitted
1/2 c papaya, frozen in chunks
1/2 c mango, frozen in chunks
1/2 c carrots
1   Tbsp honey

250 calories, 1 g fat (0 g saturated), 63 g carbohydrates

THE SMOOTH OPERATOR

The yogurt aids digestion, while the mango and juice boost immune response.

1/4 c pitted cherries
1/2 c mango
1/2 c nonfat vanilla yogurt
1/2 c pineapple orange juice
1   c ice (about 6 cubes)

260 calories, 0 g fat, 59 g carbohydrates

THE SANDMAN

Melatonin is nature's Ambien®, bestowing on even the most restless rug rat a set of heavy eyelids. Cherries, bananas, and grapes are all great sources of this sleep-inducer, and they make for a healthy encore to dinner.

1/4 c pitted cherries
1/2 banana
1/2 c grape juice
1/2 c nonfat vanilla yogurt
1   c ice (about 6 cubes)

270 calories, 0 g fat, 59 carbohydrates

THE MOOD MAKER

This one's an all-fruit smoothie, packed with carbs to boost serotonin levels. Add a handful of flaxseeds for an extra dose of mood-boosting omega-3 fatty acids.

1/2 c fresh or frozen blueberries
1/2 c fresh or frozen mango
1/2 c orange juice
1/2 c nonfat vanilla yogurt
1   c ice (about 6 cubes)
1   Tbsp ground flaxseeds (optional)

269 calories, 1 g fat (0 g saturated), 61 g carbohydrates

11 Foods That Cure

RASH RELIEVER: PAPAYA
Vitamin C and flavonoids are known to help prevent infection and the spread of rashes. They also act as a natural antihistamine that reduces swelling. Nothing on this planet carries more of both than papaya.

COUGH AND COLD CURE: CHICKEN NOODLE SOUP
More than just comfort food. Researchers at the Nebraska Medical Center proved that the compounds in chicken soup lessen inflammation, a cause of cold symptoms.

BURN AND WOUND BALM: HONEY
Researchers at the Mayo Clinic have found that applying honey directly to a wound protects it from outside contaminants. It also contains enzymes that have been shown to prevent infection and speed healing.

ATTENTION RETAINER: FLAXSEED
A 2006 study looked at the effects of flaxseed oil on children and reported that after 3 months of supplementation, children were found to be 18 percent less hyperactive and 19 percent more attentive.

CAVITY FIGHTER: CHEESE
Researchers found that eating less than a quarter ounce of Jack, cheddar, or mozzarella will boost pH levels to protect teeth from cavities. Cheese also contains casein, which combines with calcium to fill cracks in teeth.

TOOTHACHE TREATMENT: CLOVES
Cloves contain eugenol, a natural antiseptic that can be released by lightly chewing on a clove in the area where the pain is coming from. If your kid won't chew, try applying clove oil directly to the sore area.

NATURAL RELAXANT: POULTRY
Chickens and turkeys contain an amino acid called tryptophan, which is important for the production of serotinin, a brain chemical that helps regulate sleep cycles.

If some doctors had their way today, our kids would be more medicated than feedlot cattle. What most parents don't realize is that the first line of defense is found in the aisles of the supermarket, not in the drug store. Here are 11 research-backed quick cures in the form of fresh produce and reliable pantry products. Add them to your next grocery list and you might be able to save some space in your medicine cabinet.

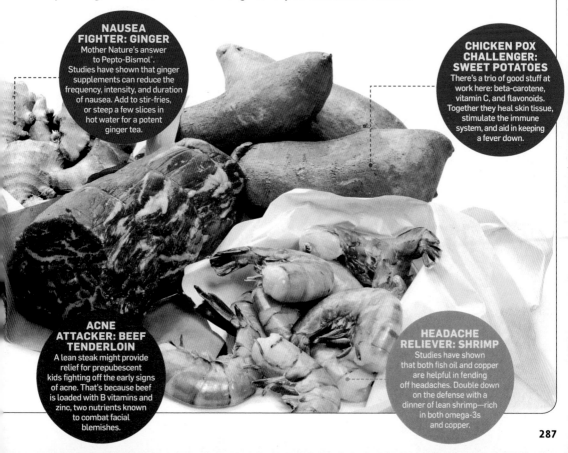

NAUSEA FIGHTER: GINGER
Mother Nature's answer to Pepto-Bismol®. Studies have shown that ginger supplements can reduce the frequency, intensity, and duration of nausea. Add to stir-fries, or steep a few slices in hot water for a potent ginger tea.

CHICKEN POX CHALLENGER: SWEET POTATOES
There's a trio of good stuff at work here: beta-carotene, vitamin C, and flavonoids. Together they heal skin tissue, stimulate the immune system, and aid in keeping a fever down.

ACNE ATTACKER: BEEF TENDERLOIN
A lean steak might provide relief for prepubescent kids fighting off the early signs of acne. That's because beef is loaded with B vitamins and zinc, two nutrients known to combat facial blemishes.

HEADACHE RELIEVER: SHRIMP
Studies have shown that both fish oil and copper are helpful in fending off headaches. Double down on the defense with a dinner of lean shrimp—rich in both omega-3s and copper.

A FITNESS LEGACY

A Fitness Legacy

I've just spent the last 297 pages telling you that it's the food our children are eating—and not a lack of exercise—that's the main culprit that's making them fat. It's true: Remember, we burn only about 15 percent of our calories by actually moving. The rest goes to digesting food and maintaining our life functions.

Still, adding exercise to a sensible diet is like adding lighter fluid to a backyard barbecue—it lights things up, big time! So by increasing the time your children spend being active, you'll turbocharge the weight-loss effect of **EAT THIS, NOT THAT! FOR KIDS!**

Only one minor problem: Kids don't want to exercise, because exercise feels like work. And as the song goes, girls (and boys) just want to have fun.

But aha: Therein lies the key.

Exercise for kids shouldn't be primarily about burning calories and losing weight. Those are just the fringe benefits. And it shouldn't be about sets and reps, or targeting specific body parts, either.

No, first and foremost, exercise for kids is about fun.

You might think that sounds overly idealistic. ("Come on, kids, strap on those sneaks! Jogging is way more fun than 'Grand Theft Auto!'") But it's not as crazy as it sounds. Children, bless their goofy little hearts, are nothing if not impressionable; the fact is, when exercise is called "fun" or "play," 83 percent of overweight children will do it consistently, report UK researchers. In a 10-week study, the scientists discovered that kids who switched their view of exercise from negative ("Exercise is work!") to positive ("Exercise is fun!") felt more confident and were more likely to engage in fitness activities again.

It doesn't take a rocket scientist (or an exercise scientist, for that matter) to conclude that you're more likely to stick with an activity if you enjoy doing it. So it's not a leap to suggest that learning to love exercise when you're young will make you far more likely to find time for it as an adult.

Unfortunately, it seems most of us missed out on this message as kids, and we're not passing it on to our children either. The evidence: Only 19 percent of Americans participate in "high levels of physical activity," according to the National Center for Health Statistics. The President's Council on Physical Fitness and Sports defines this as just three intense, 20-minute workouts per week—hardly an unrealistic time commitment.

So along with making smart nutritional choices, we can't underscore the importance of regular physical activity enough—for both you and your children. Case in point: A student who enters high school overweight has only a slight chance of reaching a normal weight by adulthood, report researchers at Baylor College of Medicine who studied more than 800 people, at age 10 and again between the ages of 19 and 35. High-school freshmen with a healthy weight, on the other hand, are four times as likely to stay slim as adults. The bottom line: Help your kids develop healthy habits early, and you'll help them grow into healthy adults.

FIT BODY, FIT MIND

Besides the ultimate payoff of a leaner, healthier body, exercise also makes kids smarter. That's not hyperbole; it's hard science from researchers at the University of Illinois at Urbana-Champaign, who studied the impact of regular physical activity on elementary-school students. Turns out, physically fit kids had a couple of advantages over those who were sedentary. Measurements of brain activity revealed that highly active children were not only able to process information faster, but that they also showed greater ability to focus. "Parts of your brain don't develop until late teenage years," says Charles H. Hillman, PhD, the study's lead author. (This may explain a lot of the dents in your car.) "These data show that those who are fit are better able to use what they have."

And it's not just teens who can muscle up their gray matter with exercise. In fact, the younger a child is, the more she may have to gain from regular activity. In a review of 44 studies examining the relationship between physical activity and cognition in children of varying ages, researchers at Arizona State University found that the youngest kids (grades one through five) improved cognitive development the most, followed by middle-school students. The California Department of Education found that the fittest students in the state scored best on academic tests. For instance, the average reading score of students who achieved one of six goals on the statewide fitness test was 38; students who achieved all six fitness goals averaged a reading score of 52.

The research is clear: Regular physical activity not only fosters a fit body, but also a fit mind. By ensuring that your child is exercising regularly, you're helping provide him with more opportunities to succeed in every aspect of his life—now and in the future.

MAKE EXERCISE A REWARD, NOT A PUNISHMENT

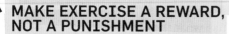

If you've ever watched "fat-to-fit" reality shows, you've witnessed running and pushups performed as punishment. But think of it this way: If you punish kids with exercise, how can they ever love it? Remember, exercise is something your kids should do for fun. Your dog wags his tail before a walk; build that sense of anticipation into activities you pursue and suggest to your kids. How? Use these simple guidelines— no matter what age your child is—to instill a love for activity that will linger for a lifetime.

GUIDE, DON'T PUSH.

What's your child interested in? Watch him in his free time and suggest new forms of active behavior. In a study of fifth and sixth graders, University of Missouri researchers found that parental encouragement is the second most important factor in determining whether or not kids exercise. Enjoyment of activity ranked first. So pick an activity your child already shows aptitude toward. If your daughter likes climbing trees, high-five her when she gets down, then take her to a rock-climbing gym. If your son is a one-man home-destructo unit, channel that excess energy into mixed martial arts.

CAP TV TIME.

Television is the enemy of activity: Studies show kids are half as likely to exercise if the tube roots them in place for more than 2 hours a day.

THINK OUTSIDE THE GYM.

Exercise doesn't have to be confined to a strict daily regimen. Gardening or driving to a local farm and picking berries, for instance, are active learning experiences. Plot your Sunday-afternoon bike ride on a map and build in extensions and diversions for the trip.

HANG A NERF HOOP.

Children are 38 percent more likely to exercise 60 minutes or more a day when exercise tools are available at home, report Australian researchers. But that doesn't mean your house has to be a jungle gym: Just make sure toys are visible and kids are allowed to move freely.

SET A GOOD EXAMPLE.

Kids are a whopping six times more likely to exercise when both Mom and Dad are active, according to a study in the *Journal of Pediatrics*. You could even exercise as a family. In fact, 76 percent of children say they'd like to exercise with their parents, according to a survey run by *Prevention* magazine. So get moving. Try this fun workout that you can do with your kids.

DIRECTIONS: Complete all sets of each task before moving to the next.

1. **RABBIT RACE:** Allow your kid a 5- to 10-yard head start for a 40-yard race, chasing him from behind. Rest 90 seconds, then repeat five times.

2. **DRIVEWAY SHUTTLES:** Place six objects—tennis balls, for instance—at the end of the driveway. Your kid starts, retrieving an object as fast as possible. You get the next one. Alternate until all of the objects have been retrieved. Rest 90 seconds, then repeat three to five times.

3. **TAG:** Mark off a 20-foot-by-20-foot area and play tag. (You're it!) Go continuously for 60 seconds, then rest for 60 seconds. Go five rounds.

The Fit Kids Toolbox

You've already discovered that this book is about giving you tools—powerful tools that will help you raise a happy, healthy child. And that's why we asked Brian Grasso, CEO of the International Youth Conditioning Association and a member of our FitSchools faculty (see "How Fit Is Your Child's School?" on page 300 to learn more), to provide you with your own toolbox of "fit kid" activities.

They'll sound like games to you—and they are. Your child will have loads of fun. But these activities will also boost your child's strength and improve her cardiovascular fitness. What's more, they'll stimulate your kid's central nervous system, the key to all bodily movements and coordination. For instance, our ability to throw and catch, kick, balance, and produce force are all dependent on our central nervous system. They're also all critical factors to develop from the ages of 5 to 12, since that's the period of life when our central nervous systems are the most "plastic," or adaptable. Help a child develop coordination, and he'll retain it for the rest of his life.

Of course, a nice side effect of participating in these games—in addition to a healthier heart, stronger muscles, and greater coordination—is that they also burn tons of calories. Paired with good eating habits, this can help any child achieve a healthy weight. So what are you waiting for? Open up your toolbox—and a world of fun and fitness for your kids.

AGES 2 TO 4

Kids are most active in their early years, between the ages of 2 and 4, since figuring out all the cool things their bodies are capable of is no small task. Unless you somehow stop them (and good luck trying), your children will be frenetic balls of relentless energy—and you'll be the one looking to take a breather.

AGES 5 TO 7

It's around age 5 that SpongeBob begins to exert his unholy pull. Don't get me wrong—I love SpongeBob, too (darn you, Mr. Krabs!). But it's now when a little parental coaching can make a difference. Here are some games that will keep your child active.

Balloon Up

DIRECTIONS FOR KIDS:
Blow up 8 to 20 balloons (depending on how many kids are participating). Start by throwing one balloon up in the air—the objective is for you to keep all the balloons from touching the ground. Every 10 seconds, throw another balloon into the mix. This is a great game to do with a group of kids.

TO INCREASE DIFFICULTY AND ADD FUN, INCORPORATE THE FOLLOWING PROGRESSIONS:
In groups, each participant is allowed to touch a balloon only once. Someone else must hit the balloon before they are allowed to hit it again.

You can use only your right hand, left hand, left knee, right elbow, and so on.

THE BENEFITS
Better Hand-Eye Coordination
Improved Agility
Cardiovascular Fitness

Tag Variations

DIRECTIONS FOR KIDS:
Standard tag isn't the only way to play the game. Try these variations:

One-Legged Tag: All participants must be on one foot the entire time.

Small Area Tag: Make the playing field a small area, so that participants must stay within close quarters during the game. Less running, but much more tactical thinking.

Monkey Tag: Each participant must squat down and stay in that position the entire time. They can run, jump, and side skip to move and avoid being tagged, but they must do so from this deep squatted position.

Crawling Tag: Each participant must be on all fours and bear crawl during the entire game.

THE BENEFITS
Cardiovascular Fitness
Improved Agility
Speed
Greater Strength and Flexibility

Wall Ball

DIRECTIONS FOR KIDS: This game is best played in groups of three or four kids. Start by facing a wall and designate an order: player 1, 2, 3, 4. Player 1 throws a tennis ball against a wall and then moves out of the way. Player 2 then tracks the ball, runs to retrieve it, and from that spot, throws it against the wall. Players 3 and 4 follow suit. Each player must retrieve the ball after only one bounce.

TO INCREASE DIFFICULTY AND ADD FUN, INCORPORATE THE FOLLOWING PROGRESSION:
Kids should learn to throw with both hands. This improves coordination, increases bodily strength, and helps avoid overuse injuries on one side of the body. So every other game played should be based on each participant throwing with his or her nondominant hand. Not only is this difficult, but tremendously fun to master.

THE BENEFITS:
Cardiovascular Fitness
Tactical Thinking
Greater Strength

Dynamic "Simon Says"

DIRECTIONS FOR KIDS: Just like tag, this conventional game is fun, but can also be a great fitness-oriented experience when played with certain rules. "Simon" should create the game so that the commands incorporate one of the following:

Running
Jumping
Crawling
Climbing
Skipping
Throwing or
Kicking

THE BENEFITS:
Cardiovascular Fitness
Improved Coordination
Greater Strength

DON'T JUST STAY IN PLACE. Make the participants move from one place to another. For example, "Simon says: Run to the nearest tree," or "Simon says: Skip for 10 seconds." Also, play the game at "warp speed." That is, have each Simon command come right after the other so that the participants are constantly moving and changing direction.

THE FIT KIDS TOOLBOX: AGES 8 TO 12

By age 8, many children begin to develop passions of their own: They may have rooted for the same team Mom and Dad did, but only because it was a family activity. Their musical taste was dictated by whatever you listened to. And their hobbies and favorite sports were whatever you signed them up for. But as their minds grow more independent, a slightly more targeted —and more challenging—fitness plan might be in order, one that begins to develop their skills in a variety of areas and prepares them for the challenges of organized sports and other group activities. Here are some of the most effective— and most fun!

Scramble to Balance

DIRECTIONS FOR KIDS: Start face down on the ground with your eyes closed. Have someone yell, "Go!" As soon as they do, stand up and balance on one leg (keeping your eyes closed). Hold that position for 5 seconds and then drop straight back to the ground. Repeat, this time standing on your opposite leg. Do this a total of 8 to 10 times per leg.

TO INCREASE DIFFICULTY AND ADD FUN, INCORPORATE THE FOLLOWING PROGRESSIONS:
While balancing on one foot, hold your hands over your head and pretend that you're reaching for something high up on a shelf.

After balancing for 5 seconds, open your eyes and perform 8 to 10 one-legged bunny hops before returning to the ground.

Rather than someone yelling, "Go!", use different auditory cues. For example, snap fingers, whistle, or clap hands.

THE BENEFITS:
Improved
Reaction Time
Better Balance
Cardiovascular Fitness
Greater Strength
Tons of Fun

Obstacle Course

DIRECTIONS FOR KIDS: This can be done in a variety of ways and virtually anywhere. For example, your backyard, the local park, or the school playground. Simply use what's available to you—stairs, swing sets, jungle gyms, playground slides, tennis balls, and so on. Then make the obstacle course diverse, fun, and spirited. Think of it in terms of shapes: That is, create a course that goes in a square or triangle pattern.

HERE ARE THREE SUGGESTIONS:
Triangle:
Side 1: Run
Side 2: Crab Walk
Side 3: Bunny Hop

Square:
Side 1: Skip
Side 2: Somersault
Side 3: Backward Jog
Side 4: Monster Walk

Playground:
Run from a tree to a bench—do 10 step-ups (each leg) on a bench
Run to the slide—climb up and slide down
Run to the swing set—do 15 swings as high as you can

THE BENEFITS:
Cardiovascular Fitness
Movement Skills
Greater Strength and Flexibility
Speed

Target Throws

DIRECTIONS FOR KIDS: Set up cones or some other type of target—for example, empty aluminum cans. Stand 10 to 20 feet away from the targets and be ready with various size balls, such as tennis balls, soccer balls, footballs, and so on. Using different kinds of throws, try to hit each target with a different ball. The throws could be overhead, underhand, a two-hand chest pass, or one-handed—it's up to your imagination. As soon as you throw the ball, chase after it and then run back to the cone and throw again. To increase difficulty and add fun, stand farther away from the targets.

THE BENEFITS:
Greater Strength
Accuracy
Cardiovascular Fitness

Hand Walks

DIRECTIONS FOR KIDS: Start in a push-up position—your hands set just wider than your shoulders, your arms straight, and your body forming a straight line from head to your ankles. Without bending your knees or back, walk forward on your hands and toes for a few feet. To make it harder, walk sideways or backward.

THE BENEFITS:
Greater Strength

How Fit Is Your Child's School?

Taking control of your kids' fitness at home is just a start. That's because most children 5 and up will spend the majority of their days from September to May not at home, but in school. Unfortunately, fewer than 10 percent of US schools offer daily physical education classes to their students, according to the Centers for Disease Control and Prevention. And in those schools that do offer regular PE, teachers and coaches around the country tell us that they simply don't have enough time, space, or equipment to provide an effective program for their students.

That's why *Men's Health* magazine established the FitSchools Foundation, a nonprofit organization designed to rescue physical-fitness programs from the budget cuts that are crippling public schools in America. We began the program in 2007 at Gettys Middle School in Easley, South Carolina, and have since instituted the FitSchools curriculum in schools across the nation. And the fact is, FitSchools works. In a recent pilot study, University of Southern California researchers found that our program significantly improved kids' fitness levels and love for physical activity. So they're not just getting healthier, they're enjoying the process—which will help them stay fit for a lifetime.

What's more, FitSchools is 100 percent free. Our ultimate mission: To inspire and enable kids, parents, and teachers to improve their lives and the world around them.

Ready to join the team? Go to **eatthis.com/FitSchools** *for more information on how you can help support this initiative.*

Index

Boldface page references indicate photographs.
Underscored references indicate boxed text and tables.

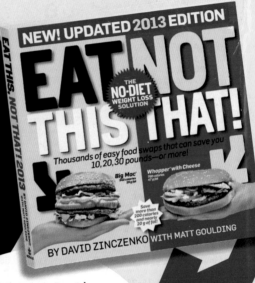